MEDICAL INSTITUTION OF GENEVA COLLEGE

GENEVA MEDICAL COLLEGE.

STATE UNIVERSITY OF NEW YORK

LET EACH BECOME ALL HE IS CAPABLE OF BEING

UPSTATE MEDICAL CENTER SYRACUSE

STATE UNIVERSITY OF NEW YORK

TO LEARN TO SEARCH TO SERVE

1834

HEALTH SCIENCE CENTER • SYRACUSE

SUNY Upstate Medical University

A Pictorial History

Eric v.d. Luft

North Syracuse, New York
Gegensatz Press
2005

Cataloging-in-Publication:

Luft, Eric v.d. (Eric von der), 1952-
SUNY Upstate Medical University : a pictorial history / Eric v.d. Luft.
p. ; cm.
"The history of medicine in Central New York has national and international as well as local and regional importance. The world's first woman physician to earn her M.D. by completing the regular course of study at an accredited medical school received that degree in Central New York. Alumni and faculty of SUNY Upstate Medical University and its precedessor institutions have achieved greatness that has enriched medicine and society around the world since 1834. This book tells their stories."
Includes bibliographical references and index.
ISBN 1-933237-34-1
1. Medical education—New York (State)—Syracuse—History. 2. Medical colleges—New York (State)—Syracuse—History. 3. Medicine—New York (State)—Syracuse—History. 4. Women physicians.
[DNLM: 1. Schools, Medical—history. 2. Education, Medical—history. 3. Physicians, Women. 4. State University of New York Upstate Medical University—history. 5. State University of New York Health Science Center at Syracuse—history. 6. State University of New York Upstate Medical Center—history. 7. State University of New York College of Medicine at Syracuse—history. 8. Syracuse University College of Medicine—history. 9. College of Medicine of Syracuse University—history. 10. College of Physicians and Surgeons of the Syracuse University—history. 11. Geneva Medical College—history. 12. Medical Institution of Geneva College—history. 13. New York. 14. Blackwell, Elizabeth, 1821-1910. W 19 U69 L83s 2005]
I. Title. II. Title: State University of New York Upstate Medical University. III. Title: Upstate Medical University.
R 747 U69 L83s 2005
610—dc22 AACR2
Library of Congress Control Number 2004099671

First edition, first printing. Printed in the United States of America by United Book Press, Inc., Baltimore.

Distributed to the trade worldwide by:
Gegensatz Press
108 Deborah Lane
North Syracuse, NY 13212-1931

Designed by the author. Printed on acid-free paper. ∞

Contents

I dedicate this book to all women physicians, to honor their brilliant tradition that began with Elizabeth Blackwell's graduation as M.D. at the predecessor of SUNY Upstate Medical University, the Medical Institution of Geneva College, on January 23, 1849.

The front cover shows a detail of Joseph Stanley Kozlowski's 1963 painting of Elizabeth Blackwell, M.D. The green lettering is the academic heraldic color of medicine.

The back cover shows Charles Schmidt's painting of neurosurgeon Robert B. King, M.D., in consultation with his health care team in the 1980s.

Except where otherwise noted, all images in this book are from the Department of Historical Collections, Health Sciences Library, SUNY Upstate Medical University.

Preface and Acknowledgments

In 1987, when the Health Sciences Library of what was then the State University of New York Health Science Center at Syracuse hired me to catalog rare books, develop preservation policies, publicize the historical aspects of the Library's collections, and generally to be the historical resource person on campus, I was immediately fascinated by this institution's history. The more of it I learned, the more fascinated I became and the prouder I grew to work here. Frankly, I thought that working for the medical school that graduated the world's first woman physician was just the most splendid twist of fate. My own physician since 1985 was a woman, Lakshmi Kavety, and she was the best doctor I have ever had. I could not imagine a reasonable or viable medical world without women in it. To think of a time when medicine was really so unreasonable and lacked such viability inspired me to learn more about the conditions that led to the most important social reform that the medical profession has ever undergone.

My colleagues just as immediately began encouraging me to write this history, and that very year the earliest plans for this book emerged. Its title was to have been *Elizabeth Blackwell's Alma Mater: A History of Geneva Medical College (1834-1871)*, but as step by step I became aware of what would need to be in such a book, and especially as I discovered noteworthy facts about the life of this institution throughout its entire span, facts that had nothing to do with Elizabeth Blackwell, my focus shifted to include its history after 1871. Just going about my daily job of answering historical reference questions provided me with an unparalleled osmotic learning experience, filling me with local medical lore and enriching my perception of the whole medical heritage of Central New York.

Even though she is is foremost in our local medical history — and deserves to be — there is more to Upstate Medical University than Elizabeth Blackwell, and to show that is my main purpose in writing this book.

Since this book is primary pictorial rather than a continuous scholarly analysis or narrative, it is necessarily episodic, or a series of stories and vignettes only loosely connected. Read it more like an album than like a treatise.

Most of the primary research resources for this history are in the Archives of Upstate Medical University or in the Special Collections of its Health Sciences Library. Among the most useful of these resources is the six-volume loose-leaf illustrated biographical history of the Syracuse University College of Medicine and SUNY Upstate Medical Center up to 1968 that J. Howard Ferguson, M.D., Class of 1926, compiled as a labor of love. In preparing it, he drew heavily upon the Medical Photography Unit, which he himself had founded in 1928 with $500 of his own money. He added material to this chronicle until his death in 1978 and many hands expanded it thereafter. I have taken so much from Ferguson's work that I consider him almost a co-author.

Through eighteen years of researching the history of medicine in Central New York, I have incurred many intellectual debts to the excellent archivists and librarians at Hobart and William Smith Colleges, Syracuse University, the Edward G. Miner Library of the University of Rochester Medical Center, the College of Physicians of Philadelphia, the New York Academy of Medicine, the Onondaga Historical Association, the Geneva Historical Society, the Episcopal Diocese of Central New York, and the New York State Library. I would like to thank them all now. Without them this book would not exist. Most particularly I would like to recognize the contributions and support of three of my librarian colleagues at Upstate, Suzanne H. Murray, Patricia W. Onsi, and Peter A. Uva.

I also thank Julia Boyd of the University of Cambridge for her wonderful friendship and her unique British perspective on Elizabeth Blackwell; *Syracuse Post-Standard* columnist Dick Case for his encyclopedic knowledge of Central New York; Upstate Medical University President Gregory L. Eastwood, M.D., Provost Kenneth L. Barker, Ph.D., Dean of Student Affairs E. Gregory Keating, Ph.D., and Vice Provost for Research John J. Lucas, Ph.D., for their continuing and dependable support; portrait artist Susan Keeter for her creative spark and her keen interest in Sarah Loguen Fraser; Christine Ruggere of the Johns Hopkins University, formerly of the College of Physicians of Philadelphia, for having awakened my interest in the history of medicine in the first place; Susan K. Rishworth of the American College of Surgeons for helping me learn how to study the medical women of the late nineteenth and early twentieth centuries; Lloyd F. Novick, M.D., M.P.H., and Sally M. Sutphen, M.Sc., M.P.H., of the Upstate Preventive Medicine Program for information they supplied about the 1918-1919 influenza epidemic; the extended Ecker family for their concern with many kinds of historical phenomena; Max Kutzer, M.D., and Howard Weinberger, M.D., Class of 1958, for identifying photographs; Upstate physical plant administrator Douglas Joseph for all his little historical surprises, and anyone else who kindly answered my questions or gave me data.

I am especially grateful for the suggestions and enthusiasm of Carole Novick, Executive Director of the Syracuse Medical Alumni Association from 1996 to 2005; and the members of the *ad hoc* Alumni Editorial Advisory Committee for this book: the late David W. Brewer, M.D., Class of 1941; Ellen Townley Cook Jacobsen, M.D., Class of 1950; Stanley D. Leslie, Class of 1951; Robert W. Daly, M.D., Class of 1957; Patricia J. Numann, M.D., Class of 1965; Andrew J. Rurka, M.D., Class of 1970; Gregory A. Threatte, M.D., Class of 1973; Ruth Hart, M.D., Class of 1980; and Kirsten P. Magowan, M.D., Class of 1987. My particular thanks go to Bob Daly, Carole Novick, Andy Rurka, and my wife Diane, who each read the manuscript before it went to press. Of course, all its faults are mine, not theirs.

I also want to express my admiration and affection for the late Kenneth W. Wright, M.D., Class of 1938. Unfortunately he did not live to see his own dream of a history of Upstate Medical University properly realized.

1

The Dawn of Medical Education in Upstate New York

Early American medical education was spotty. A colonial American who wanted to become a physician or surgeon could either serve as a doctor's apprentice, take private lessons from a doctor, or travel to Europe for formal medical education. The first American medical school was founded at the University of Pennsylvania in 1765 but by the early nineteenth century there were still only a handful. London, Paris, and especially Edinburgh remained popular places of study for the best American medical students. American medical schools were poorly and inconsistently regulated, usually by local medical societies, if at all. The apprentice and tutorial systems persisted well into the nineteenth century.

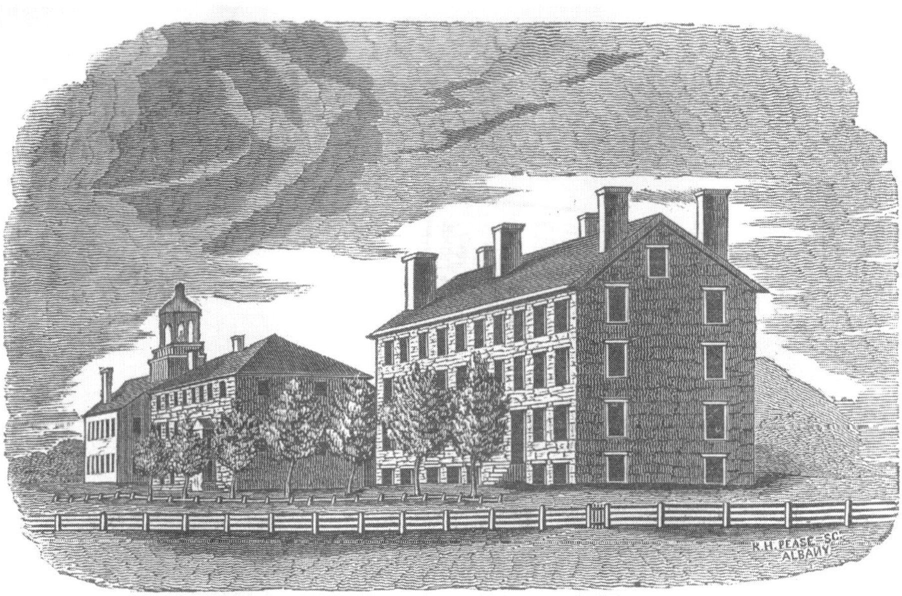

MEDICAL COLLEGE, FAIRFIELD, N. Y.

To fill a perceived need for a medical school to serve the rapidly growing population of Upstate New York, Lyman Spalding, Westel Willoughby, and James Hadley incorporated the College of Physicians and Surgeons of the Western District of the State of New York on June 12, 1812 in Fairfield, replacing the Medical School of Fairfield Academy, which had been founded in 1809. Its first set of *Ordinances*, published in 1813, stated four requirements for the M.D.:

1. Study three years with a "reputable practitioner" in a tutor/preceptor or apprentice/master relationship.
2. Attend two semesters of a full course of lectures. One semester lasted three months.
3. Pass exams in anatomy, surgery, obstetrics, chemistry, materia medica, minerology, and the institutes of medicine.
4. Write and defend a thesis.

A bachelor's degree was not necessary to matriculate. A candidate only had to demonstrate proficiency in Latin, English, and natural science, and be of "fair moral character." Such requirements were typical of American medical education nationwide for the first half of the nineteenth century.

Despite its small size and remote location, the medical school in Fairfield counted a disproportionate number of eminent physicians among its alumni, including obstetrician Charles Brodhead Coventry, botanist Asa Gray, American Medical Association founder Nathan Smith Davis, orthopedic surgeon Frank Hastings Hamilton (who attended Fairfield but received his M.D. at the University of Pennsylvania), and surgeon Frederick Hyde. Coventry, Hadley, Hamilton, and Hyde would later play important roles in the development of Geneva Medical College.

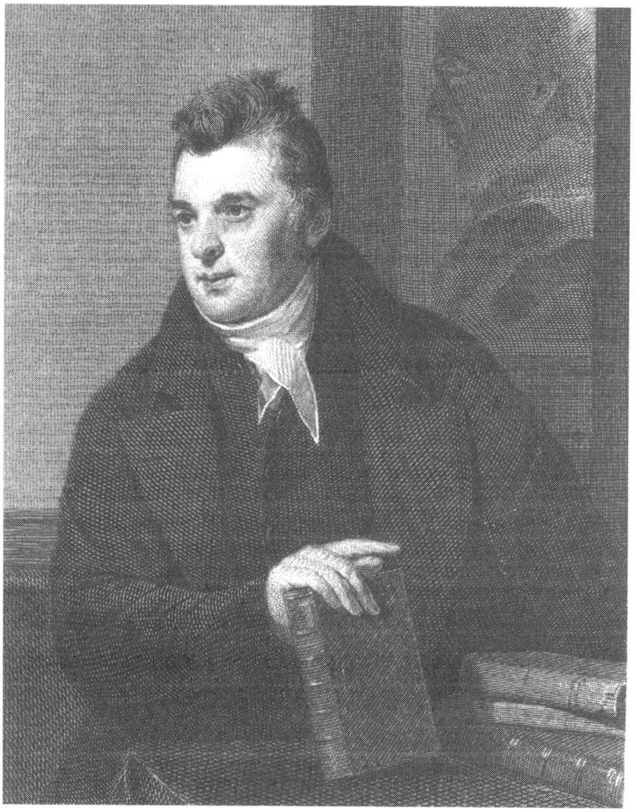

David Hosack (right) was among the most brilliant, prominent, controversial, and irascible physicians in New York City in the early nineteenth century. He taught medical botany at Columbia, founded the Elgin Botanical Garden, was the attending surgeon at the famous duel between

Alexander Hamilton and Aaron Burr, contributed to the progress of Bellevue Hospital, and for thirty years tried to establish himself as the prime mover of medical education in New York. In 1826 he spent $20,000 of his own money to establish a regular medical school at 68 Duane Street, Manhattan. This school had a weak affiliation with Rutgers College in New Jersey, which was supposed to grant the M.D., but in 1827 Hosack's many political enemies in New York and disgruntled colleagues at Columbia exploited a technicality to gain passage of a law which would deny his graduates the right to practice medicine in New York State on the grounds that their degrees would be granted in New York by an out-of-state institution that had no such authority. Unfazed, Hosack then persuaded his friend, Episcopal Bishop John Henry Hobart, who had founded Geneva College in Geneva, New York, in 1822, to reaffiliate the medical school within New York State. Again Hosack's enemies sought to enact new legislation to their advantage and took their case to court, but under Hobart's auspices Hosack created the Rutgers Medical Faculty of Geneva College, which trained physicians at Duane Street until the New York State Supreme Court closed it in 1830, ruling that Geneva College, even though an in-state institution, had no right to maintain a medical school off-site. Hosack finally admitted defeat and retired from medical education shortly after the court handed down this decision. Hosack's departure from these intrigues enabled the New York County Medical Society, dominated by his enemies, to found the short-lived New York School of Medicine in 1831.

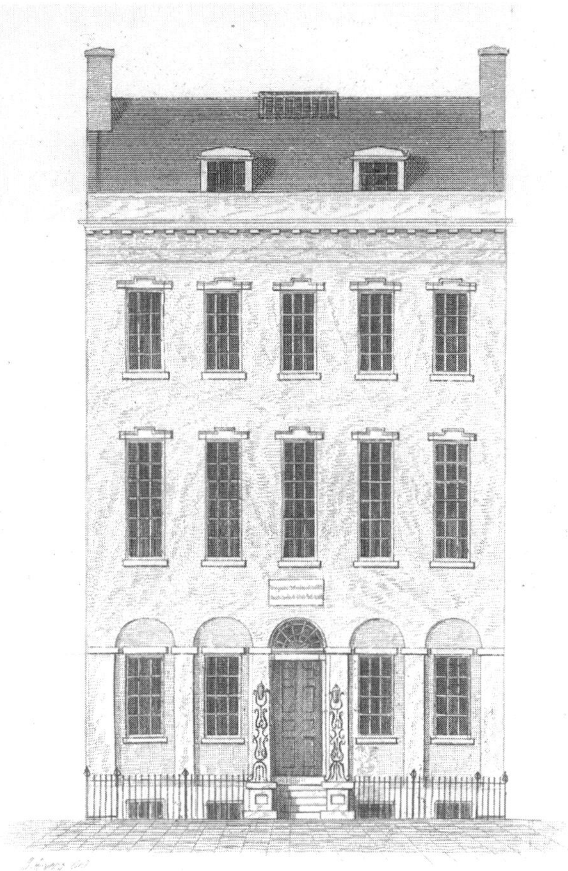

RUTGERS MEDICAL COLLEGE.

INSTITUTED OCT. 26TH 1826.

The founding in 1834 of the Medical Institution of Geneva College, the earliest direct forerunner of Upstate Medical University, resulted in an oblique way from the imperious policies of President Andrew Jackson, satirized in this cartoon from 1832.

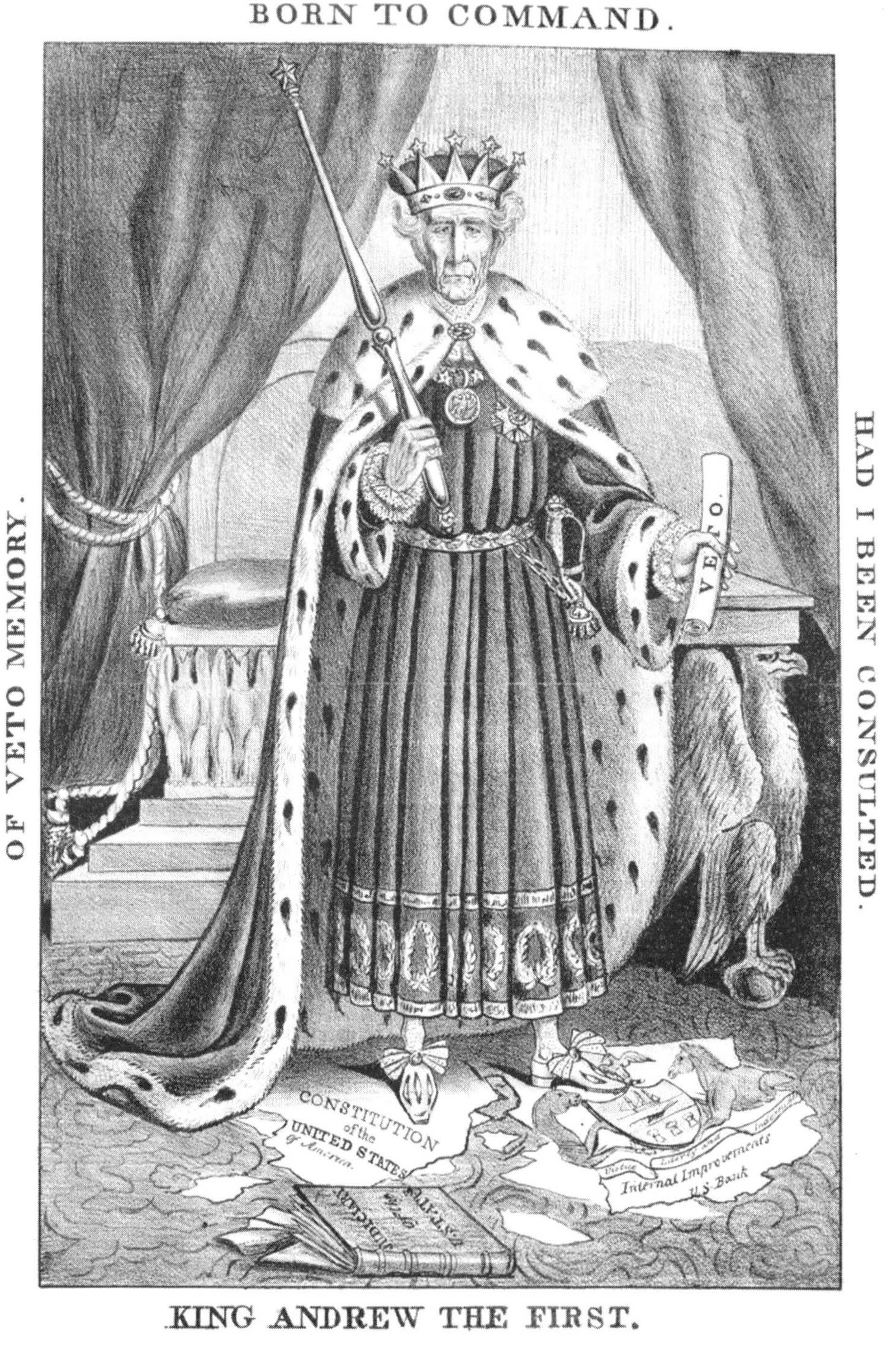

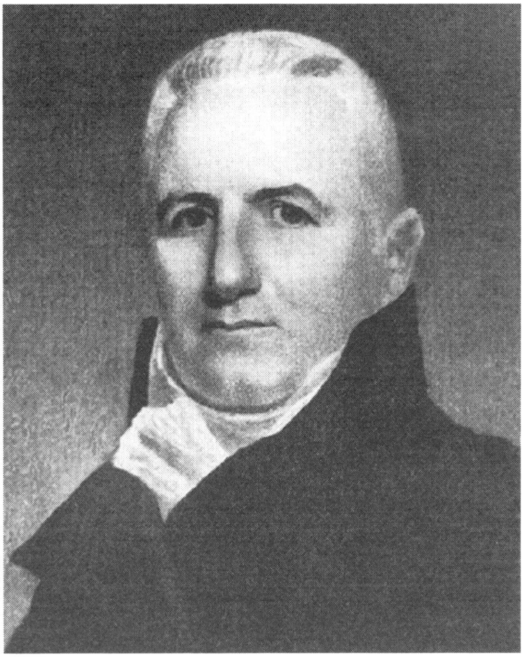

Edward Cutbush, Jr. (right) was born in Philadelphia on January 5, 1772, the eldest son of immigrants from Wokingham, Berkshire, England. In 1784 he entered the College of Philadelphia, later renamed the University of Pennsylvania. It was not unusual then for such young boys to be college students. Even degrees as high as the M.D. were sometimes granted to teenagers.

Because of his father's financial setbacks, Cutbush had to quit college after two years. He then worked as a draft artist for his father, a sculptor. After the deaths of his mother in 1789 and his father in 1790, Cutbush assumed responsibility for his three younger siblings, James, later a surgeon and chemist at West Point, William, later an army engineer, and a sister. While raising these children, he nevertheless found time for medical studies at what is now the School of Medicine of the University of Pennsylvania. Among his medical teachers were such prominent early American physicians as Abraham Chovet, John Foulke, Adam Kuhn, Benjamin Rush (left), James Hutchinson, Thomas Parke, William Shippen, and Caspar Wistar.

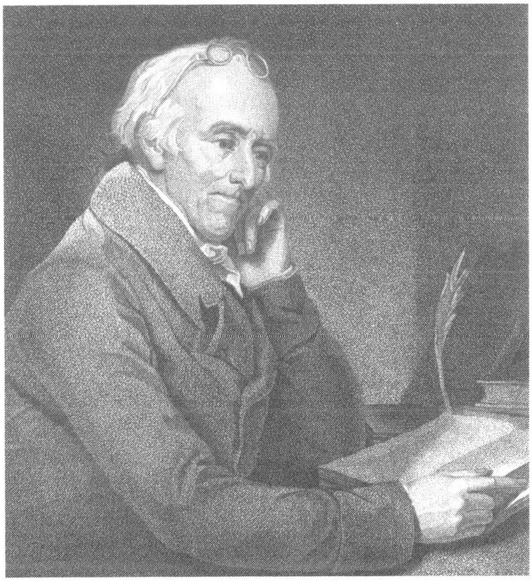

In the summer of 1793, while Cutbush was still in medical school, two events occurred which had profound effects on his understanding of medicine. First, an encounter off the Delaware coast between British and French frigates in the French Revolutionary Wars resulted in a number of wounded sailors from both sides being brought to Pennsylvania Hospital in Philadelphia for treatment. As one of few on rounds who could speak French, Cutbush found himself able to treat the

French wounded better than many senior staff who could not communicate with them. Second, the worst of several yellow fever epidemics hit Philadelphia. Cutbush and his patients were all quarantined inside the hospital. After the crisis passed, Cutbush received the official thanks of both the city and the hospital for his exemplary service. In later years, he especially valued the June 1794 certificate from his colleagues and supervisors at Pennsylvania Hospital as witness to his character and achievements.

Cutbush received his M.D. on May 19, 1794, with a dissertation on insanity which explicitly followed Rush's theories and therapeutics. In August 1794, shortly after he set up private practice at Second and Chestnut in Philadelphia and became a charter member of the Philadelphia Medical Society, the Whiskey Rebellion broke out in western Pennsylvania. Because of Cutbush's superior hospital experience, Pennsylvania Governor Thomas Mifflin appointed him, at the age of twenty-two, Surgeon General of the Pennsylvania Line. During this uprising he met Major James Rees, who lived in Upstate New York at the head of Seneca Lake. The two became lifelong friends. Cutbush's wife Ann ("Nancy"), whom he married 1795, and Rees's wife Elizabeth ("Betsy") were sisters, née Reynolds.

Cutbush tried to resume his civilian medical practice after the rebellion, but since the largely Quaker population of Philadelphia had turned increasingly hostile toward him because of his military adventures, he decided to take a different career path. He visited Rees in Central New York in 1798 and fell in love with the countryside, but saw no professional opportunities there. The Village of Geneva would not be incorporated until 1806. Returning to Philadelphia in March 1799, he decided to join the U.S. Navy. He was appointed navy surgeon on May 28 and commissioned on June 24. He shipped out first under Commodore John Barry in the frigate *United States* on July 2. Nancy, William, and several of his other close relatives lived in Geneva with Rees.

From 1802 to 1803 he saw service in the Tripolitan War aboard the frigate *Constellation*. Back stateside on furlough at half-pay, he was ordered to the ill-fated frigate *Philadelphia* in March 1803, but was too sick to make the voyage. It was just as well, for in a famous incident, Captain William Bainbridge ran the *Philadelphia* aground near Tripoli on October 31, 1803. Bainbridge and his entire crew, including Cutbush's replacement, surgeon Jonathan Cowdery, were prisoners-of-war for the next eighteen months.

In 1804 Cutbush sailed under Commodore Samuel Barron aboard the frigate *President* to establish a naval hospital in Syracuse, Sicily. He directed this hospital until 1806, then was assigned to the Philadelphia Navy Yard. There, in 1807, he translated Francesco Calcagni's *Lettera sulla inoculazione della vaccina practicata in Sicilia* from Italian and wrote his masterpiece, *Observations on the Means of Preserving the Health of Soldiers and Sailors and on the Duties of the Medical Department of the Army and Navy, with Remarks on Hospitals and Their Internal Arrangement*. Published in 1808, this 350-page book included a reprint of Rush's *Directions for Preserving the Health of Soldiers, Addressed to the Officers of the Army of the United States* (1777).

Cutbush remained at the Philadelphia Navy Yard until 1813, when he was ordered to Washington, D.C. to direct the naval hospital. During the Battle of Bladensburg, Maryland, and the subsequent burning of Washington by the British on August 24, 1814, Cutbush was on the field evacuating and treating the wounded. After the war, he returned full-time to administration. In 1816 he co-founded the Columbian Institute for the Promotion of Arts and Sciences, forerunner of the Smithsonian Institution. In 1824 he was appointed senior member of the Board of Naval Medical Examiners. From 1825 to 1827 he was the original professor of chemistry at the Columbian College Medical Department, now the George Washington University School of Medicine.

When Andrew Jackson won the presidency in 1828, he and his appointees were determined to use the spoils system to their perceived advantage at every turn. Cutbush was an old Federalist in the spirit of George Washington, Alexander Hamilton, and John Adams, and was well known in Washington as preferring the cultural and intellectual elite to the vulgar Jacksonian mob. Although he had long been the senior medical officer in the Navy, had an unblemished service record, and had spent thirty years in tireless efforts to improve conditions for patients, surgeons, and hospital staff alike, he was a marked man. On June 6, 1829, Jackson's new Secretary of the Navy, John Branch, ordered the 57-year-old Cutbush back to sea: "Proceed to Norfolk Va. and report to Comm. Barron for duty in the Constellation." Cutbush scribbled on the back of this order: "... to the Constellation as a Surgeon!! A ship in which I had acted as Surgeon 27 years ago. — A retrograde movement in Public Service." He resigned rather than obey.

Rees was shocked when he heard this news. By then a successful banker in Geneva and a founding trustee of both Geneva Academy in 1813 and its successor, Geneva College, in 1822, Rees invited Cutbush in the fall of 1829 to become professor of chemistry at Geneva College. On March 3, 1830, the trustees appointed Cutbush Professor of Chemistry, Agriculture, and the Mechanic Arts at a salary "not exceeding four hundred dollars." Cutbush accepted, and moved to Geneva that spring.

Because of the Erie Canal, which had opened in October 1825, Central and Western New York were growing rapidly in the late 1820s and early 1830s. Cutbush became discouraged that the nearest medical school was Fairfield, over a hundred miles away in Herkimer County. He asked the Geneva College trustees to create one. On September 15, 1834, they approved his suggestion and soon thereafter appointed him its first dean. Earlier, on May 19, 1834, they had approved the plan proposed behind Cutbush's back by trustee J.C. Spencer, whom Cutbush considered duplicitous, for a medical school to be led jointly by two physicians, the respected Philadelphia medical scholar Thomas Spencer (no relation to the trustee) and John George Morgan, a practitioner in Auburn whom Cutbush considered incompetent. But eventually it was Cutbush who sparked the enterprise, with Spencer and Morgan among the original six medical professors.

As the founder of the Medical Institution of Geneva College on September 15, 1834, Cutbush was *ipso facto* the founder of the present State University of New York (SUNY) Upstate Medical University.

Cutbush insisted that all who practice medicine should be broadly educated. He emphasized above all the need for physicians to have command of many languages, especially Latin, French, and German, so as to be conversant with the medical literatures of many cultures. At the official opening of the medical college on February 10, 1835, he expressed his own ideals for medical education: "If I possessed the power, no man should be permitted to enter on the exercise of the profession, who has not been engaged in studying the various branches for at least five years; and even after that period, the life of a conscientious practitioner should be a life of *study*, *research*, and *reflection*." That quotation is from the printed version of his speech, *A Discourse Delivered at the Opening of the Medical Institution of Geneva College, State of New York, February 10, 1835* (p. 15), but the original manuscript, preserved in the Archives of Hobart and William Smith Colleges, says: "If I possessed the power, no man should be permitted to enter the medical profession who has not been engaged in studying its various branches for at least four years, and even after that period, the life of a conscientious practitioner should be a life of study, research and reflection." Whether he wanted five years or only four, Cutbush did not have that power, and the earliest medical curriculum at Geneva was nearly identical to Fairfield's, except that each semester was sixteen weeks long. The curriculum remained a two-year program until the first medical courses were offered at Syracuse University in 1872.

Neither Hosack nor other New York City physicians had anything directly to do with the founding of medical education in Geneva, but had only planted in the minds of Geneva College administrators and trustees the seeds that germinated under Cutbush's care. Besides Cutbush, the other five original medical faculty members were Willard Parker, from

New Hampshire with a Harvard M.D.; Thomas Spencer, from Massachusetts with a Fairfield M.D.; John George Morgan, from Missouri wih unknown medical credentials; Charles Brodhead Coventry, from Upstate New York with a Fairfield M.D.; and Anson Colman, an Upstate New Yorker with a University of Pennsylvania M.D.

The medical school held its first classes in February 1835 in Geneva Hall and graduated its first six physicians later that year. Cutbush laid the cornerstone of its first separate medical education building on September 2, 1835. This "Middle Building" (below) opened in 1836, housed the medical school for five years, and burned in 1885. In 1841 the medical school moved into new and larger quarters on the west side of South Main Street. That second building (shown on page 17) burned in 1877.

MEDICAL INSTITUTION

OF

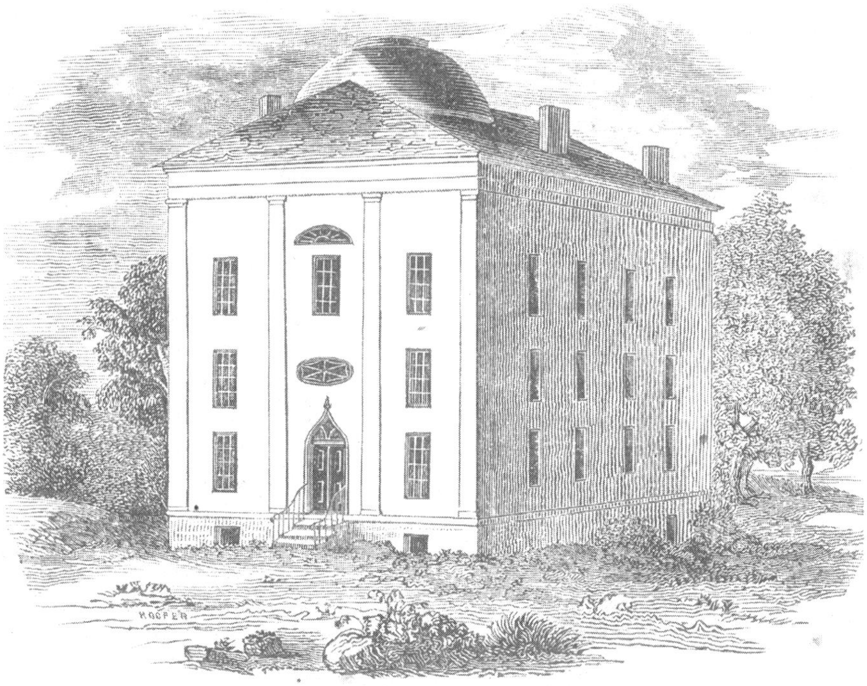

GENEVA COLLEGE.

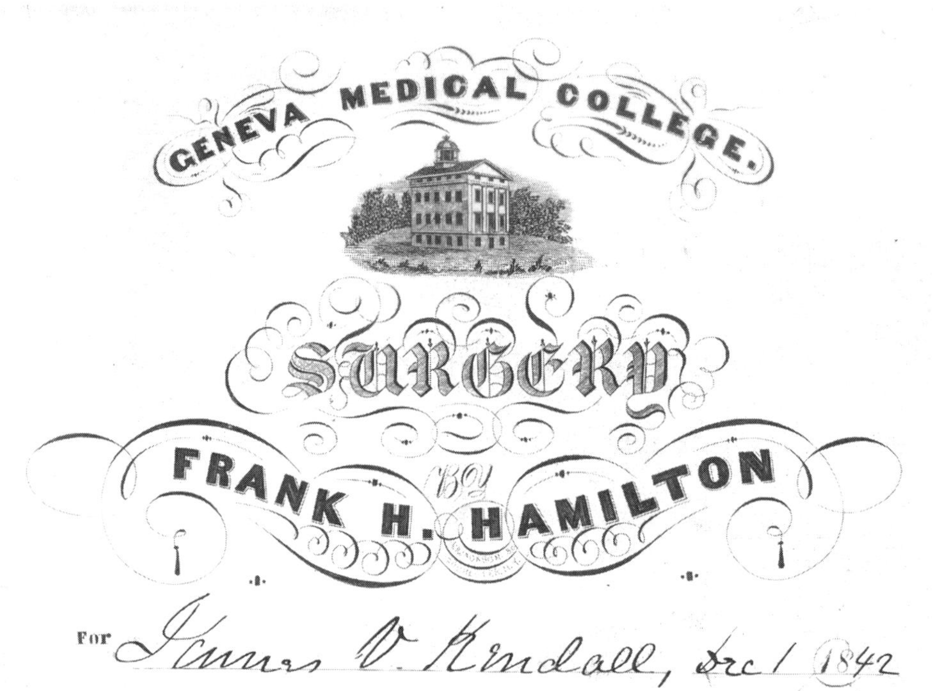

Early nineteenth-century medical students bought tickets authorized by professors to gain admission to lectures. Professors' pay was determined by the number of students.

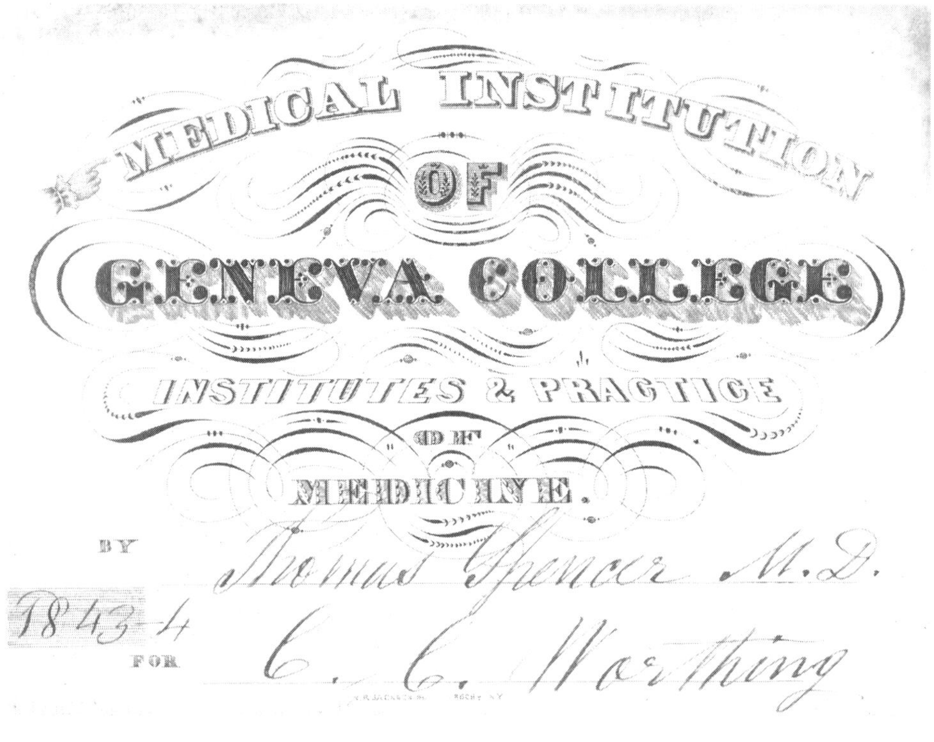

Twenty-nine medical schools were founded in North America by 1833. Fifteen survive.

The fourteen extinct schools are the Faculty of Physic of Queen's College; New York (1787-1794; 1812-1816); the Medical College of Transylvania University (1799-1857); the Medical School of Fairfield Academy (1809; 1812-1841 as the College of Physicians and Surgeons of the Western District of the State of New York); Brown University Medical School (1811-1831); Castleton Medical Academy (1818-1861); the Medical School of Maine of Bowdoin College (1820-1921); Berkshire Medical Institution of Massachusetts (1823-1869); Auburn Medical School, Cayuga County (1824-1839); the College of Physicians of the Valley of Virginia at Winchester (1825-1829); Washington Medical College of Baltimore (1826-1852); Rutgers Medical College in the City of New York (1826, 1827-1830 as Rutgers Medical Faculty of Geneva College); Clinical School of Medicine, Woodstock, Vermont, or Vermont Medical College (1827-1856); Miami University Medical Department (announced 1831 but never established); and the New York School of Medicine (1831-1833).

The fifteen survivors are the School of Medicine of the University of Pennsylvania (1765), the College of Physicians and Surgeons of Columbia University (1767), Harvard Medical School (1782), Dartmouth Medical School (1797), the University of Maryland School of Medicine (1807), Yale University School of Medicine (1810), the University of Cincinnati College of Medicine (1819), the University of Vermont School of Medicine (1822), Jefferson Medical College of Thomas Jefferson University (1824), the Medical University of South Carolina College of Medicine (1824), the University of Virginia School of Medicine (1824), George Washington University School of Medicine and Health Sciences (1825), the Medical College of Georgia School of Medicine (1828), McGill University Faculty of Medicine (1829), and the University of Louisville School of Medicine (1833).

Cutbush founded the seventh medical school in New York State. It is the second oldest surviving in the state, behind only Columbia. Also founded in 1834 were Tulane University School of Medicine and the Ohio State University College of Medicine, but since the Medical College of Louisiana was founded on September 23 and Willoughby Medical College was founded in November, Upstate Medical University can claim priority over both Tulane and Ohio State as the sixteenth oldest surviving medical school in North America.

The faculty of Geneva Medical College, shown chronologically within each subject taught, included some of the most important names in nineteenth-century American medicine, such as Flint, Hamilton, Parker, and Delamater, although most of them made their reputations elsewhere:

Anatomy
1834-1836 Willard Parker
1836-1854 James Webster
1840-1841 Sumner Rhoades
1842-1849 Corydon La Ford (below)

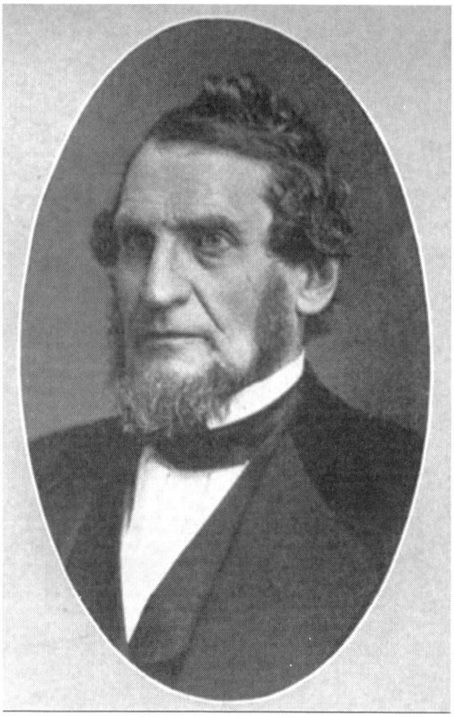

1849-1853 George White Field
1853-1855 Charles ap Arthur Bowen
1854-1855 Augustine Boyer Hawley
1855-1859 James Henry Jerome
1855-1856 Charles Nathaniel Hewitt
1856-1857 Elias de Long Cone
1859-1867 Lyman Warren Bliss
1867-1870 Orin W. Smith
1870 Daniel Swift Burr
1870 Miles Goodyear Hyde

Botany
1834-1836 Anson Colman

Chemistry
1834-1839 Edward Cutbush
1839-1840 Benjamin Hale
1840-1869 James Hadley
1853-1868 John Towler

Diseases of Women and Children
1865-1872 Hiram Newton Eastman

General Pathology
1840-1843 John Delamater
1842-1845 Thomas Rush Spencer
1844-1853 Charles Alfred Lee
1853-1854 Thomas Rush Spencer
1855-1862 Caleb Green

Institutes and Practice of Medicine
1834-1848 Thomas Spencer
1853-1855 William Sweetser

Materia Medica
1834-1853 Charles Brodhead Coventry
1840-1843 John Delamater (below)

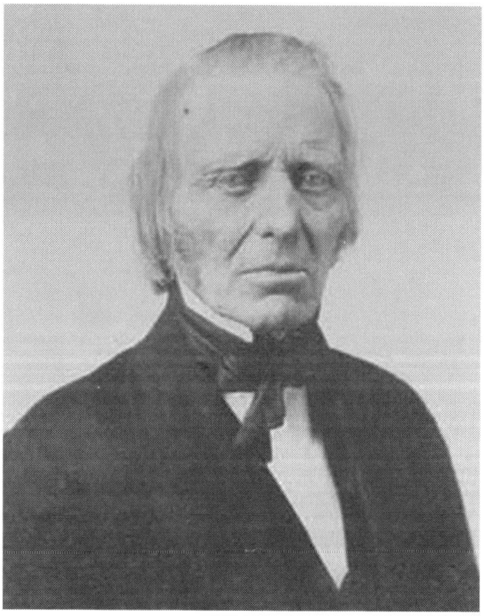

1842-1845 Thomas Rush Spencer
1844-1853 Charles Alfred Lee
1853-1854 Thomas Rush Spencer
1855-1859 Caleb Green
1859-1862 Hiram Newton Eastman
1864-1872 Ezra Pascal Allen

Medical Jurisprudence
1834-1836 Anson Colman
1840-1853 Charles Brodhead Coventry
1854-1855 Frederick Hyde

1855-1859 George Burr
1859-1862 Joseph Beattie

Microscopic Anatomy
1862-1872 Nelson Nivison

Obstetrics
1834-1853 Charles Brodhead Coventry (below)

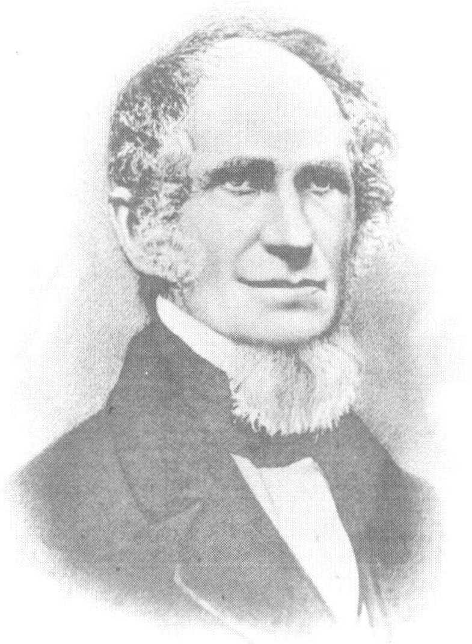

1854-1855 Frederick Hyde
1855-1859 George Burr
1859-1862 Joseph Beattie
1864-1872 Ezra Pascal Allen

Ophthalmology
1870-1872 Charles Everts Rider

Pathology
1859-1862 Caleb Green
1862-1872 Nelson Nivison

Pharmacy
1834-1839 Edward Cutbush
1840-1869 James Hadley
1853-1868 John Towler

Physiology
1834-1836 Willard Parker
1836-1854 James Webster
1853-1855 Charles ap Arthur Bowen
1855-1859 James Henry Jerome
1859-1862 Caleb Green
1862-1872 Nelson Nivison

Practice of Medicine
1859-1872 Hiram Newton Eastman

Principles and Practice of Surgery
1834-1836 John George Morgan
1837 James Webster
1838-1840 David L. Rogers
1840-1848 Frank Hastings Hamilton
1849-1853 James Bryan
1853-1854 Joel Edwin Hawley
1854-1872 Frederick Hyde

Theory and Practice of Medicine
1847-1849 Austin Flint
1847-1849 Edwin Robinson Maxson
1849-1855 William Sweetser
1856-1858 Alfred Bolter
1865-1872 Hiram Newton Eastman (below)

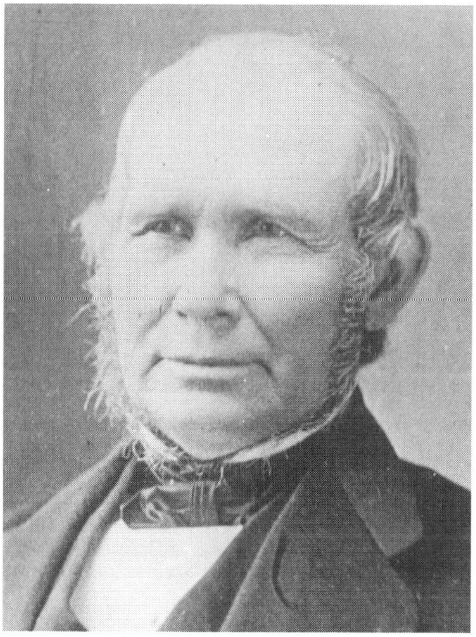

Cutbush retired in January 1839, died on June 23, 1843, and is buried in Glenwood Cemetery, Geneva. Besides his 1794 dissertation, his 1807 translation, his 1808 book, and his 1835 inaugural speech, his publications include *An Address Delivered Before the Columbian Institute for the Promotion of Arts and Sciences at the City of Washington on the 11th January, 1817*; and *An Address Delivered Before the Domestic Horticultural Society of the Western Part of the State of New York at the Semi-Annual Meeting Held at Canandaigua on the 30th Day of June, 1831.*

In 1851 Geneva College changed its name to Hobart Free College. To correlate with that name change, the Medical Institution of Geneva College in 1852 officially assumed the name by which it had been commonly known for years: Geneva Medical College.

George W. Cook, a native of Camillus, New York, enjoyed a long career practicing medicine in Syracuse. He began medical school in the spring term of 1852 at Geneva, then transferred to the New York University School of Medicine, where he received his M.D. in 1853. Forty-three years later he presented a speech called "Some Reminiscences of my Medical College Days; Read Before the Syracuse Academy of Medicine, April 21, 1896," which included humorous vignettes of his Geneva professors. His favorite was the pudgy little James Webster:

> The term had already opened [when I arrived], and I was soon ushered into the college amp[h]itheatre where from forty to fifty students were assembled, and Prof. James Webster, Professor of Anatomy, was holding a surgical clinic.
>
> On the operating table was lying a man with the bloody stump of one of his thighs projecting over the end, an amputation having just been performed. That was the "first blood" for me. Soon after — I think the same week, Prof. Webster essayed to make an extensive plastic operation to remove a large and tense cicatrix from the lower face, chin and neck of a young man, such cicatrix having been caused by a burn. The lesion was a formidable one, and the contracted tissues drew the chin so firmly to the sternum as to preclude rotation of the head. The Professor proposed to dissect out the cicatricial tissues, make a flap from one shoulder and upper arm, and turn it, on a narrow isthmus, into the space vacated by the cicatrix.
>
> Those were early days in the use of chloroform, and a Dr. Smith, I think of the village, was called in to administer the anaesthetic. Having done so, at the supposed proper moment, the Professor made a sweeping incision through the skin from under one ear to the same relative point under the other ear. And immediately the incision was made, the patient made a lunge which placed the surgeon and his assistants perfectly "hors du combat." He was promptly seized, and several stalwart students enlisted to restrain the now crazed and refractory subject.

More chloroform was administered, and at last by means of sheer force and vigorous fighting, the Professor succeeded in dissecting nearly all of the cicatrix he had intended, when the patient made another terrific spring, thus clearing himself and the arena, a second time.

To me, "A tenderfoot," this sight, with blood flowing, and the bloody flap a flapping, was simply horrible; and I suddenly thought that I would go down town to the post-office, and see if there was any mail for me — in short, I preferred to be an outside member for a while. It being Saturday, I went a few miles into the country and spent Sunday with relatives, returning to the college on Monday. I never saw or heard any more of the immolated victim. ...

James Webster was one of the most brilliant and thoroughly accomplished anatomists then known. He followed the celebrated Doctor [John D.] Godman's system of teaching; i. e. dissecting and demonstrating as he delivered his lectures. He was, indeed, to my mind, a most wonderful man; versatile and rapid; he could reel off more anatomy in his lecture of one hour, than I could digest in a week; and, as was his habit, cut short his hour, by telling a good story that would set the boys shouting and cheering, during which the wily Professor would covertly slip out of the lecture room. Poor Old Prof. Webster! He had his many enviable and good qualities, and some weak ones, the lat[t]er proving his physical wreck.

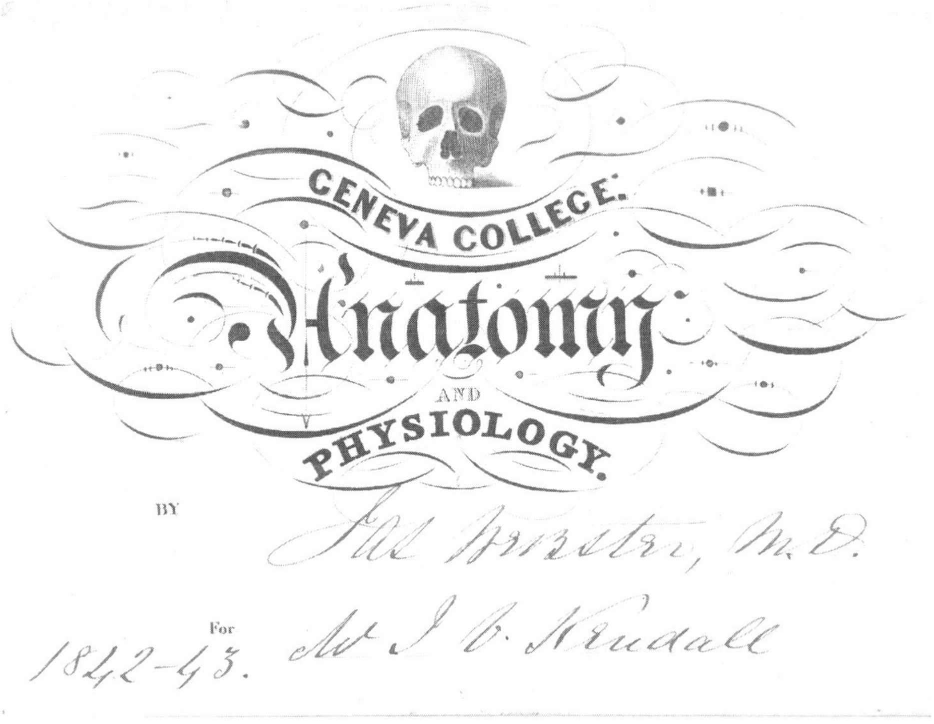

Cutbush's retirement in 1839 placed a great strain on the ability of the medical faculty to teach effectively a scope of material broad enough to justify awarding medical degrees. Only four qualified medical teachers were left, Coventry in obstetrics, Rogers in surgery, Spencer in medicine, and Webster in anatomy. President of the College Benjamin Hale, a minister by profession, had to be pressed into service until Hadley arrived in 1840 so that chemistry could still be offered to medical students. Neither physiology nor pharmacy was given in 1839-1840. No one had taught medical jurisprudence since Colman, nor would until Coventry took up the subject in 1840. There was no instruction in pathology at Geneva before Delamater's course in 1840-1841. Webster had to handle all the anatomical chores himself; he had no demonstrator until Rhoades was hired in 1840.

A branch canal connected Geneva to the Erie Canal in 1829, but the railroad bypassed the town. As the community became a rural backwater instead of an outpost of civilization, more and more isolated from the growing industrial and commercial corridor along what is now the New York State Thruway, clinical experience for medical students became more difficult to obtain. Not medical schools themselves, but independent preceptors and nearby hospitals, were expected to provide clinical experience for medical students. Finding such practitioners and such hospitals was not usually a problem for schools in urban areas, but for schools in more remote locations, such as Fairfield, Auburn, and Geneva, neither enough doctors nor a wide enough variety of clinical cases existed to give students adequate bedside training. Some Geneva students became disappointed and even angry about this.

In view of the meager offerings of the competent but overworked crew of teachers in 1839 and the lack of local opportunities for hands-on clinical learning, the most savage and serious of all student complaints against Geneva Medical College was asserted during the 1839-1840 term.

Andrew Boardman of the class of 1840 presented as his senior thesis in January 1840 an attack on the governance of the school. His charges were not merely the grumblings of a malcontent. On the contrary, they were substantial, to the point, and farsighted. Concerned to eliminate the disparity of qualifications among medical graduates at different institutions, he proposed in some detail the establishment of a national medical university with uniform standards for its many branches. He offered cogent suggestions to improve the quality of teaching, to guarantee the character of teachers, and to deny medical degrees to those who just paid fees and kowtowed but did not attend lectures. Moreover, he accused the school of deceiving prospective students with promises of adequate clinical facilities.

Boardman's thesis caused a scandal on campus, with the majority of the medical faculty obstinately refusing to consider any change at all on his account, despite the fact that all his charges were well founded and well documented. Only one professor stood by him, his preceptor, surgeon David L. Rogers. When Rogers failed to persuade even a single one of his colleagues to agree with him and Boardman that reform was necessary, he resigned from the faculty in protest on January 20, 1840.

Boardman revised his diatribe and published it in the April 1840 of *The Eclectic Journal of Medicine* as “An Essay on the Means of Improving Medical Education and Elevating Medical Character.” Later that year another version appeared as a book, *An Essay on the Means of Improving Medical Education and Elevating Medical Character; Presented to the Faculty of Geneva College, January, 1840; Extracted from The Eclectic Journal of Medicine, for April, 1840* (Philadelphia: Haswell, Barrington, and Haswell, 1840), with Rogers’s letter of resignation quoted in full in the introduction.

After graduating from Geneva, Boardman had an uneven career and eventually became an apologist for phrenology. Rogers continued as a successful surgeon and published a book on surgery.

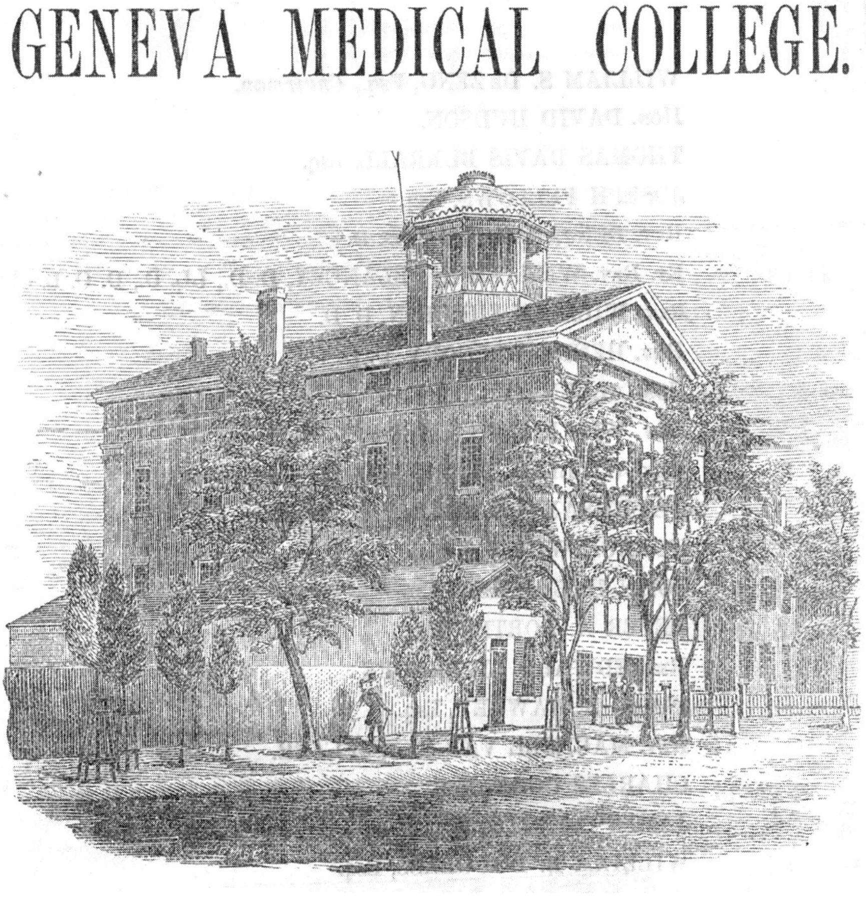

The quality of the original six Geneva professors ran the gamut from well-deserved national reputation (Cutbush, Parker) to regional recognition (Spencer, Coventry) to a promising career tragically cut short (Colman) to questionable character (Morgan).

Parker received both his B.A. and his M.D. from Harvard, in 1826 and 1830 respectively. Before coming to Geneva, he taught at the Berkshire Medical Institution of Massachusetts from 1830 to 1833; and after leaving Geneva, at Daniel Drake's famous but ill-fated Medical Department of Cincinnati College until 1839, when he accepted the chair at the College of Physicians and Surgeons in the City of New York that he held until 1869. He was a surgical pioneer, with major publications on cystitis, vascular surgery, and appendicitis.

Spencer was a member of the New York State Legislature in 1824, President of the Medical Society of the State of New York from 1832 to 1833, and author of works on cholera, biochemistry, and metabolism.

Coventry was President of the Medical Society of the State of New York in 1854 and holder of several other important offices, but he was apparently not much of a teacher. Cook described him as a "peculiar man ... evidently a master of his specialty, and in his lectures, the embodiment of care and deliberation ... excessively modest and unobtrusive. His lectures were never chargeable with being embellished by flights of oratory, brilliant digressions or tedious verbosity. He would be the last man that any one would suspect of the least levity; but one day while lecturing on 'The Conduct of Labor', he remarked, "Now, gentlemen, after the labor has been accomplished, the placenta delivered, and the mother properly cared for, you must not neglect or forget the child."

Colman, born in 1795, learned medicine by apprenticeship in his native village of Richfield Springs, Otsego County. He opened a medical practice in Rochester with John B. Elwood in 1817 and co-founded the Monroe County Medical Society in 1821. Prompted by the worldwide cholera epidemic of 1831 to get better medical training, he went to Philadelphia, where in 1832 he earned his M.D. at the University of Pennsylvania. He continued medical studies in Montreal, New York City, London, and Paris until returning to Rochester in 1834. Cultured and generous, he donated to the new medical school's library the medical books he had acquired in Europe, including the copy of Thomas Hodgkin's *On Some Morbid Appearances of the Absorbent Glands and Spleen* that the author had inscribed to him in London on May 4, 1833. Colman resigned because of chronic poor health in 1836 and died in 1837.

Morgan served as Bishop Hobart's personal physician and was attending surgeon at the state prison in Auburn, from which, it is said, he acquired cadavers for the medical school. After leaving Geneva in 1836, he may have practiced medicine in New York, San Francisco, New Orleans, or St. Louis. He died on October 4, 1878 in Philadelphia.

2

The World's First Woman Doctor

In 1847 Harvard-educated Austin Flint began a two-year term at Geneva Medical College as Lecturer on the Theory and Practice of Medicine. In the late 1840s and early 1850s Flint quickly became a major force in American medicine. The prominent Philadelphia surgeon Samuel David Gross called him "The American Laënnec" for his work in thoracic diagnosis. He served as President of the New York Academy of Medicine from 1872 to 1885 and President of the American Medical Association in 1884. But his most noteworthy achievement with respect to Geneva Medical College was his support of Elizabeth Blackwell. In an era when few medical men would even speak in favor of women doctors, Flint not only spoke, but acted.

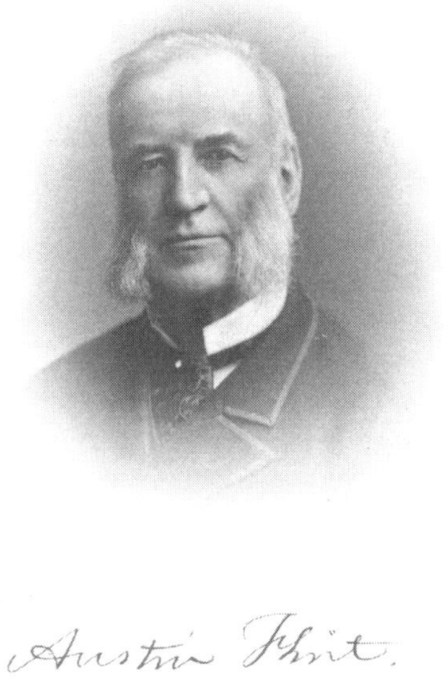

Women have practiced medicine since antiquity, but until the mid-nineteenth century were generally denied the M.D. degree and the other formal credentials of the profession. Some, like Dorothea Christiane Leporin Erxleben in Germany in 1754, received their M.D.'s as flukes, by passing examinations. Others pretended to be men. The woman whose real name may have been Miranda Stuart disguised herself as "James Barry" and earned her M.D. at the University of Edinburgh in 1812, but then was committed to passing herself off as a man for the rest of her life. Others, like Marie Colinet in seventeenth-century Germany, married into the profession and occasionally surpassed their physician husbands. Others, like Marie Anne Victoire Boivin in nineteenth-century France, achieved levels of skill as midwives that made them superior to most of their contemporary male obstetricians. Still others, like Harriot Kesia Hunt in nineteenth-century Boston, just practiced medicine openly without an M.D.

The first woman in the world to earn a regular M.D. from an accredited medical school by satisfying the usual requirements of a full course of study according to modern educational and credentialing standards was born in Bristol, England, on February 3, 1821, the third daughter among the nine children of a sugar refiner, Samuel Blackwell, and his wife, Hannah. The Blackwell family was very close-knit, and all felt a spirit of reform, dissent, and progressive political thinking. For example, they believed in free and equal education for both sexes, a radical notion in those days. Most of the children, not just Elizabeth, later became leaders in social reform movements. Her brother Henry married Lucy Stone, an important suffragist, and her brother Samuel married Antoinette Brown, the first woman the United States to be ordained a member of the clergy.

When Elizabeth's father's business collapsed in 1832, the family left England to start over in America. By the mid-1840s she had lived in New York, New Jersey, Cincinnati, Kentucky, North and South Carolina, and Philadelphia, mostly under adverse financial circumstances. She eked out a living by teaching a variety of subjects to children, but also, encouraged by Rev. John Dickson of Asheville, North Carolina and Dr. William Elder of Philadelphia, studied medicine privately under Dr. Samuel H. Dickson in Charleston, South Carolina and Dr. Joseph Warrington in Philadelphia. Her circle in Philadelphia consisted mainly of Quakers, abolitionists, and other liberal reformers, who noticed her talent for medicine and urged her to try to break the gender barrier in that profession. Warrington, an obstetrician, an 1828 University of Pennsylvania M.D., and a Fellow of the College of Physicians of Philadelphia, was the most prominent of her early supporters. He, Elder, and other liberal Quakers risked their careers by helping her to apply to medical schools.

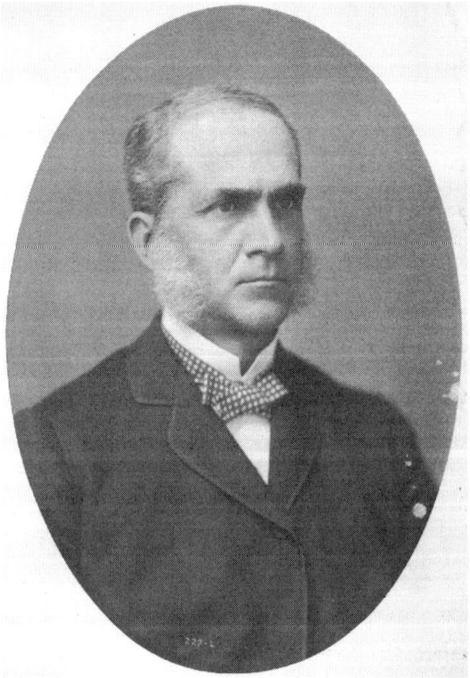

Stephen Smith (left) began his illustrious career in Homer, New York, as the medical apprentice of Caleb Green, who would later teach at Geneva Medical College. Smith attended the medical schools in Geneva and Buffalo before receiving his M.D. in 1850 at Columbia University. A Bellevue Hospital surgeon for the rest of his life, he became a zealot for sanitation reform and was the founding president of the American Public Health Association.

When Elizabeth Blackwell's application reached Geneva in the October 1847, Smith was a student there. As he told the tale in the "Woman as Physician" chapter of his 1872 book, *Doctor in Medicine*, in a letter to the *New York Church Union* in 1892, and again in his appendix to her 1895 autobiography, her rejection was a foregone conclusion. The faculty saw in the situation an opportunity to improve their relations with the students, which had been strained since the Boardman incident and for several other reasons. They submitted the decision to the students, but with the stipulation that the decision must be unanimous. The students, for their part, saw a great opportunity to play a tremendous practical joke on the faculty by letting the woman in. They achieved unanimity by beating up the lone holdout until he capitulated. The astonished faculty, against their will but bound by their word of honor, had no choice but to admit her. Dean of the Faculty Charles Alfred Lee wrote to her on October 20:

> ... A quorum of the Faculty assembled last evening for the first time during the session, and it was thought important to submit your proposal to the class, who have had a meeting this day, and acted entirely on their own behalf without any interference on the part of the Faculty. I send you the result of their deliberations and need only add that there are no fears but that you can, by judicious management, not only "disarm criticism," but also elevate yourself without detracting, in the least, from the dignity of the profession. Wishing you success in your undertaking, which some may deem bold in the present state of society. ...

Blackwell arrived in Geneva to begin her medical studies on November 11, 1847. Immediately (as Smith reported in his 1892 letter) the usual boorish, boisterous, and macho atmosphere of the medical college became more civilized as the male students, shamed by her dignity and intelligence, settled down to serious work. Yet the story of her fifteen months as a student in Geneva epitomizes the nature of small-town mid-nineteenth century prejudice against women medical students. With few exceptions, the Geneva community treated her terribly. Doctors' wives refused to speak to her. Townies stared at her as if she were an exotic animal. Many regarded her as either a lewd woman, or insane, or both, and in any event someone sure to be a bad influence on children. Hadley, the Registrar, promised her letters of recommendation but never sent them.

Besides Flint, Webster was her only other champion among the faculty. He supported her forthrightly, personally, and actively. Having been there only four days, and after only two days of lectures, she wrote to one of her sisters on November 9, 1847, "I feel sunshiny and happy, strongly encouraged, with a grand future before me, and all owing to a fat little fairy in the shape of the Professor of Anatomy."

Webster's colorful vulgarity made him exceedingly popular. Prior to Blackwell's arrival, he enjoyed a grand reputation among the students for his jovial manner and especially for the ribald jokes he would tell in connection with his dissections of the male reproductive system. Although he had welcomed Blackwell from the start, he politely suggested that she not attend that particular session. But when she offered him sound reasons why she should attend, he relented, and confessed to the whole class that he had been justly rebuked. Smith believed that her influence on the culture of Geneva was entirely positive, and especially that her presence in Webster's course lifted the minds of professor and students alike out of the gutter and forced the students to concentrate instead on actually learning the material.

Blackwell was luckier than most Geneva students at finding adequate clinical experience. While most of them had to rely on the volunteer spirit of local practitioners in Upstate New York, she had the resources of a large segment of the Philadelphia Quaker community at her disposal. From March to September 1848, with Elder as her preceptor, she walked the hospital rounds at Blockley Almshouse in Philadelphia, where her patients were mostly women suffering from sexually transmitted diseases. This experience horrified her, and committed her to a lifetime fight against prostitution.

On January 23, 1849, not only did Blackwell became the world's first official woman doctor, but she also she ranked first in her class.

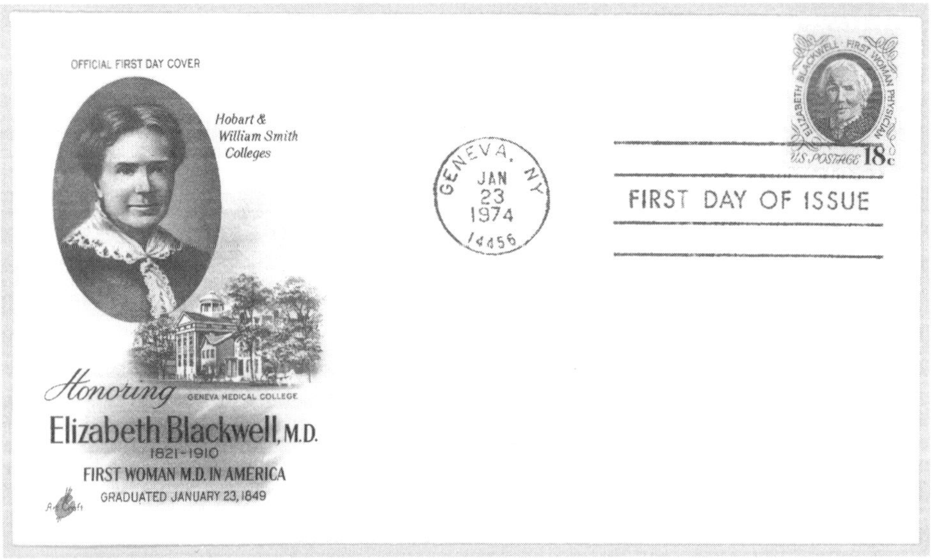

The first day cover issued on the 125th anniversary of her medical graduation repeats a common understatement about her — "First Woman M.D. in America." She was, in fact, the first in the world to earn that degree.

An eyewitness to the ceremony at the Presbyterian Church in Geneva, Margaret Munro DeLancey, wrote in a letter to her sister-in-law Josephine DeZeng DeLancey on January 29:

> I thought I would scribble a few words to you about the graduation of "the female Student." The Medical Commencement took place last Tuesday, a bright Sunshiny day. ... Annie and I went down early to the "Presbyterian House" but though there a full hour before the exercises commenced yet we were unable to get a *front* seat in the gallery. We sat in the Second tier. About half past ten or eleven the procession entered the building. The Lion*ess* of the day, Miss Blackwell met them at the door and entered with the Medical Students, *without* hat or shawl. She wore a black silk dress — and cape — lace collar and cuffs and her *reddishly inclined* hair was very nicely braided. She sat in a front side pew with old Mrs. Waller until she received her Diploma. After President Hale "made a prayer" the choir and fiddles struck up, and the audience were favored with some *extraordinary* performances in *Presbyterian* church music. One woman in the choir was (next to Miss Blackwell) the most conspicuous individual in the meetinghouse. Most alarmingly loud were the tones she uttered, and the *very* peculiar emphasis of the words in the anthem (or whatever they called it) excited any feeling *but* that of solemnity! Take it altogether—*the ladies*—carried the day! ... Nothing but a vast expanse of woman's bonnets and curious eyes. The noise on the "Singer's bench" completed, *President* Hale made a brief Address to the graduating class, then donned the velvet cap and seated himself in the large chair. *As usual,* he did not know his lesson, and had *to read* his few words in Latin as he called up the graduates. Four at a time they came on the stage. The Doctor spoke. They *looked* Knowing. One of them grasped the bundle of sheepskins, all four bowed and vanished. Last of all came "Domina Blackwell"! She ascended the steps. The President touched his cap and rose. You might have heard a pin drop. He *stood* while he conferred the Degree on her, handed her the diploma and bowed, evidently expecting she would bow also and retreat. Not so, however! She seemed embarrassed and after an effort, said to the Dr., "I thank you kind Sir. It shall be the effort of my life, by God's blessing, to shed honor on this Diploma," then bowed, blushed scarlet, left the stage and took her seat in the front pew among the Graduates, amid the Enthusiastic applause of all present. Her color left her cheek in a few moments and she sat calm and composed through the address of Dr. Lee. This was long but very interesting and ably written. And at the conclusion he alluded in a dignified manner to the fact that one of the present class was a female, complimented the sex generally

> and Miss B. in particular, and told us that she was fully qualified to practice as Physician, and that the degree was *fully merited.* The applause was again *loud* though brief. The music "*audiantur"ed,* according to the Presidents order, a short prayer made, the benediction given, and *Elizabeth Blackwell M.D.* and her classmates were turned adrift on the Streams of time each "to paddle his own canoe"! The Faculty of Arts, the Medical professors, Father, and sundry others, as they passed out stopped and congratulated her. When nearly all the crowd had gone she put on her hat and shawl, took the arm of her brother (who came from N.Y. to be present) and so escorted, *Miss Blackwell, M.D.* mingled with the mass and disappeared and so ended Medical Commencement January 23d, 1849 — a day to be remembered — being the first instance the world has ever had, where the degree of M.D. was conferred on *a Woman.*

Another eyewitness, Elizabeth's brother Henry, wrote in a letter to their family on January 23:

> ... The important crisis is past — the great occasion over — the object of so much & so justifiable anticipation has been attained ... About half past 10 o'clock E. & I walked up to the church ... it was arranged that Eliz. & I should sit down at the entrance of the left aisle and join the procession as it came up ... We found the church — galleries and all, crowded with ladies, they only having been as yet admitted & of course when we came in there was a general stir & murmur & everybody turned to look at us. By the time the procession came up — all the pews except those reserved for them were filled ... After a short discourse by Dr. Hale the President - the diplomas were conferred — 4 being called at a time — and ascending the steps to the platform the President addressed them in a latin formula — taking off his hat, but remaining seated — & so handed them their diplomas, which they received with a bow & retired. Eliz. was left to the last & called up alone — the President taking off his hat, rose & addressing her in the same formula — substituting Domina for Domine, presented her the diploma — whereupon our Sis. who had walked up & stood before him with much dignity bowed & half turned to retire but suddenly turning back replied Sir I thank you — by the help of the Most High, it shall be the effort of my life to shed honour upon your diploma — whereupon she bowed & the President bowed — the audience gave manifestations of applause — little Dr. Webster rubbed his hands — the learned curators & faculty nodded grave approbation at each other upon the platform & our Sis. descending the steps took her seat with her fellow-physicians in front. ...

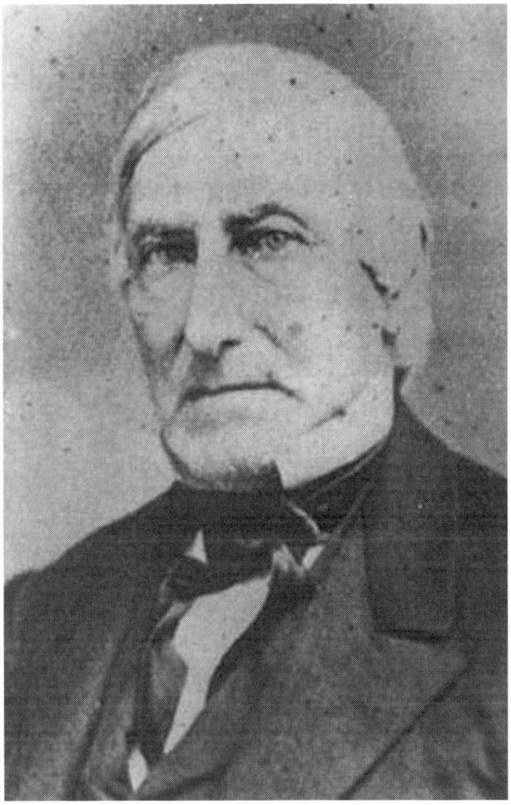

Lee (right), in his valedictory speech, invariably called his audience just "Gentlemen" — as if alluding to the fact that not all of the people in his audience were physically capable of ever becoming gentle "men." Yet his rhetoric, if it was sincere (and Blackwell apparently thought it was), may have been applauded even by feminists, for he lavishly and specifically praised the thoroughness and integrity of her study of medicine. But then he added: "Such cases must ever be too few, to disturb the existing relations of society, or excite any other feeling on our part than admiration at the heroism displayed, and sympathy, for the sufferings voluntarily assumed!" In other words, Lee and most of his colleagues would have been quite happy if Blackwell had been not only the first, but also the last woman ever to receive a degree in medicine. They considered her a talented freak.

Immediately after Blackwell's graduation, a vigorous debate about whether women should be physicians arose nationwide. The leading American medical journal of the era, the the *Boston Medical and Surgical Journal* (now the *New England Journal of Medicine*), simply reported the facts of Blackwell's graduation, without editorializing, in an anonymous announcement, "Doctress in Medicine," on February 7, 1849. Reaction was swift and almost entirely negative. The journal published two pseudonymous attacks, "The Late Medical Degree to a Female" by "D.K." on February 21, 1849, and "The Late Medical Degree at Geneva" by "Justus" on February 28. Since "D.K." is pronounced like the Greek *dikê* (δικη), both pseudonyms are puns on the word "justice." D.K.'s letter to the editor was particularly vitriolic:

> ... I am sorry that Geneva Medical College should be the first to commence the nefarious process of amalgamation. Hitherto an intuitive sense of propriety has induced all civilized nations to regard the professions of law, medicine, and divinity as masculine duties ... The course of "*domina* Blackwell" cannot be justified by any urgent necessity. The profession was quite too full before, and could well

> afford to dispense with her services. ... Would either of the other two learned professions have received and graduated a female? ... Certainly not. Then why desecrate the profession of medicine, and publicly disparage it?

Justus argued that occasionally some "masculine women" are called to medicine and that the profession should find places for them as obstetricians and gynecologists. The last paragraph of his response to D.K.'s letter is: "Even admitting the correctness of D.K.'s remarks in general, with respect to woman's unfitness for engaging in the practice of medicine, it would be strange indeed if exceptions did not occasionally occur. From all we have been able to learn respecting Miss B., she is emphatically an exception. *Exceptio probat Regulam.*" In the published version of his valedictory speech, Lee added this footnote, referring to D.K.:

> ... an article has appeared in the *Boston Medical and Surgical Journal*, condemning in very severe terms, the conduct of the Faculty of Geneva College, in allowing Miss B. admission to their courses of lectures, and of the Trustees in conferring upon her the degree of M.D.
>
> The writer, while he acknowledges the validity of the argument, so far as it is founded on the general physical disqualifications of the sex for the medical profession, and the incompatibility of its duties, with those properly belonging to the female portion of society, believes, nevertheless, that instances occasionally happen, where females display such a combination of moral, physical, and intellectual qualifications for discharging creditably and skilfully the duties belonging to our calling, that it would seem equally unwise and unjust, to withhold from them those advantages and those honors, which are open to nearly all others, whether deserving of them or not. While he holds this opinion, he at the same time feels bound to say, that the inconveniences attending the admission of females to all the lectures in a medical school, are so great, that he will feel compelled on all future occasions, to oppose such a practice, although by so doing, he may be subjected to the charge of inconsistency.

Defending his institution for having admitted and graduated a woman and apologizing to male medical students for having "inconvenienced" them with her, Lee admitted that he would rather be both "unwise and unjust" than participate in creating any further "inconveniences" for men. Plainly the greatest obstacle that Blackwell had to overcome was neither the alleged physical, intellectual, and moral limitations of her sex nor even the open hostility of conservatives such as D.K., but rather the entrenched hypocrisy or crypto-misogyny of liberals like Lee and Justus, who believed that the only way for a woman to become a doctor legitimately would be first to "defeminize" herself and assume instead the purely "masculine" moral and intellectual characteristics of medical men. The rub was that such a process of "defeminization" is contrary to nature, and should thus be condemned.

Reacting to the general outrage of the medical community, Geneva Medical College immediately shut its doors to women. In the early 1850s not even Blackwell's sister Emily could persuade Geneva to relax its new policy (although there is a record of a Martha A. Rogers receiving an M.D. from Geneva in 1865). Emily Blackwell received her M.D. from Cleveland Medical College in 1854, after having been rejected by several other American medical schools besides Geneva, and after having been expelled from Rush Medical College in Chicago because of her gender.

Flint published Blackwell's doctoral dissertation on epidemic louse-borne typhus ("ship fever") in the February 1849 issue of the *Buffalo Medical Journal* and offered her other support, but America in general was against her. Wanting to become a surgeon, she decided — correctly — that she could best pursue postgraduate medical education in Europe. She arrived in Paris in May 1849 to begin her residency at La Maternité in June. In November of that year, while syringing the eyes of a child with purulent ophthalmia, she accidentally splashed her own eye and contracted the disease herself. The resultant blindness of her left eye precluded a career in surgery.

She left Paris to continue postgraduate studies briefly at St. Bartholomew's Hospital in London, then returned to America in 1851, but not before she had begun a lifelong friendship and collaboration with Florence Nightingale. She became increasingly interested in social causes, especially those regarding the political and educational status of women.

Unable to overcome the prejudice against her, unable to attract any patients except the truly desperate, and unable to establish herself in New York City either in private practice or as a hospital-affiliated physician, she resolved to found her own infirmary. Her sister Emily and Marie Elizabeth Zakrzewska (pronounced "zak-SHEFF-ska"), a superbly trained German immigrant midwife who earned her M.D. at Cleveland Medical College in 1856, helped her with this project. The result was her greatest achievement. The New York Infirmary for Women and Children, later known as the Beekman Downtown Hospital, was chartered in 1854 and opened in May 1857 with "Dr. Zak" as chief resident and Emily as chief of surgery. It grew steadily, developing programs of medical social work and nurses' training as well as caring for pediatric, obstetrical, and gynecological patients. Under Emily's administration, it ran a medical school for women from

1868 to 1899. Emily closed the school only after she was satisfied that Cornell University Medical College would give equal training to both sexes and after she had arranged for all of her students to transfer to Cornell.

In 1854, when Elizabeth was 33 and had already determined not to marry, she adopted Katharine ("Kitty") Barry, a 7-year-old Irish-American orphan. She probably felt that having a dependent would help her to fight the loneliness and isolation which her chosen profession had imposed on her. Kitty became absolutely devoted to her, always living with her, always calling her "Doctor," and not changing her own name to "Blackwell" until after Elizabeth's death.

From the late 1850s until she finally settled in England in 1869, Blackwell was back and forth across the Atlantic. One curious consequence of her seeking professional refuge in Europe was that, in addition to being the first woman doctor in America, she was also the first woman doctor in Great Britain. In 1858, principally through the influence of Sir James Paget, who had secured her internship at St. Bartholomew's eight years

ADDRESS

ON THE

MEDICAL EDUCATION OF WOMEN,

PREPARED BY

DRS. E. AND E. BLACKWELL,

READ BEFORE A MEETING HELD AT THE

NEW YORK INFIRMARY,

DECEMBER 19TH, 1863.

16

NEW YORK INFIRMARY

FOR

WOMEN AND CHILDREN,

126 SECOND AVENUE.

This Institution was incorporated in 1854. Its objects are to aid the sick poor; to give to female students an opportunity of taking part in practical medicine; and to train nurses for the sick. During the past seven years it has relieved 26,000 patients.

Trustees:

CHAS. BUTLER, *President.*	MARCUS SPRING.
STACY B. COLLINS, *Vice-President.*	CYRUS W. FIELD.
ROBERT HAYDOCK, *Treasurer.*	CHAS. A. DANA.
MERRITT TRIMBLE, *Secretary.*	MRS. HENRY BAYLIS.
SAMUEL WILLETS.	" ROBT. CAMPBELL.
CHAS. B. TATHAM.	" PETER TOWNSEND.
RICHD. H. BOWNE.	" JAS B. WRIGHT.
SIMEON DRAPER.	" W. H. HUSSEY.
HENRY J. RAYMOND.	" E. BLACKWELL.

Consulting Physicians:

VALENTINE MOTT, M. D. S. L. D.

WILLARD PARKER, M. D. JAS R. WOOD, M. D.

GUSTAVUS A. SABINE, M. D. AUSTIN FLINT, M. D.

Attending Physicians:

ELIZABETH BLACKWELL, M. D. EMILY BLACKWELL, M. D.

Assistant Physician:

FRANCES A. COOK, M. D.

earlier, she became the first woman to be entered in the *British Medical Register*. Such listing is tantamount to being licensed to practice medicine in Great Britain.

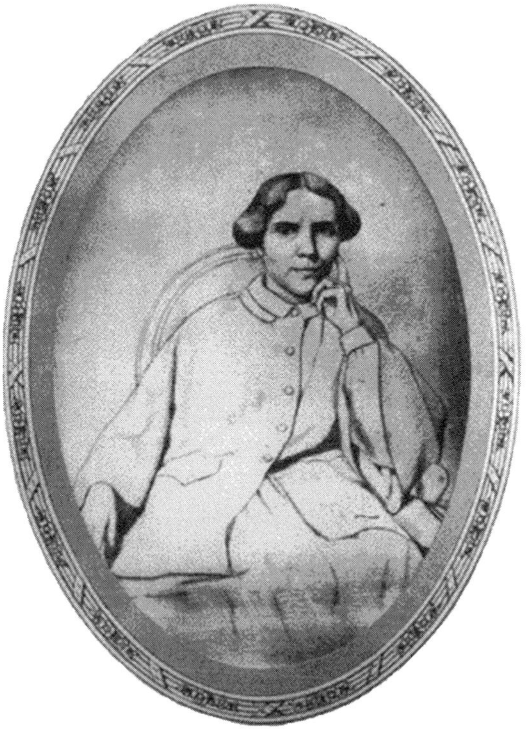

Elizabeth Blackwell in 1859, drawn by Claire d'Agoult, Marquise de Charnacé

In 1859 the young British feminist Elizabeth Garrett Anderson was inspired by meeting Blackwell to try to become the first woman to earn a medical degree in Britain. She was refused admission by every British medical school but found a loophole in the British Society of Apothecaries regulations, sat for their qualifying examination, passed it in 1865 and thus became in 1866 the second woman in the *British Medical Register*. The Society of Apothecaries immediately changed its regulations specifically to bar women. A third woman did not appear in the *British Medical Register* until 1877 when Sophia Jex-Blake and four other women, all with Swiss M.D.s, were added.

In the American Civil War, with Nightingale's guidance and support, Blackwell organized relief efforts, promoted sanitary services, and trained nurses. She established a prosperous private practice in England in the 1870s, helped to found the British National Health Society in 1871, and held the Chair of Gynecology at the London School of Medicine for Women from 1875 until she retired in 1907 at the age of 86. She died at her home, Rock House, in Hastings, England, on May 31, 1910, and is buried in Kilmun, Scotland, a place that she and Kitty particularly enjoyed visiting in later life.

Blackwell became a prolific author. Among her published books and pamphlets are *Medicine and Morality* (1850); *The Laws of Life with Special Reference to the Physical Education of Girls* (1852); *An Appeal in Behalf of the Medical Education of Women* (published anonymously, 1856); *Address on the Medical Education of Women* (1856); *Medicine as a Profession for Women* (co-authored with Emily, 1860); *Address on the Medical Education of Women* (co-authored with Emily, 1864); *How to Keep a Household in Health* (1870); *Lectures on the Law of Life* (1871);

The Religion of Health (1878); *Counsel to Parents on the Moral Education of Their Children* (1878; second edition published in 1879 as *The Moral Education of the Young in Relation to Sex, Under Medical and Social Aspects*); *Christian Socialism* (1882); *Rescue Work in Relation to Prostitution and Disease* (1882); *Wrong and Right Methods of Dealing with Social Evil, as Shown by English Parliamentary Evidence* (1883); *The Human Element in Sex* (1884); *On the Decay of Municipal Representative Government* (1885); *A Medical Address on the Benevolence of Malthus, Contrasted with the Corruptions of Neo-Malthusianism* (1888); *The Influence of Women in the Profession of Medicine* (1889); *Why Hygienic Congresses Fail* (1892); *Pioneer Work in Opening the Medical Profession to Women* (1895, her autobiography and masterpiece); *Scientific Method in Biology* (1898); and *Essays in Medical Sociology* (1899).

After 1849 the percentage of women physicians in America steadily increased, up to a high point of about 10 percent in 1914. The situation had improved so much by 1889 that Blackwell could write in *The Influence of Women*: "The avenues by which all may enter into the profession are now so much more widely thrown open, that there is little difficulty in the way of any man or woman who may wish to acquire a legal right to practice medicine." Ever the optimist, she painted perhaps too rosy a picture of the reality. After 1914 began a decrease and a leveling off that did not rebound until the 1970s. Women were only about 6 percent of all American physicians in 1924, 7.8 percent in 1970, 9.1 percent in 1975, 11.6 percent in 1980, and 22 percent in 1997. These percentages continue to rise in women's favor, and in 2005 half of American medical students are women.

By the 1870s, women were well established as co-educational medical students in the United States. America was slightly ahead of Europe in this regard. At the College of Medicine of Syracuse University, for example, no fewer than eleven women received the M.D. between 1873 and 1878. Sarah Van Tuyl was the first of these, and there is no indication that she was the victim of any sort of sustained or systematic gender prejudice as a medical student. Syracuse University, founded by socially progressive Methodists, was co-educational in all departments from the start.

Blackwell wrote in *The Influence of Women* in 1889 that the duty of medical women was not to imitate medical men, but to define ever more clearly what is morally right and wrong in medicine. For her, the entrance of women into medicine made the profession in general more moral, i.e., more responsive to a wider variety of human needs than men alone recognize. This is because the "high moral life, enlarged by intelligence" is the natural "ideal of womanhood." "It is through the moral, guiding the intellectual, that the beneficial influence of women in any new sphere of activity will be felt."

3

Geneva Medical College and its Competition

In 1851, Sumner Rhoades, an alumnus, curator, and former faculty member of Geneva Medical College, publicly advocated closing the medical school and substituting a school of agriculture. He was not only disgusted by declining enrollments and prestige following the hostile reaction of the medical community at large to the graduation of Elizabeth Blackwell, but also convinced that little headway had been made since the Boardman scandal and that the apparently permanent lack of nearby hospitals would soon make competition with urban medical schools impossible. Geneva's problem with providing adequate facilities for clinical training was getting worse. Medical and surgical science, especially in the wake of the dawn of dependable surgical anesthesia in October 1846, was beginning to make rapid advances. With that grew the demand among medical students for the type of teaching hospitals which only large metropolitan areas could offer. This problem was a major factor in overpowering at the time not only Geneva, but many other rural or small-town medical schools.

Rhoades's plea was not without reason. Flint, La Ford, Hamilton, and the elder Spencer all left in 1848 or 1849 and, with the exceptions of William Sweetser, John Towler, and Frederick Hyde (left), those who replaced them were not up to the standards of quality that they had established. In 1848-1849 there were 106 students enrolled in the medical program, the next academic year, 101; but in 1851-1852, 79, and in 1852-1853, only 43. The Class of 1848 graduated 27 (all with earned degrees), the Class of 1849, 36 (32 earned, four honorary), the Class of 1850, 32 (31 earned, one honorary), the Class of 1851, 31 (28 earned, three

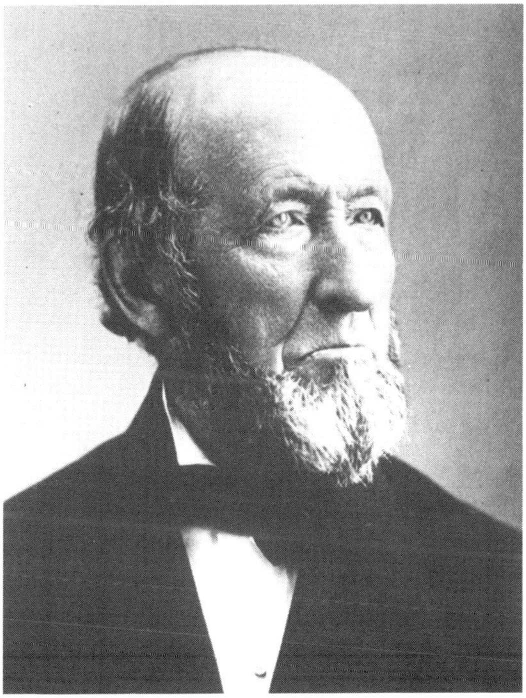

honorary); but the Class of 1852, only 21 (15 earned, six honorary), and the Class of 1853, 15 (12 earned, three honorary). Even as early as 1854 the attractiveness of Geneva Medical College had deteriorated to such an extent that no medical degrees of any kind were conferred that year. Specifically because Geneva had admitted and graduated a woman, many students refused to go there and many professors refused to teach there.

Small, unregulated, proprietary medical schools, representing a wide variety of medical philosophies, flourished nationwide in the early nineteenth century, especially in areas of burgeoning population such as the Erie Canal corridor. Competition among them for medical students and disciples, not to mention patients, was fierce. Regular or "allopathic" medicine, although scientific, was at that time impotent to cure most diseases and thus could easily lose its popular support to the scientific alternative of eclecticism and even to such pseudoscientific alternatives as hydropathy, homeopathy, Thomsonianism, and various botanical or herbal theories of healing. Standards of medical education were almost non-existent. Practitioners and medical educators alike ranged from upright and virtuous physicians to well-meaning fools to utter quacks and scoundrels.

To bring order out of this chaos and thereby to solidify respect for regular medicine was the main reason that Nathan Smith Davis — just ten years out of Fairfield — founded the American Medical Association at the Academy of Natural Sciences in Philadelphia in 1847. Immediately the AMA established clear standards for awarding the M.D. degree, appointed a standing Committee on Medical Education, and wrote a code of medical ethics. The aim of the new organization was nothing less than eradicating irregular and defining and controlling regular medicine.

The proximate cause of the closing of the medical schools in Auburn in 1839 and Fairfield in 1841 was the founding and initial success of Geneva Medical College. Despite this, Geneva never dominated the market for medical students in Upstate New York. Its competition came from both regular medicine and the plethora of alternative theories of medicine. Regular medical education was enhanced at each end of the Erie Canal by the founding of Albany Medical College in 1839 and the Department of Medicine at the University of Buffalo in 1846.

Alden March, a private teacher of surgery in Albany, and his student and brother-in-law, James Harvey Armsby, professor of anatomy and physiology at Castleton Medical Academy in Vermont, co-founded Albany Medical College with $800,000 that Armsby raised. Ten years later they co-founded Albany City Hospital, thus putting the clinical foundation of medical education in Albany on solid ground.

The medical school in Buffalo was Flint's brainchild. Its main advantage over Geneva was the excellence of its faculty. Seven of the eight

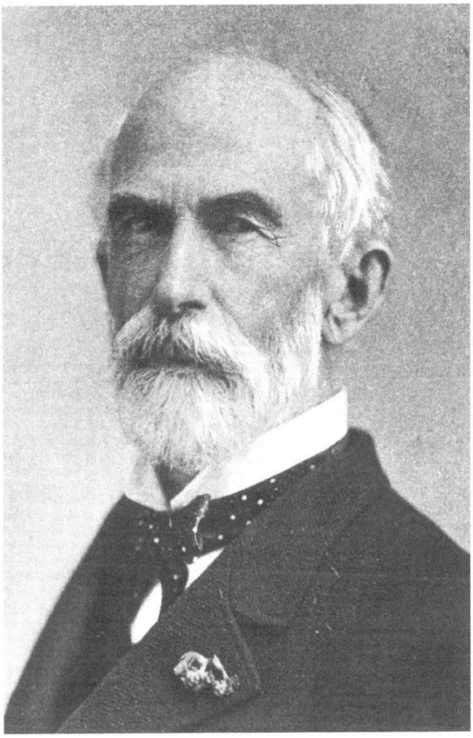

founding faculty members in Buffalo (Coventry, Flint, La Ford, Hadley, Hamilton, Lee, and Webster) were either present or past members of the Geneva faculty. The eighth, obstetrics professor James Platt White, an 1834 Jefferson graduate, later became a nationally prominent gynecologist. Flint was especially fortunate at being able to attract Frank Hastings Hamilton (right), who, after his eight-year term teaching surgery at Geneva, achieved great fame as a military surgeon, an orthopedic surgeon, and an advocate of sanitation and antisepsis. Flint made sure that the clinical and pedagogical resources and equipment in the rapidly growing urban area were state-of-the-art.

Geneva Medical College could not acquire or maintain the same level of educational quality that the new medical schools in Albany and Buffalo had quickly developed in the 1840s, mainly because it could not provide the variety of clinical experiences that they could. Nevertheless, throughout its existence from 1834 to 1871, it graduated some stellar physicians, including Corydon La Ford, Class of 1842, lecturer and author on anatomy and physiology and dean of the Medical School of the University of Michigan; John Preston Mann, Class of 1842, pioneer in non-invasive orthopedic treatment of clubfoot and other abnormalities; Alfred Mercer (right), Class of 1845, outstanding surgeon, medical educator, and public health administrator in Syracuse, father of histologist Alfred Clifford Mercer, Class of 1878, and great uncle of pathologist Herman Gates

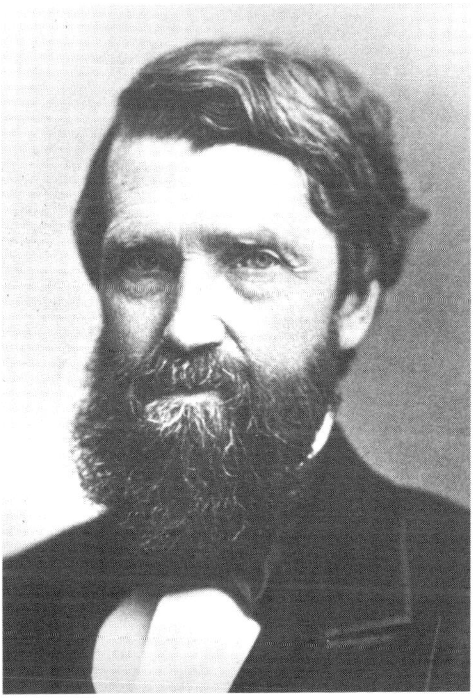

Weiskotten, Class of 1909; Moses Gunn, Class of 1846, dean of the Medical School of the University of Michigan; Geneva Medical College Dean John Towler, Class of 1855; Cornelius Wilson Larison, Class of 1863, New Jersey clinician, teacher, and administrator, advocate of spelling reform, and publisher of the *Jurnal of Helth*; and Charles Leonard Wells, Class of 1869, president of the Minnesota Academy of Medicine.

While many Geneva Medical College alumni made their careers far from Upstate New York, most of them stayed nearby. This demographic had its benefits and drawbacks. One symptom of the decline of any institution of higher learning is what could be called "professional inbreeding," that is, the policy of hiring too many of the school's own recent graduates to be its teachers. Without diverse faculty backgrounds, students lose much of the advantage had by being able to compare a wide variety of shared experiences. Geneva Medical College fell heavily into this error in the 1850s. Of the final twenty new professors hired by Geneva, eleven had Geneva medical degrees (seven earned, four honorary), and an additional two had Geneva or Hobart College baccalaureates. These figures do not count Thomas Rush Spencer, rehired in 1853, who was a Geneva undergraduate alumnus.

Even after the energetic early days of the AMA, educational and credentialing reform was slow in coming. For much of the nineteenth century, licensing agencies did not require medical practitioners to have either a medical degree or any formal education at all. In many jurisdictions, especially on the frontier, practicing medicine without a license was acceptable. American medical schools in general until the 1870s asked students for little more than paying the fees, attending two years of lectures, and writing a dissertation in order to receive a degree.

All of the above-mentioned factors combined to make Upstate New York in the mid-nineteenth century fertile ground for all kinds of medicine. Despite the growth of the Albany and Buffalo regular medical environments, regular medicine between these two points did not make much headway, and non-allopathic systems continued to attract the popular imagination. Regular medicine in those days was violent, invasive, and insensitive, with frightful procedures such as bloodletting, cupping, leeching, purging, inducing emesis, chilling, steaming, and scarifying all more or less typical. Patients' abhorrence of these mostly ineffective methods contributed to the rise of gentler therapeutics at the hands of unconventional practitioners.

A great many varieties of herbal or botanic therapeutic systems have appeared throughout American history. The naturalness of the healing properties of plants appeal intuitively to patients who distrust artificial or extraordinary remedies and instead find solace in familiar substances. The best known is probably Thomsonianism, founded in the late eighteenth century by a New Hampshire farmer, Samuel Thomson, whose basic premise was that normal bodily functions, when obstructed, cause illness, which can then be cured by restoring these functions to normal. But unlike his mainstream medical contemporaries, who would accomplish this "unclogging" by aggressive means, he relied on a vegetable materia medica and a milder set of purgatives and emetics. His books include an autobiography and *New Guide to Health, or Botanic Family Physician*, his major work, which appeared first in 1822 and in many subsequent editions, some legitimate and some pirated, until 1894.

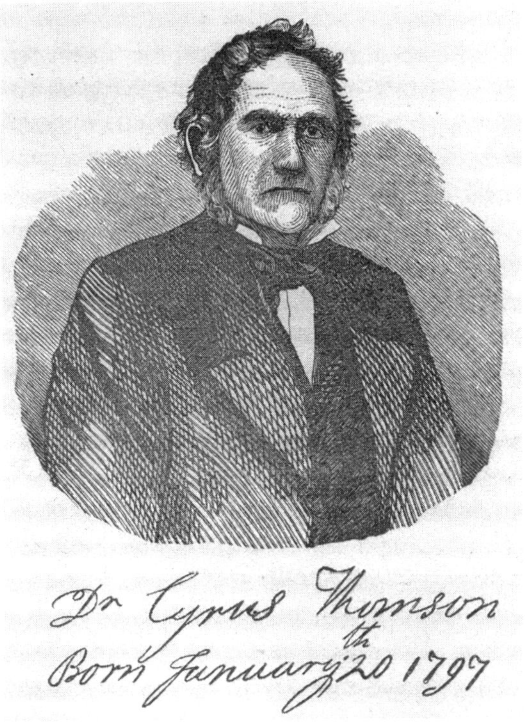

Thomson's son Cyrus lived in Upstate New York as an itinerant botanic healer. Briefly in the 1830s he ran Syracuse's first hospital, a botanic infirmary on West Genesee Street near the Erie Canal. He followed his father's principles, but expanded them, and to some degree supported them with his own interpretation of Benjamin Rush's medical philosophy. By prescribing various foods of mostly vegetable origin, and steam baths, he sought to keep patients warm, stabilize body heat, and restore the balance of body fluids. Taking "Every man his own physician" as his motto, he strived to educate patients about self-care. His four books were all published in either Syracuse or Geddes: *Learned Quackery Exposed; or, Theory According to Art, as Exemplified in the Practice of the Fashionable Doctors of the Present Day* (1843); *An Abridgement of the Life of Dr. Samuel Thomson, Founder of the Thomsonian System* (1846); *A Brief Narrative and Life of the Author: Comprising his Views of Medicine and the Theory of Diseases* (1860); *Dr. Thomson's Materia Medica: A Book for Everybody ... Designed to be a Substitute for [Samuel Thomson's] "The Family Physician"* (1863). The first two are compilations of his father's works; the second two are his own.

The younger Thomson generally agreed with Rush on the issue of disease classification. He wrote in his autobiography: "I think this system when reduced to plain language, may be expressed in few words. My father taught, and I his successor maintain, the principle of the *Unit[y] of Disease*, and that it is the result of *cold* — the negative of heat — which is life and health." "I think every disease takes its name from the effect it produces." "I believe that unnatural heat, cold, pains, aches, and all bad feelings, are the *effects* of disease, but not the *cause*." While Rush held that all disease was fever, Thomson held that it was all the result of cold, but they agreed about the essential unity of disease and its single ultimate cause, despite the diversity of its clinical manifestations. Thomson specifically attacked the nosologists (who were by his time rather *passé*): "... all diseases are brought on by derangement of the fluids of the body, and ... all diseases can be cured by restoring order and regularity to said fluids. ... It is thought by some, that unless the physician knows the name which has been given to the disease by others, he cannot treat it successfully."

But Thomson was not unqualified in his praise of Rush. On some issues, such as bloodletting, Thomson lumped Rush together with those he thought were quacks: "Where are the theories of Paracelsus, of Cullen, Rush, Brown and others? Alas, for the instability of the inventions of men, they were not founded upon truth and experience." "Seventy years ago, Samuel Thomson discovered that Heat was Life and Cold was Death. ... Nearly forty years ago, I (Cyrus Thomson) told the people that the Blood was the Life of the body, and in proportion as they take the Blood they take the Life." Bloodletting was central to Rush's therapeutics but Thomson believed it to be unfounded and pernicious. He lambasted Rush's methods of violent purges in a chapter called "The Scourge of Pennsylvania," yet was never slow to cite Rush favorably whenever he thought they would agree, especially on questions of heat and cold: "Dr. Rush, in his luminous lecture on Animal Life, says, that heat is an uniform and active stimulus in promoting life."

Cyrus Thomson's knowledge of botany was substandard, even for his time. For example, his 1863 *Materia Medica* contains this illustration, easily recognizable as the beautiful wildflower, the trillium. Thomson identified it, both in the text and in the caption, as an orobanchacea, or broomrape, a leafless root-parasitic herb that does not at all resemble trilliums.

MATERIA MEDICA. 615

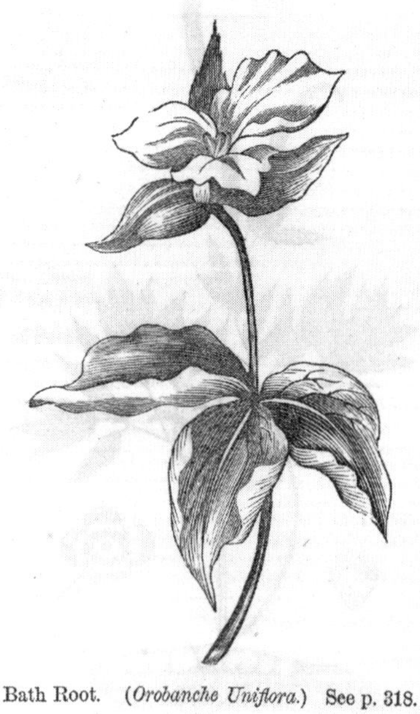

Bath Root. (*Orobanche Uniflora.*) See p. 318.

Starting in the 1830s the diagnostic pseudoscience of phrenology became popular for a few decades in America. Phrenologists claimed to be able to discern facts about individuals by studying the lumps on their skulls. Although phrenology was seen as chiefly diagnostic, not therapeutic, its findings typically had therapeutic implications. Founded by Viennese anatomist Franz Joseph Gall about 1800 and popularized in Europe by German physician Johann Gaspar Spurzheim and Scottish law clerk George Combe, its main exponents in America were Lorenzo Niles Fowler, his wife Lydia Folger Fowler, his brother Orson Squire Fowler, and their friend Samuel R. Wells. Together in New York City they ran a publishing house that at first specialized in phrenological works. Sometimes known as Fowler and Wells and sometimes as Fowlers and Wells, it became the leading American publisher of alternative medicine in the nineteenth century.

Homeopathy, invented in the early nineteenth century by German physician Samuel Hahnemann, is medicine based on the "like cures like" principle. To cure a given disease, homeopathic physicians prescribe infinitesimal doses of substances that in larger doses would cause the same symptoms as that disease. Allopathic medicine has always disliked and distrusted homeopathy, accusing it of offering only placebos, claiming that it relies too much on its patients' faith in its remedies, and arguing that its so-called cures are really just nature taking its course.

In Upstate New York, homeopathy was popular among the people and had many practitioners but was not represented by any educational institutions. The most prominent nineteenth-century homeopathic physician in Upstate New York was Frederick Humphreys, a native of Marcellus, New York, and an 1850 graduate of the Pennsylvania Homoeopathic Medical College in Philadelphia. He taught briefly at his alma mater, lived and practiced in Auburn, New York, founded the Humphreys Homoeopathic Medicine Company, was active in the Central New York Homoeopathic Medical Society and the New York State Homoeopathic Medical Society, was the founding editor of the *Journal of Specific Homoeopathy* from 1856 to 1859, and wrote at least seven books: *The Cholera and its Homoeopathic Treatment* (1849); *Homoeopathic Treatment of Diseases of the Sexual System* (1850); *Dysentry and its Homoeopathic Treatment* (1853); *Manual of Specific Homoeopathy for the Administration of Medicine and Cure of Disease* (1855); *Manual of Veterinary Specific Homoeopathy* (1860); — It was not unusual in those days for physicians of any school to treat both humans and farm animals. — *Homeopathic Mentor; or, Family Adviser in the Use of Specific Homeopathic Medicine* (1872); and *Guide for Humphreys' Homoeopathic Veterinary Specifics* (1885). Most of these books appeared in multiple editions and the *Homeopathic Mentor* was translated into Spanish, Portuguese, and French.

Much of the impetus for the nationwide hydropathy or "water cure" fad in the mid-nineteenth century came from Upstate New York. Russell Thacher Trall and Joel Shew opened their hydropathic spa in Lebanon Springs, New York, between Albany and Pittsfield, Massachusetts, in 1845. The principle is that water is naturally soothing and promotes healing. Trall's two-volume *Hydropathic Encyclopedia*, which went through several editions in the early 1850s, and Shew's *Hydropathic Family Physician* (1854) were the basic literature of the movement. Hydropathy is a narrower version of hydrotherapy, which consists of using large quantities of mineralized or purified water for drinking, bathing, showering, steaming, cold wraps, etc.

The illustration on this page and the top illustration on page 39 are from Trall. The bottom illustration on page 39 is from Shew.

CHAPTER II.

WATER-CURE PROCESSES.

THE hydropathic appliances embrace all the usual methods of vapor, warm, tepid, cool, and cold bathing, besides a variety of processes which have had their origin in the development of Water-Cure as a system.

Fig. 164.

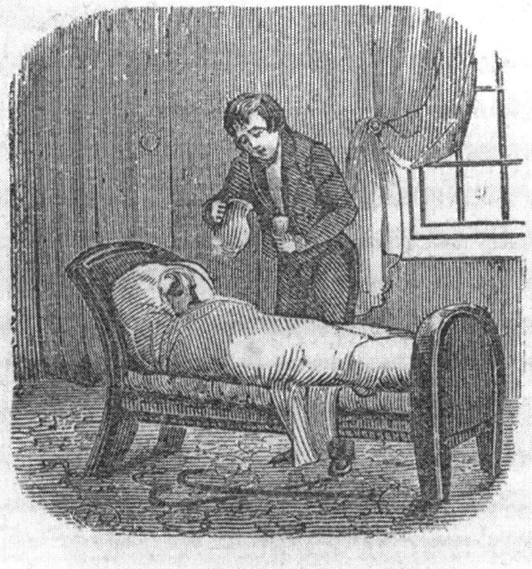

THE WET-SHEET PACKING.

THE WET-SHEET PACKING.—This process, the *lien tuch* of the Germans (fig. 164), is admirably calculated to answer two general indications, which are manifestly leading ones in a long catalogue of maladies, both acute and chronic, viz., to reduce the heat of the body and the force of the circulation, and, as an alterative, to correct morbid and restore healthy secretions. It produces also, incidentally, a powerfully detergent or cleansing effect, and generally exerts a wonderfully sedative or soothing influence on the whole nervous system. The first disagreeable sensation of cold is usually soon followed by a pleasurable warmth over the whole surface. It is capable of superseding, to advantage, bleeding, antimony, salts, hydriodate of potassa (iodide of potassium), calomel, and opium, and a hundred other more or less injurious agents.

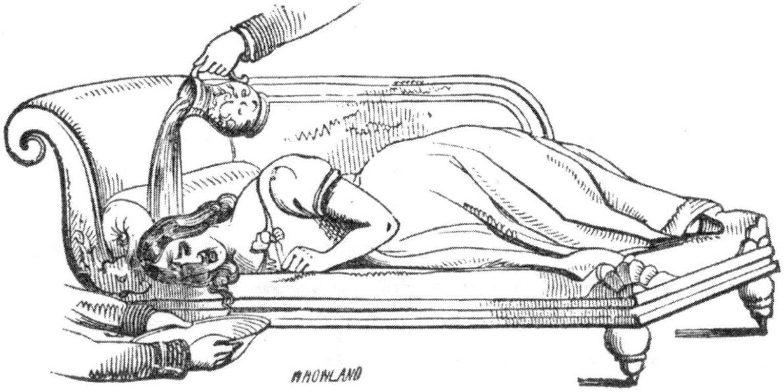

TREATMENT OF HYSTERIA.

"Place the head over a basin, and pour water from a jug over the head and chest till the patient becomes chilly and revives. Never use any thing but cold water for the hysterical fit, unless the party turn very cold, when you should discontinue it, and apply warmth to the feet. I once saw the cold applied for three hours, but the patient was quite well the next day."

To correct the condition on which the hysterical paroxysms depend, we must, during their intervals, employ the abdominal bandage, frequent hip-baths, and occasional dripping-sheets or packs. In almost all cases the bowels are more or less constipated, and the diet must be regulated accordingly.

LEG-BATH.

This is useful in cases of ulcers, swellings, eruptions, gout, or rheu-

Fig. 241.

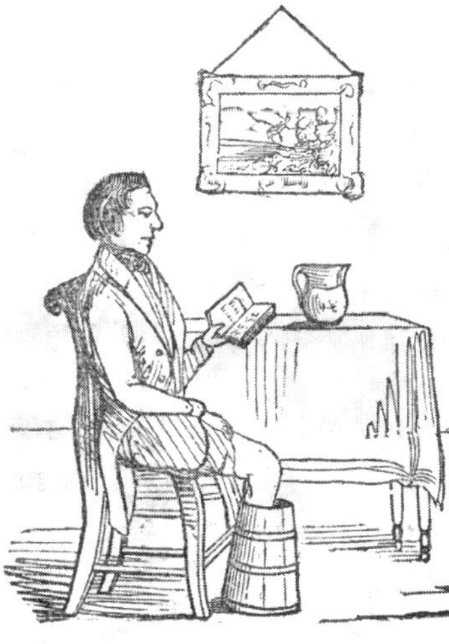

LEG-BATH.

Fig. 242.

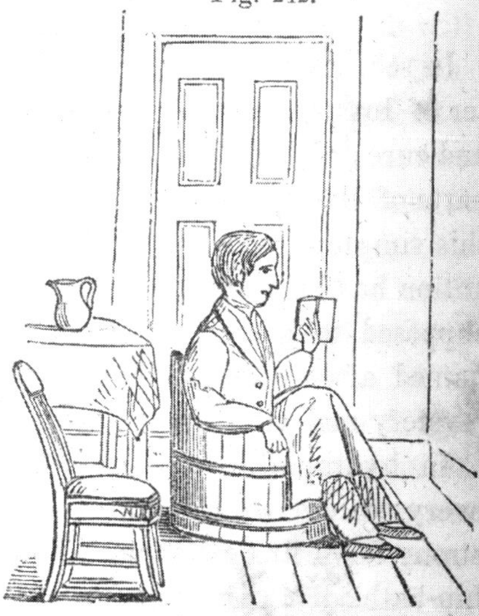

SITTING-BATH.

BEACH'S

FAMILY PHYSICIAN

AND

HOME GUIDE

FOR THE TREATMENT OF THE DISEASES OF

MEN, WOMEN AND CHILDREN,

ON

REFORM PRINCIPLES,

BY WOOSTER BEACH, M. D.,

MEMBER OF THE MEDICAL SOCIETY OF THE CITY AND COUNTY OF NEW YORK; OF THE MEDICAL AND PHYSIOLOGICAL SOCIETY OF WETTERAU, GERMANY; OF LEIPSIC, SAXONY; OF THE MEDICAL SOCIETY OF BAMBERG, BAVARIA; MEMBER OF THE ROYAL COLLEGE OF PHYSICIANS AND SURGEONS OF BERLIN, PRUSSIA, ETC., ETC.

ILLUSTRATED WITH NEARLY TWO HUNDRED ENGRAVINGS.

FORTY-FIFTH THOUSAND, REVISED AND ENLARGED,

WITH AN APPENDIX, FROM EMINENT WRITERS, GIVING

THE LAWS OF HEALTH,

AND IMPORTANT SUGGESTIONS FOR THE ATTAINMENT OF COMFORT, PROSPERITY AND HAPPINESS.

CINCINNATI:
MOORE, WILSTACH, KEYS & CO.,
25 WEST FOURTH STREET
1860.

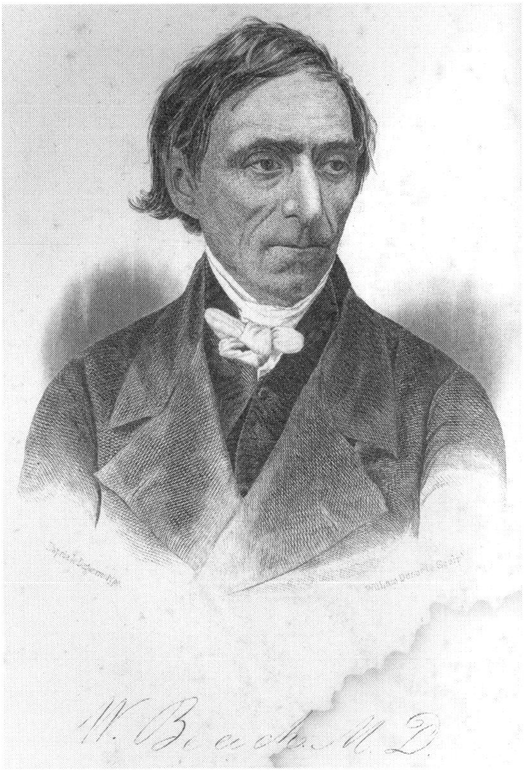

Besides botanic medicine, in the nineteenth century homeopathy and eclecticism were the stiffest challenges to regular medicine.

Wooster Beach, a New York City physician who had received both Thomsonian and non-Thomsonian botanic medical training but had also earned a regular M.D. degree, founded eclectic medicine around 1829 or 1830. His basic idea was that whatever worked was valuable for patients, regardless of its source or ideological underpinnings. His goal was to combine the best aspects of homeopathic, botanic, and allopathic medicine, and to study each of them carefully and without bias. The word 'eclectic' comes from the Greek infinitive *eklegein* (ἐκλέγειν), which means to pick out, to single out, or to select. The eclectic principle, which is familiar in disciplines as diverse as philosophy and agriculture, as well as in medicine, is that anything true, useful, or beneficial can legitimately be taken from anywhere, even from contradictory sources. Systematic thinkers may argue against eclecticism's lack of consistency, but even its staunchest opponents have difficulty challenging the open-mindedness of its precept.

Beach correctly noticed that botanic practitioners tended to be poorly educated but well versed in folk remedies, some of which actually worked, while allopathic practitioners tended to be well educated but prejudiced against any remedy that was not sanctioned by their textbooks. Both groups were keen observers and could usually diagnose patients accurately to the extent that diseases, injuries, and their causes were then understood. But they could cure practically nothing. Ironically, the adoption of some eclectic findings improved late nineteenth-century botanic medicine.

Beach was a particularly thoughtful physician. He was well aware of the most significant physiological, pathological, anatomical, chemical, and botanical advances of his day, and applied whatever he could from this science to his therapeutics. His books, the three-volume *American Practice of Medicine* (1832-1833) and the gigantic one-volume *Family Physician* (1842) contained some of the best practical medical advice of the day. Both were very popular, the former with practitioners, the latter with the laity, and went through many editions and title changes. Beach moved to Ohio in 1845, but eclectic medicine thrived in New York State, especially Upstate New York, for the next several decades.

Unlike Thomsonian books, eclectic botanicals dealt scientifically with the chemical, toxicological, pharmacological, and therapeutic properties of plants, as well as their specific physiological actions, side effects, and adverse interactions. Eclecticism was radically empirical. Its patients often found themselves used as guinea pigs for massive doses of untried remedies. The results were unpredictable, sometimes disastrous, but in general no worse than those of the regular medicine of the time. As the trend in eclectic research moved more toward chemistry, eclecticism gradually disappeared as a separate movement, with some of its practitioners going to regular medicine and some to various schools of herbalism or naturopathy.

Of all the alternatives in the mid-nineteenth-century marketplace of American medicine, eclecticism was the closest in theory to allopathic medicine, even to the extent that regular practictioners and licensing authorities commonly accepted eclectic M.D. degrees as legitimate. Eclecticism was more pragmatic than ideological, and that made it respectable. The Onondaga County Medical Society explicitly condemned homeopathy in 1845, but never made any such move against eclecticism.

The same year that Elizabeth Blackwell received her M.D., Stephen Hollister Potter, a native of Solon, Cortland County, New York, founded in Syracuse the world's first medical school whose policy from the start was co-education. This school, Syracuse Medical College, was eclectic.

In the 1840s and 1850s Potter tried to run three medical schools more or less simultaneously, in Syracuse, Rochester, and Cincinnati, and had difficulties with both finances and public relations in all three locations. In essence, his Syracuse Medical College, Central Medical College (in Rochester), and American Medical College (in Cincinnati) were just three different campuses of the same institution.

Potter published one book, *Notes of Lectures on the American Practice of Medicine, Delivered in the American Medical College at Cincinnati, O[hio]* (Syracuse: Potter & Volk, 1855). He also published his own medical journal under various titles. It consisted mostly of his own ideological essays and those of other authors, letters to and from him, articles culled and reprinted from other journals, case reports, and publicity for his and other eclectic medical schools. The April 1855 issue of his *American Medical and Surgical Journal* carried a detailed account of the Syracuse Medical College commencement exercises held on February 22, 1855, including full texts of all the speeches. One of the speakers was Mary Edwards Walker, the only woman among the twelve students who received the M.D. that day.

JULY, 1854.

THE SYRACUSE MEDICAL & SURGICAL JOURNAL:

EDITED BY

S. HOLLISTER POTTER, M. D.,

PROFESSOR OF SURGICAL DISEASES AND THEORY AND PRACTICE IN SYRACUSE MEDICAL COLLEGE,

AND PUBLISHED BY

DR'S J. N. BETTS AND JESSE WATSON,

AT THE SYRACUSE PHARMACY AND ECLECTIC DISPENSING STORE 37, EAST GENESEE ST., SYRACUSE, N. Y.

PUBLISHED MONTHLY.

☞ Letters on the business of the Journal, should be addressed (post-paid) to F. W. Walton, Esq., No. 37, East Genesee Street, Syracuse, N. Y.

Fourth Series,--Vol. I. Whole Series,--Vol. VI.

SYRACUSE.

PRINTED AT THE EVENING CHRONICLE OFFICE, No. 18, DILLAYE BUILDINGS.

TERMS--ONE DOLLAR A YEAR, IN ADVANCE.

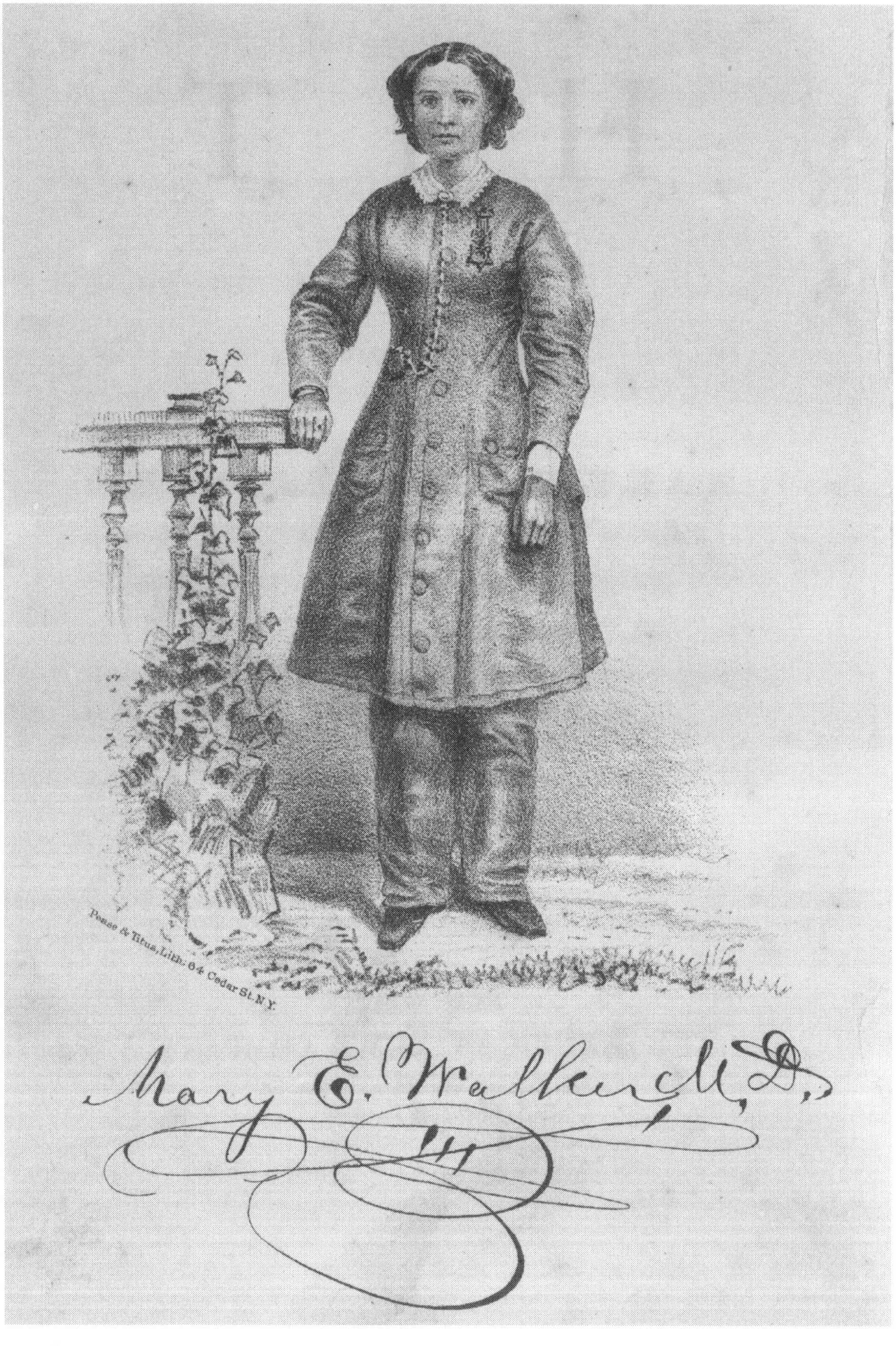

Walker, shown here in the frontispiece of her 1871 autobiography, *Hit*, is the most famous of all Potter's graduates. She practiced medicine first in Columbus, Ohio, then, with her classmate and husband, Albert Miller (whose name, scandalously for her time, she never took), in Rome, New

York. In the late 1850s she became the first American woman to practice general surgery. When the Civil War broke out, she immediately offered her services to the Union Army as a battlefield surgeon. At first she was allowed to be only a nurse, but was soon hired as Contract Acting Assistant Surgeon and saw action at First Bull Run, Chickamauga, and in the aftermath of the burning of Atlanta. From April 10 to August 12, 1864, she was a prisoner-of-war in Richmond, Virginia. On the recommendations of Generals William Tecumseh Sherman and George Henry Thomas, she was decorated with the Congressional Medal of Honor in 1865.

After the war Walker practiced medicine in her hometown of Oswego, New York, but dedicated her life mostly to social and political reform, lecturing widely but with little success. Her major issues were dress reform (she always wore pants), hygiene, and social morality. She was such a radical and controversial feminist that other suffragists shunned her. Both *Hit* and her other book, *Unmasked* (1878), were notorious polemics.

Potter can also take credit for graduating, about a year and a half after Blackwell earned her degree, the second woman physician in America. Lydia Folger Fowler was talented in science, especially mathematics and astronomy, and became interested in medicine through the efforts of her husband and his partners to publicize phrenology, hydropathy, and other medical innovations. Even before she received her M.D. at Potter's Central Medical College in June 1850, she was already lecturing and writing on hygiene, physiology, and astronomy, mostly for audiences of women and children. As professor of midwifery, gynecology, and pediatrics at Central during the 1851-1852 academic year, she became the first female faculty member of an American medical school. Her career thereafter was mediocre, but along with Blackwell she was an important catalyst in encouraging other women to take up medicine.

An even more prominent graduate of Central Medical College was Sarah Read Adamson Dolley, a polymath who received her M.D. there in 1851 as the third woman physician in America. She had close blood ties to the Quaker medical establishment in Philadelphia. Two of these physicians, her uncle, Hiram Corson, and his friend, Isaac Pennypacker, obtained for her a one-year staff position at Blockley. When she returned to Rochester to begin her medical practice in 1852, she thus became the first woman in America to complete a full hospital internship. Besides her successful career as an obstetrician/gynecologist, she taught obstetrics, worked alongside Susan B. Anthony and other prominent suffragists for women's rights, organized a women's clinic and dispensary, co-founded the Rochester Chapter of the American Red Cross, founded the Practitioners' Society of Rochester (a group of women physicians who later changed their name to the Blackwell Society) and the Rochester Society of Natural Sciences, and in 1907 became the first president of the Women's Medical Society of the State of New York.

Another of Potter's graduates was Clemence Sophia Lozier, who received her M.D. from Syracuse Medical College in 1853. She founded the New York Medical College and Hospital for Women in 1863 and ran it as a homeopathic rival to the Blackwell sisters' New York Infirmary.

Women applicants were more likely to be admitted to eclectic, homeopathic, botanic, women-only, or other so-called "irregular" medical schools in the mid-nineteenth century than to schools approved by state medical societies and the AMA. But Elizabeth Blackwell's case was not the only attempt in the 1840s to give allopathic medical education to a woman. Hezekiah Joslyn, a freethinking physician in private practice since 1823 in Cicero, New York, tried in the 1840s to get his daughter Matilda into Geneva Medical College, but there is no record of her ever applying for admission. She married merchant Henry H. Gage in 1845, settled eventually in Fayetteville, and spent the rest of her life urging society to consider women the equal of men in every way.*

As all these developments were unfolding, the town of Geneva was becoming more marginalized and the city of Syracuse was gaining recognition as the economic and cultural hub of Central New York.

The Syracuse area was a bustling and growing metropolis throughout the nineteenth century. Onondaga County was established in 1794 and the Onondaga County Medical Society was founded in 1806, but Syracuse was not incorporated as a village until 1825 or as a city until 1848. The present downtown area was first called Webster's Landing when it was settled in the 1780s, and the present North Side was first called Salt Point in the 1790s. Salt Point soon changed its name to Salina. Webster's Landing combined with Bogardus Corners, Cossit's Corners, and other tiny communities to form the community of Corinth in 1819. The following year, when the Syracuse population was 600 and that of the county 47,000, and — notably — when the first Erie Canal boat arrived, the village changed its name to Syracuse to avoid confusion with the Corinth in Saratoga County. In 1850, the year that the Syracuse Medical Society was founded, the population of the city was 22,000, and in 1870, the year that Syracuse University was founded, it was 48,000. The 1857 edition of *Appleton's Handbook for American Travel* described Syracuse as a "large and elegant city."

Onondaga County in general and Syracuse in particular were early pacesetters in socially progressive attitudes and accomplishments that would eventually influence the whole nation. The county prohibited corporal punishment in schools in 1807 and public whipping in 1813. Public libraries were founded in Salina in 1818 and in Syracuse in 1852. The local

* Known to friends and family as "M.," her son-in-law L. Frank Baum immortalized Matilda Joslyn Gage and her husband as "Aunt Em" and "Uncle Henry" in *The Wizard of Oz*, changing only one letter in their surname to create the heroine Dorothy's surname, "Gale."

stations of the Underground Railroad probably began operating in the 1820s. Gerrit Smith and William Lloyd Garrison organized abolitionists in Syracuse in 1835 and the Rev. Jermain Wesley Loguen moved to Syracuse in 1841. Resistance to the Fugitive Slave Law was so strong in Syracuse that Senator Daniel Webster chose this city as the place to give a speech that labelled as "traitor" anyone who broke that law. But just four months later, on October 1, 1851, a violent mob defied it to save William ("Jerry") Henry from re-enslavement. Such a hotbed of liberal, abolitionist, and proto-feminist thought and action was naturally receptive to many kinds of new ideas, including those that would advance education and medicine.

Among the reforms gaining momentum in New York State in the mid-nineteenth century was the redesigning of treatment for the insane. A physician in Utica, Amariah Brigham, founder of *The American Journal of Insanity* in 1844, was a nationally recognized leader in this field. As the original superintendent of the New York State Asylum for Lunatics at Utica, which opened in 1843, he sought to create a model institution of humane, patient-centered care. Unlike the old almshouses that housed the insane and mentally deficient in a harsh, prison-like conditions, the Utica Asylum was established as a treatment facility.

In this atmosphere of reform the New York State Legislature, acting on a recommendation contained in the 1846 annual report of the New York State Asylum for Lunatics, authorized the New York State Asylum for Idiots in 1851. Hervey Backus Wilbur (left), an 1843 Berkshire Medical College graduate, was appointed its first superintendent and remained in that position until his death in 1883. First located on rented land in Albany, it admitted its first "pupils" in 1851. The cornerstone was laid on September 8, 1854, for a new building in Syracuse, and the institution moved there in 1855. Wilbur collaborated with Edward Seguin, the originator of the physiological method of training. Maria Montessori was Seguin's student. The "Montessori Method" is partly based on Wilbur's and Seguin's work.

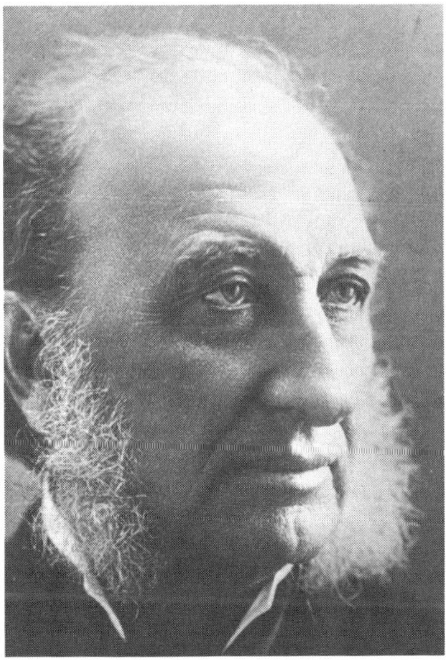

The new asylums offered clinical possibilities. As a last desperate effort to obtain the use of local clinical facilities, Geneva Medical College struck a deal in 1865 with the appointed trustees of the proposed Willard State Psychiatric Hospital in Ovid. This measure proved to be too little and too late. Enrollments continued to slip into the single digits. When the Willard Asylum, as it was known, opened in October 1869, Geneva Medical College had no expectations remaining.

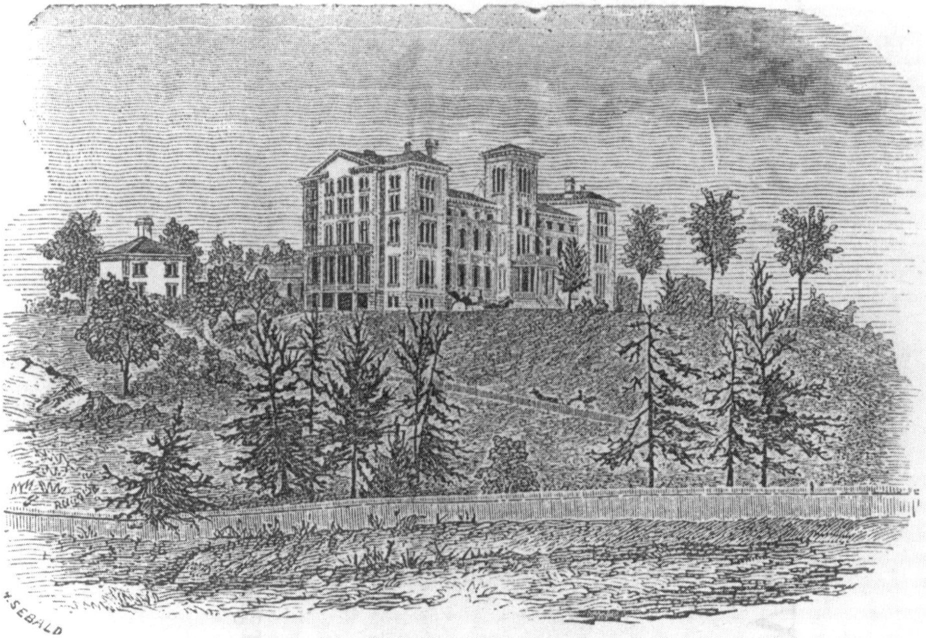

STATE IDIOT ASYLUM, AT SYRACUSE.

No clinical facility in or near Geneva could compete with the oldest general hospital in Syracuse, St. Joseph's Hospital (below), which was founded on April 12, 1869 by the Franciscan Sisters. One of the main reasons that the medical school was able to revive itself at Syracuse University in the early 1870s rather than become extinct was the existence of St. Joseph's, which would provide adequate clinical teaching for medical students.

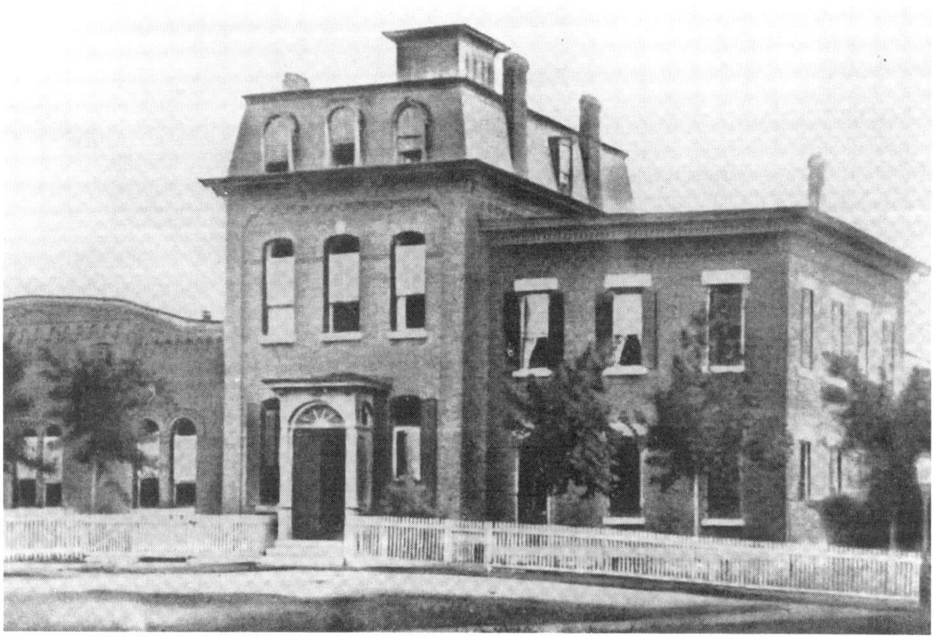

4

The College Moves to Syracuse

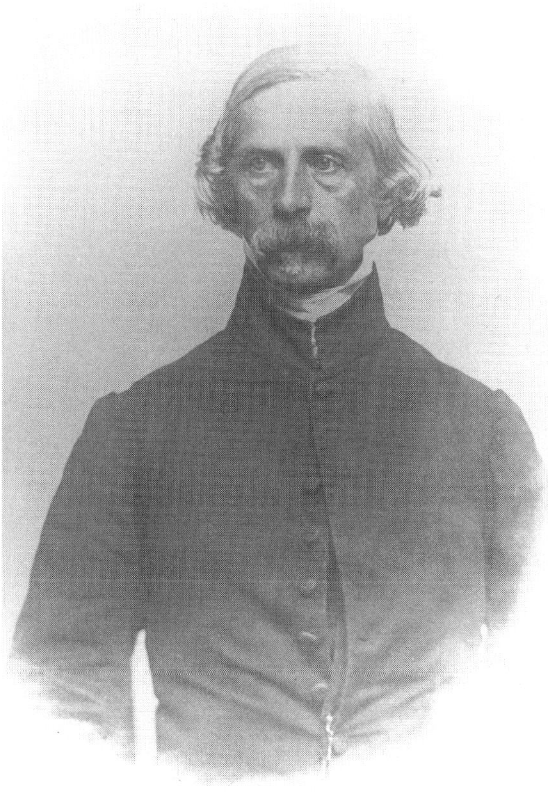

On March 25, 1870 the Methodist Church chartered Syracuse University as a liberal institution of higher learning, dedicated from the start to the education of all qualified students, including women, minorities, and people of color. In 1871 Hobart College dissolved its medical faculty and sold its medical library, pathological cabinet, and anatomical museum to Dean John Towler (right). These two apparently unrelated events soon began a new chain of events, thanks to Towler's vision and initiative.

In August 1871 Towler and Frederick Hyde approached Syracuse University as private citizens, offering to donate to the university all the Geneva Medical College property that Towler had acquired, in exchange for Syracuse University establishing and maintaining a regular medical college consistent with American Medical Association standards. The Syracuse University Board of Trustees gave provisional approval at its August 30, 1871 meeting and appointed a committee to study the matter further. One member of this committee was the Rev. Jesse Truesdell Peck, a Methodist minister, later a bishop, one of the five founders of Syracuse University, and from 1870 to 1873 President of the Board of Trustees. On November 1, 1871, Peck presented the plan to a special session of the Onondaga County Medical Society, which, after some discussion, approved its general principles. The society agreed with Hyde and Towler that a golden opportunity here presented itself to make a clean break with past deficiencies in medical education in Central New York and to re-establish a medical school in Syracuse on the most up-to-date pedagogical and scientific basis. That would entail creating a graded curriculum, one of the first in the nation. Syracuse University and the Onondaga County Medical Society then appointed several joint committees to work out the details. The committee of the Board of Trustees reported to the whole Board as follows, transcribed in full from the minutes of the December 4, 1871 meeting:

The committee of five, W[ilfred] W. Porter M.D., Hon. Geo. F. Comstock, Rev. Jesse T. Peck D.D., Rev. Geo. L. Taylor A.M., Hon., C[harles] Andrews, appointed by the Board Aug. 30th 1871 to confer with the representatives of the Medical College of Geneva and to report to the Board for consideration at its next session, presented the following report:

Whereas: it is deemed desirable to establish a Medical College in Syracuse, State of New York as a Medical Department of the Syracuse University under the government and protection of the same; and,

Whereas: the Dean of Geneva Medical College has stated to the Trustees that he has purchased the contents of the Anatomical museum and library of said College from the Trustees of the self same medical institution and has proposed to transfer said museum and library to the Syracuse University on certain conditions, viz: 1st That a Medical College be instituted under the government, influence and protection of the said Syracuse University. 2nd. That the Medical College to be thus instituted in Syracuse and incorporated with the Syracuse University shall be a regular school of medicine and surgery as recognized by all the State Medical Societies of the United States and the American Medical Association. 3rd. That the Board of Trustees of the Syracuse University shall cooperate with the medical faculty in furnishing suitable rooms for a medical institution, the responsibility for the same resting with the Medical Faculty. ~~Finally~~ Therefore: as a joint-committee we recommend the following plan of organization:

1st. This Institution shall be denominated the College of Physicians and Surgeons of the Syracuse University.

2nd There shall be nine or more Professorships in the Medical Department of the Syracuse University and these professorships shall be respectively denominated as follows viz:

1st — Chemistry, Pharmacy and Toxicology
2nd — Anatomy, general, special and surgical
3rd — Physiology and Pathology
4th — Theory and Practice of Medicine
5th — Materia Medica, Therapeutics and Botany
6th — Obstetrics and Diseases of Women and Children
7th — Principles and Practice of Surgery
8th — Mental Diseases and Medical Jurisprudence
9th — Ophthalmology and Diseases of the Ear.

3rd The Faculty of the Medical Department of the Syracuse University

hereby appointed and elected to fill the chairs under this organization shall be as follows:
1st. John Towler, M.D., Prof^{r} of Chemistry, Pharmacy & Toxicology
2nd. Geo. K. Smith, M.D., Prof^{r} of Genl Special & Surg^{l} Anatomy
3rd. Nelson Nivison M.D., Prof^{r} of Physiology, Pathology & Hygiene
4th, Hiram N. Eastman M.D., Prof^{r} of Principles and Practice of Medicine
5th, Edwd B. Stevens, M.D., Prof^{r} of Mat. Med., Therapeutics & Botany
6th, Caleb Green M.D., Prof^{r} of Obstetrics & Diseases of Women & Children
7th, Fred^{k} Hyde M.D., Prof^{r} of Principles & Practice of Surgery
8th, Hervey B. Wilbur M.D., Prof^{r} of Diseases of mind and Nervous system
9th, Chas E. Rider M.D., Prof^{r} of Ophthalmology & dis. of the Ear.
Adjunct Professors:
1st. John Van Duyn M.D. — Prof. of Histology, Microscopy & Ass^{t} to Chair of Anatomy
2nd, Joseph P. Dunlap M.D., Prof^{r} of Clinical Medicine
3rd. Henry D. Didama M.D., Prof^{r} of Clinical Medicine
4th. Roger W. Pease M.D., Prof^{r} of Clinical Surgery
5th, Alfred Mercer M.D., Prof^{r} of Clinical Surgery
6th. J. Otis Burt M.D., Prof. of Materia Medica
7th, Wilfred W. Porter M.D., Prof. of Clin^{l} Midwifery, & dis. of Women & Children
8th, William T. Plant M.D., Prof. of Med. Jurisprudence
9th, John W. Lawton M.D., Prof. of Clin. Ophthalmology & dis. of Ear.

Statutes of the Medical Department.

1st The Faculty of the Medical Department of the Syracuse University shall consist of nine Professors and nine Adjunct Professors; but this number may be increased by the Board of Trustees on the recommendation of the Faculty

2nd The different branches of the curriculum may be divided differently by the Faculty to meet any emergency or to suit the capacity of the different members of the Faculty

3rd All vacancies in the Faculty shall be filled by persons recommended by a majority of the Faculty and elected by the Trustees.

4th The Faculty shall annually appoint a Dean and Registrar from their own members to serve the ensuing year.

5th They shall appoint a Curator of the Anatomical Museum and a Librarian whose duties shall be to see that the Anatomical specimens are kept in good condition and that the books be not lost.

6th — The Dean shall be the Representative of the College of Physicians & Surgeons in the Faculty of the University

7th — The Dean shall preside at the meetings of the Faculty and at the conjoint meetings of the Faculty and Censors during the examination of candidates for the degree of Doctor of Medicine.

8th — The Registrar shall keep in a book for this purpose an accurate list of students who are admitted:

In this book each student shall write his name, age, plan of abode, and the name of the medical practitioner with whom he may have studied medicine.
The Registrar shall also take minutes of all transactions entered into at the meetings of the Faculty and shall transcribe them into a book of Records kept for the purpose: Both of these books shall be open at any time to any member either of the Faculty or of the Board of Trustees.

9th — The Trustees shall make such rules and regulations, subject to the laws of the University, regarding the admission of students, the course of study, the attendance on lectures, the examinations, the number of terms, the fees for instruction and the conduct of students, as they shall think most conducive to the prosperity and interest of the Medical Department.

10th — The Faculty shall appoint their own Demonstrator and Janitor.

11th — The Faculty shall bear all expenses for fuel, lights, anatomical material, advertising, printing of circulars, and their distribution and for everything else required in the course of Medical instruction. They shall also pay a fair annual insurance on the Medical College building and shall keep said building in repair.

12th — Three censors shall be appointed annually at the request of the Faculty: one by the New York State Medical Society; one by the Central New York Medical Association; and the third, by the Onondaga [County] Medical Society. The censors shall be invited to be present at the examination[s] for [the] Degree of Doctor of Medicine.

13th — Each censor, if he is present at the examination, shall receive one dollar out of each graduation fee.

14th — Each censor shall have an equal vote with a member of the Faculty in recommending a candidate for the Degree of M.D.

15th — The Faculty shall draw out a form for the Medical Diploma in latin for [the] Degree of Doctor of Medicine and shall have the same engraved at their own expense.

16th — The Medical Diploma shall be signed by the Chancellor of the University, the Secretary of the Board of Trustees and the Members of the Medical Faculty.

17th — The medical Faculty shall have the power of recommending men of distinction in all countries for their attainments in Medicine, Science, Art and Literature, to the Board of Trustees for [the] honorary degree of M.D.

18th — The Diploma for an Honorary Degree shall be written in latin on parchment and signed by the Chancellor of the University and the Dean of the Medical Faculty.

19th — No candidate for graduation in course shall be recommended to the Board of Trustees unless said candidate shall have fulfilled every provision required by the laws of the State in reference to graduation in Medicine.

20th — At the end of each academic year, the Dean shall make out and present to the Board of Trustees a report of all transactions of importance; but especially of the number of students that have attended the last Medical course as also the number of candidates for graduation who have satisfactorily passed their

Examinations before the Faculty and censors, and also a report to the Regents of the University. Copies of these two Reports shall be handed to the Registrar for insertion in the records of the Medical College.

21st — The statutes may be amended by the Board of Trustees on the recommendation of a majority of the Faculty.

The Committee referred to on Page 54 (University minutes) made the following additional Report:

The Committee appointed to consider the proposition made to remove Geneva Medical College to Syracuse to be organized under authority of Syracuse University would respectfully report:

That at their instance the Onondaga County Medical Society came together in extra session and thoroughly investigated the whole subject.

They appointed a committee to present the results of their inquiries to you and to deliberate with your committee and the Professors from Geneva Medical College as to the action which ought to be recommended.

The joint Committee met and adopted a report which we herewith transmit to the Board.

We submit the following:

1st Resolved: that we accept the proposition of Profs Towler and Hyde to transfer to the University the Museum and Library of Geneva Medical College with the understanding that this virtually removes the College to Syracuse without expense to the Syracuse University.

2nd Resolved: that we approve and authorize the plan of organization submitted by the joint committee as above.

3rd Resolved: that nine Professors of the College of Physicians and Surgeons be now elected with the understanding that this Board does not become responsible for the salaries of said Professors or any part thereof; and that the professors elected shall accept these conditions.

4th Resolved: that the privilege be given to announce the organization and opening of said College of Physicians and Surgeons when this Board shall receive satisfactory evidence that the provisions made by the Faculty elect are such as to afford suitable guarantees to the University of creditable standing and success

(Signed)

Com. W.W. Porter, Chairman
George F. Comstock
Jesse T. Peck

The Board of Trustees approved this plan at this December 1871 meeting, thereby bringing into existence what they called the College of Physicians and Surgeons of the Syracuse University. No direct negotiations between Hobart College and Syracuse University for the transfer of Geneva Medical College ever occurred. If Towler and Hyde had not made their proposal, the medical school would have become extinct.

Syracuse in the 1870s was a vital and rapidly changing medical environment. Besides the Onondaga County Medical Society, which existed mainly to regulate the local profession, there was another group whose purpose was to facilitate discussion of scientific and clinical topics. First organized informally in 1847, it was named the City Medical Association in 1858 and renamed the Syracuse Medical Association in 1866. Its most frequent topics were cholera, smallpox, and other infectious diseases.

At its first meeting, on January 6, 1872, the faculty of the medical school elected Hyde the dean. He served in that capacity until his death fifteen years later.

On May 22, 1872, the medical faculty signed a lease for rooms at the Clinton Block adjacent to the Erie Canal. The rent was $400 a year. The photograph below, looking northwest up West Genesee Street, shows the property in which the medical school was housed. The photograph on page 55, looking west, shows the same area and the south side of the Erie Canal, including the Amos Block at 210-216 West Water Street.

At its June 24, 1872 meeting, even as it was instituting a three-year graded curriculum for new students, the faculty "grandfathered" returning students from Geneva Medical College who expected to receive their degrees after just attending three years of lecture courses and writing a thesis.

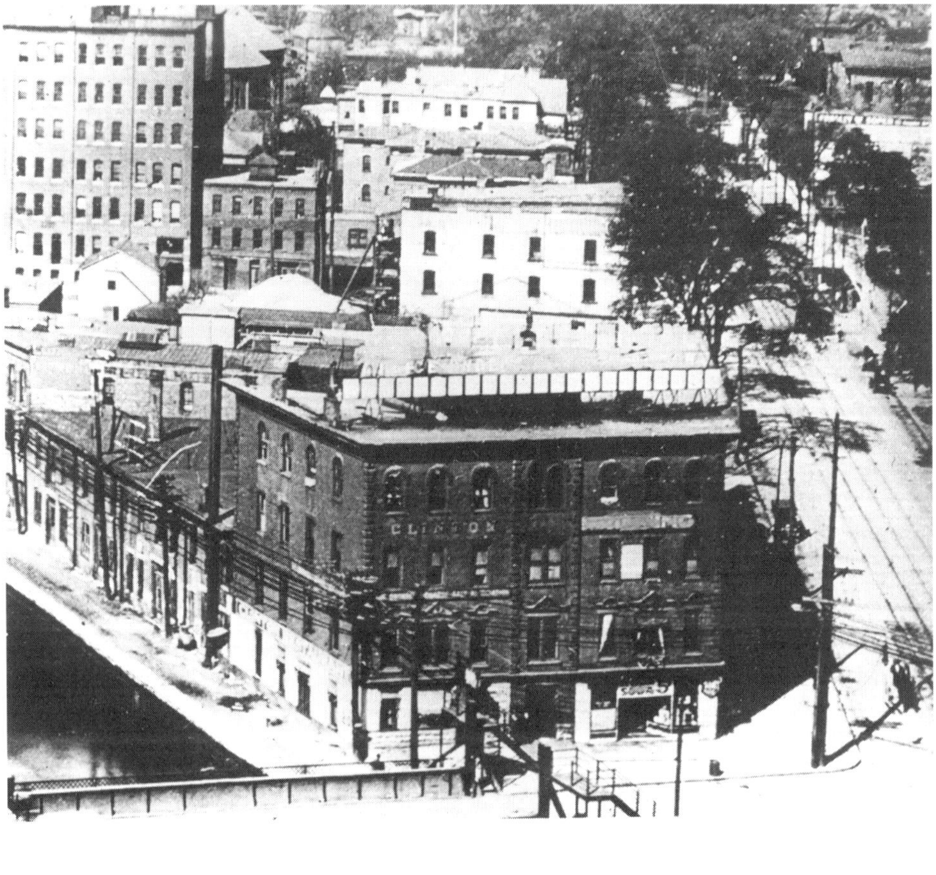

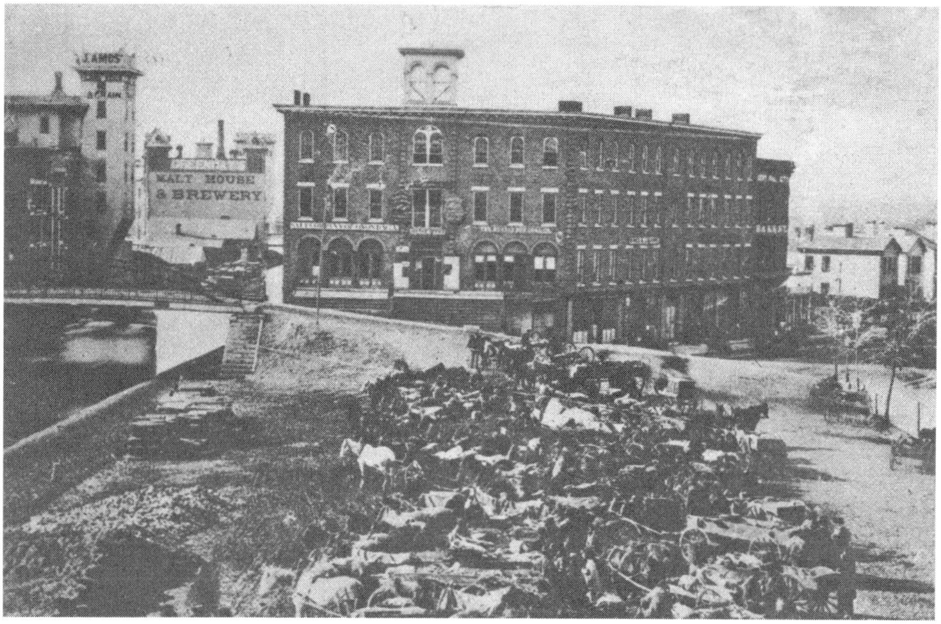

The original graded curriculum was anatomy, physiology, and general chemistry in the first year; medical chemistry (later called biochemistry), materia medica (later called pharmacology), pathological anatomy, theory and practice of medicine, clinical medicine, and surgery in the second year; and pathological anatomy, therapeutics, obstetrics, medical jurisprudence, theory and practice of medicine, clinical medicine, and surgery in the third year. Students had to pass examinations in each subject in order to advance to the next year. In addition to successful examinations in all third-year subjects, each student also had to write a thesis in order to graduate. In the quest to assure high standards of excellence among new physicians, Geneva Medical College had been one of the first medical schools to open final examinations to outside monitors. Syracuse University kept this policy and strengthened it.

The first classes were held on October 3, 1872. The tuition was $100 a year, compared with $60 for the undergraduate college. This income and the various associated fees were not enough either to meet expenses or to pay the faculty. The university provided little financial support or incentive. The faculty, acting as a body almost independent of the university, solicited its own funds, paid its own way, and generally lost money, both as a school and as individuals.

In 1875 the faculty pooled its money to buy an old carriage factory on Orange (later called South McBride) Street and to remodel it into a serviceable and permanent medical school building to replace the temporary quarters in the Clinton Block. A new pathology laboratory opened that year and in 1876 a new chemistry laboratory and the college's first dispensary.

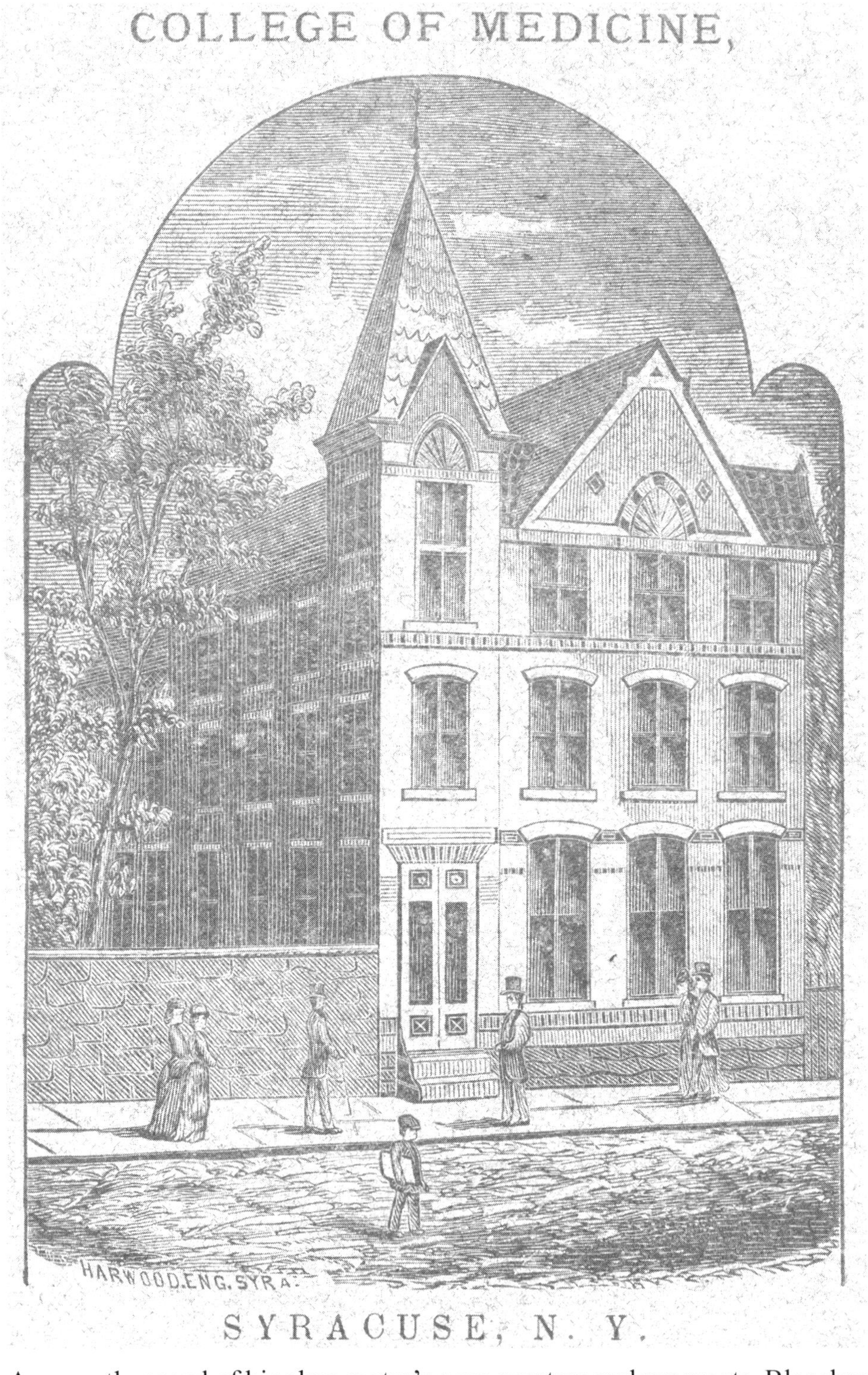

Apparently proud of his alma mater's new quarters and prospects, Bleecker Lansing Hovey, Class of 1842, a physician practicing in Dansville, New

York, and holding prominent offices in several medical societies, founded the Syracuse and Geneva Medical Alumni Association on February 19, 1875. This association was active through the 1940s. After a brief hiatus during the early years of the college's affiliation with the State University of New York, the Syracuse Medical Alumni Association was legally incorporated in May 1955, mainly as a formality to secure the release of medical alumni endowment and loan funds from Syracuse University.

The 1870s witnessed major growth in hospitals in Central New York. The City of Syracuse created the City Hospital for Communicable Diseases in 1874 in reaction to a smallpox epidemic of 97 cases in January 1872. The following year it moved to a large lot on Teall Avenue just in time to battle a worse outbreak of smallpox, which killed 200 between July and October. Also noteworthy in 1875 was the firm establishment of St. Joseph's Hospital on the North Side and the House of the Good Shepherd on University Hill as clinical facilities available to medical students. Good Shepherd was founded in 1872 by the Episcopal Diocese of Central New York under Bishop Frederic D. Huntington. After existing first at 90 East Fayette Street then at 80 Hawley Avenue, it moved in 1875 to a building (now Huntington Hall of Syracuse University) on the southwest corner of Marshall Street and University Avenue, where it soon became known as the Hospital of the Good Shepherd and in the twentieth century (below) as University Hospital of the Good Shepherd. In 1885 it began training nurses.

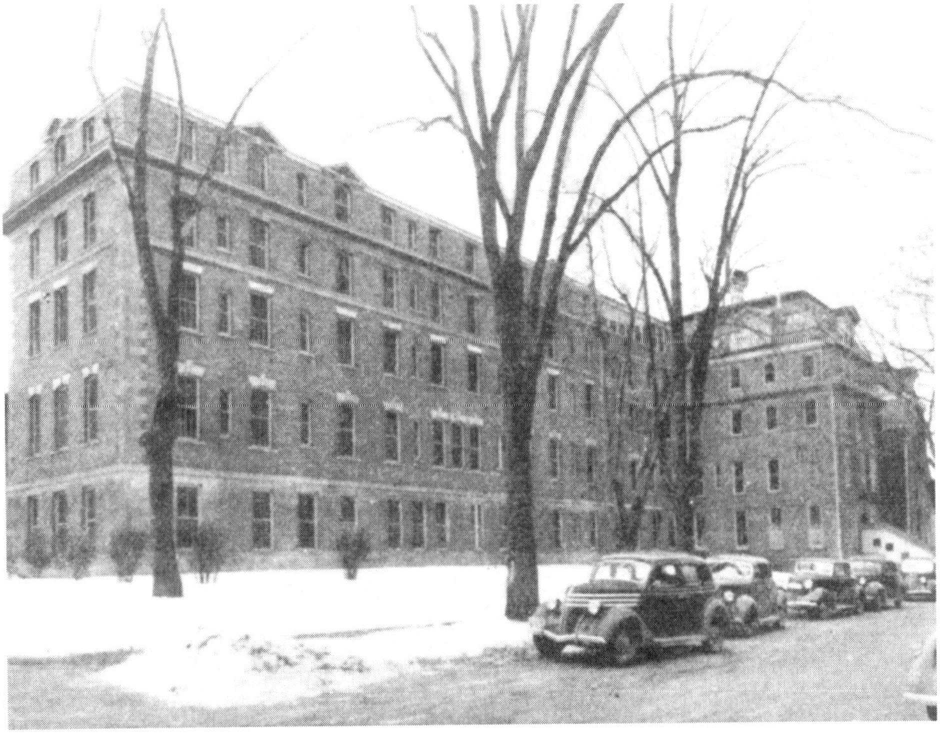

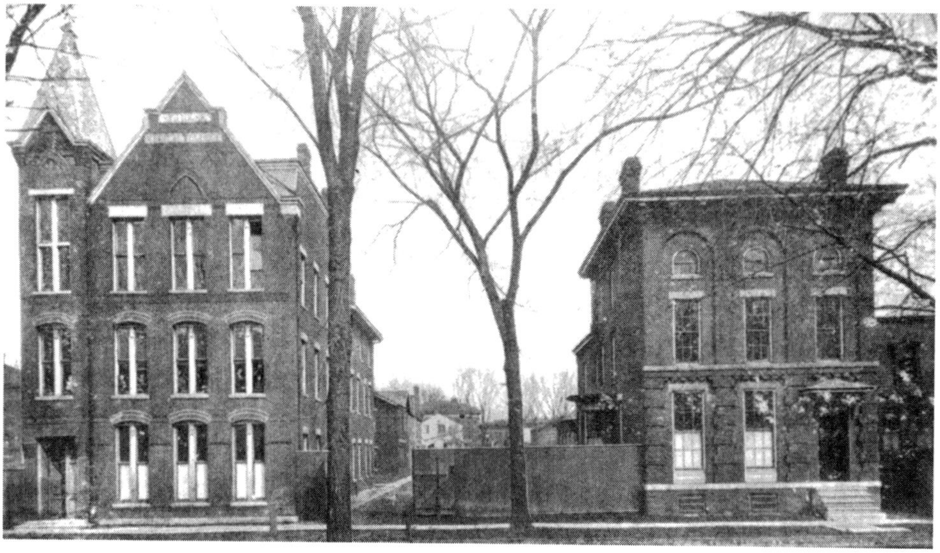

Just south of the remodeled carriage factory was the Smith Building (right), which contained the library, the janitor's room, and a smoking lounge.

The medical school's move to its permanent campus on McBride Street was accompanied by several important changes in curriculum and policy. In 1875, student participation in autopsies became mandatory. In 1876, the requirement to write a dissertation was abolished. For most of the nineteenth century, the irrelevance and inappropriateness of a doctoral dissertation for medical education was typically not recognized. Geneva Medical College required a thesis throughout its existence. (Recall that Austin Flint thought highly enough of Elizabeth Blackwell's essay on epidemic louse-borne typhus to publish it in his *Buffalo Medical Journal and Monthly Review of Medical and Surgical Practice*.) The initiative for change came from the students. According to the minutes of the April 7, 1876 medical faculty meeting: "The Registrar read a communication signed by seven or eight of the nine candidates for the degree, asking to be relieved from the writing of theses and stating succinctly and respectfully their reasons for making this request. Prof. Van Duyn moved the discontinuance of the requirement of a thesis as a preliminary to graduation. The motion was recorded by the Registrar and after remarks by several of the Faculty was passed unanimously." The next College of Medicine catalog, 1876-1877, duly reported: "The custom of requiring the candidate for the degree to submit and defend a thesis, has been abolished in this school, as being a profitless expenditure of the student's time, and void of significance in determining his fitness for graduation."

One of the most accomplished and best liked teachers in the history of the College of Medicine began his monumental 54-year academic career in 1872 as an anatomist and histologist. After graduating from Princeton

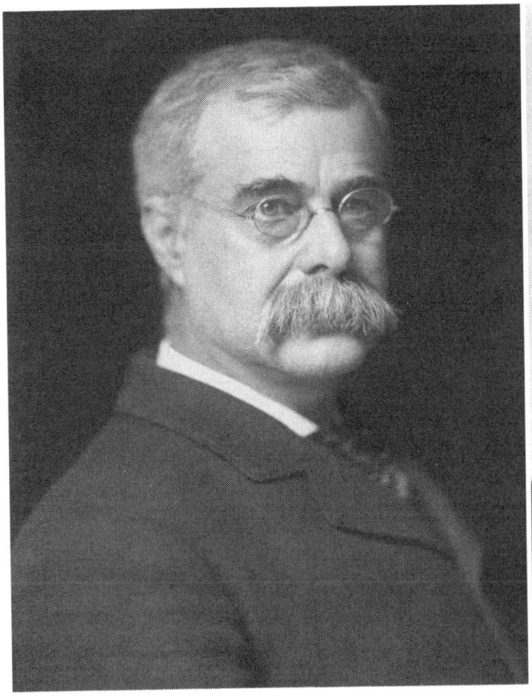

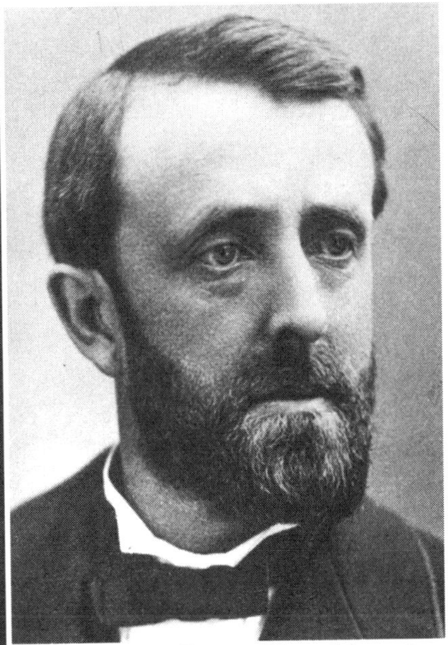

William Tomlinson Plant (above).
John Van Duyn (left).

University in 1862, John Van Duyn had immediately enlisted in the Union Army but was ordered to study medicine because he was unfit for combat. Having received a large part of his medical education on the battlefield, he earned his M.D. in Louisville from the Kentucky School of Medicine in 1865. He moved to Syracuse in 1868 and set up private practice. At the College of Medicine he eventually taught ophthalmology, otology, the history of medicine, and surgery, and chaired the Department of Surgery from 1888 to 1906. Colleagues, students, and patients all delighted in his wry sense of humor. George Birney Broad, Class of 1896, would tell a story of how Van Duyn was called to consult on a diagnosis that had stumped the other doctors. After carefully examining the patient and studying the chart, Van Duyn solemnly declared, "Gentlemen, this is a very rare disease. I will write down its name for you." Then he wrote, "damdifino."

Another early luminary in the College of Medicine was William Tomlinson Plant, who received his M.D. in 1861 from the University of Michigan, served as a U.S. Navy surgeon in the Civil War, then entered private practice. He was Professor of Medical Jurisprudence from 1872 to 1879 then Professor of Pediatrics until he retired in 1895. In 1879 he was President of the Onondaga County Medical Society. As one of the pioneers of American pediatrics, he wrote the first article in the first issue (January 1884) of *Archives of Pediatrics* and thereafter was a member of its editorial board. This journal, having merged in 1962 with *American Practitioner* and *Quarterly Review of Pediatrics*, survives as *Clinical Pediatrics*.

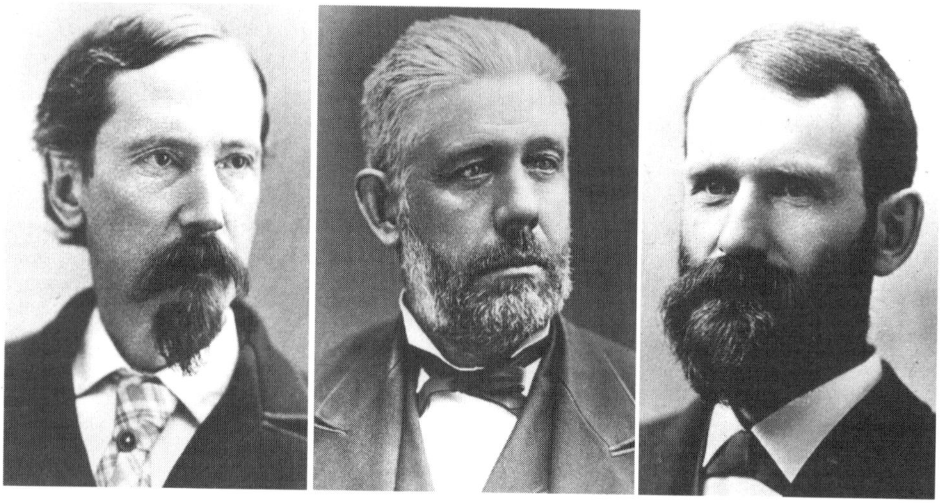

John Otis Burt (left) was a tragic example of the "impaired physician" who allowed substance abuse to ruin a brilliant career. With a Harvard baccalaureate, a Columbia M.D., and U.S. Navy service during the Civil War, Burt was a promising new faculty member in 1872, being the first to teach dermatology in the College of Medicine and sharing the duties of teaching materia medica with Edward B. Stevens. In 1876 an *ad hoc* committee of the faculty accused both Stevens and Burt of "personal habits" inconsistent with their status as professors of medicine, particularly their use of alcohol and narcotics. They were ordered to either reform or resign. Stevens resigned in 1877 but Burt apparently tried to rehabilitate himself, failed, and finally resigned in 1879. Dermatology disappeared from the curriculum from 1877 to 1886.

Wilfred Wickliffe Porter (center) worked in Geddes, New York, as a public school administrator as well as an obstetrician and gynecologist. In 1869 he was President of the Onondaga County Medical Society and from 1872 until his death in 1885 a trustee of Syracuse University. Through these offices he contributed significantly to the plan of the reborn medical school. He taught obstetrics and gynecology from 1872 until 1885 and pediatrics until 1874, when Burt briefly assumed responsibility for that subject.

Charles Everts Rider (right), an ophthalmologist and otologist practicing in Rochester, gave the last valedictory address at Geneva Medical College before it moved to Syracuse, using the occasion mainly to attack, from an ethical perspective, homeopathy and other forms of medicine not approved by the AMA. As he could not reconcile teaching in Syracuse with practicing in Rochester, the faculty declared him emeritus in 1880 and replaced him with Van Duyn. His son, Wheelock Rider, Class of 1885, became an even more distinguished ophthalmologist than his father. The two, however, apparently had a stormy relationship. The son legally changed his name to Edward Wheelock two years after the father's death.

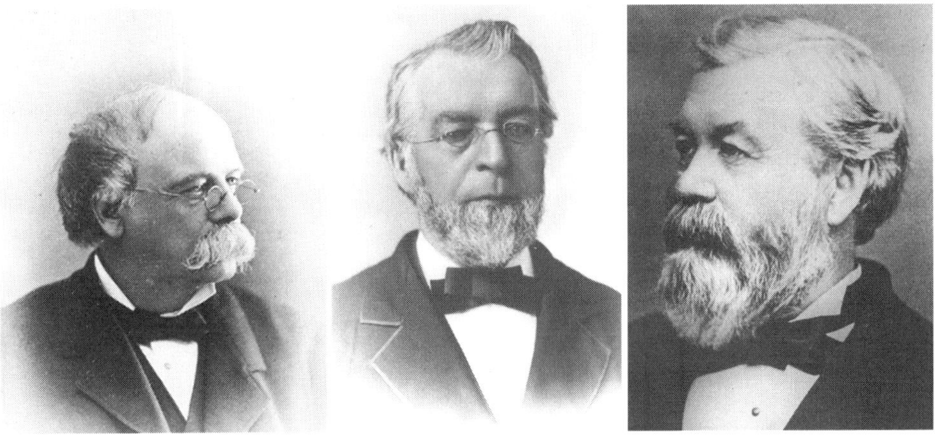

Roger Williams Pease, Class of 1848 (left), practiced medicine in Liverpool, New York, and taught surgery at the College of Medicine from 1872 until his death in 1886. When Towler, with Pease's support, was holding out in 1872 for a $500 laboratory in order to teach chemistry properly, the medical faculty hired the Rev. John J. Brown (center) as the College of Medicine's professor of chemistry. The medical students, who had to share Brown with Syracuse University undergraduates, soon expressed their dissatisfaction, complaining to the faculty in November 1872 that Brown's approach to chemistry was "not sufficiently practical." Towler and Pease meanwhile managed to raise $400 of the needed $500, and Towler took over from Brown in February 1873.

Nelson Nivison (right), who began teaching at Geneva Medical College in 1862, was doggedly attached to the pedagogical methods that dominated medical education before the advent of the graded curriculum in the 1870s. From his home and practice in Burdett, New York, at the south end of Seneca Lake just northeast of Watkins Glen, he would drive his buggy into Geneva on a schedule planned around his own convenience, give a cluster of lectures on physiology, pathology, or microscopic anatomy, then return home. This worked fine in the 1860s, but when the medical school moved to Syracuse and instituted longer sessions with three or four regularly scheduled lectures per week, Nivison found himself inconvenienced, unwilling to give up either his practice and move to Syracuse or his professorship and stay in Burdett. He managed to cope until about 1875, when he began pawning his teaching duties off on young unpaid instructors while he continued to receive full pay. Because these instructors were not really volunteers, but were coerced by Nivison, and because the quality of their instruction was inferior to his, students and faculty gradually became displeased. By 1884 matters reached crisis. An *ad hoc* faculty committee voted to cut Nivison's fees in half and use the money to pay his instructors. Nivison quit teaching pathology in 1886 and physiology in 1887.

Graduates.

GRADUATES OF 1873.

Name.	*State.*	*Name.*	*State.*
H. G. Buckingham,	New York.	George P. Reynolds,	New York.
J. E. Kelsey,	"	A. D. Simonds,	"
John S. Niles,	Vermont.	Sarah VanTuyl,	"

GRADUATES OF 1874.

E. A. Ainsworth,	New York.	Asa G. Henry,	New York.
C. O. Baker,	"	H. F. Hatch,*	"
Charles W. Bowen,	"	H. D. Hunt,	"
A. S. Edwards,	"	E. A. Overhiser,	"
J. A. Griffin,	"		

GRADUATES OF 1875.

William T. Burdick,	New York.	A. F. Vadeboncoeur,	New York.
John R. Eaton,	"	Harriet A. Woodward,	"
Owen C. Hall,	"	D. D. Wickham,	New Jersey.
J. Morris Jenkins,	"	C. H. Whiting,	New York.
C. E. Preston,	"	Louise L. Woodin,	"
J. T. Potter,	"	A. Quivey,	"

GRADUATES OF 1876.

Darwin H. Bliss,	New York.	John S. Marshall,	New York.
Eugene M. Crabb,	"	Miller K. Reading,	New Jersey.
William H. Dwight,	"	J. Erwin Reed,	New York.
David Dunham, Jr.,	"	Charles James Russell,	England.
Judson S. Gibbs,	"	Margaret Stanton,	New York.
J. H. Graves, M. D.,	"	David M. Totman,	"
George R. Kinne,	"	Frances G. Wheelock,	"
Brace W. Loomis,	"	Phebe Willet,	"
Sarah M. Loguen,	"		

GRADUATES OF 1877.

John S. Clark,	New York.	Charles H. Kingman,*	New York.
Nathan Jacobson,	"	Carrie A. Hatch,	"
Nettie E. Jenkins,	"		

All following names are arranged according to relative rank as determined by average of examinations :

GRADUATES OF 1878.

A. Clifford Mercer,	New York.	Millie E. Dann,	New York.
William H. Dunlap,	"	Seth B. Allen,	"
Newton H. Curtis,	"	A. B. Chidester,*	"
Horace D. Babcock,	"	Jennie S. Elder,	"
James D. Owen,	"	M. Virginia Glauner,	"
Garrison L. Brown,	"	Morris H. Conner,	"
Milton A. Curtiss,	"	William H. Forsyth,*	"

GRADUATES OF 1879.

Albert L. Hall,	New York.	Charles A. Boyce,	New York.
George W. Sargent,	"	A. Adelbert Young,	"
Harry Gifford, Jr.,	"		

GRADUATES OF 1880.

Gaylord P. Clark,	New York.	Peppino Melfi,	Italy.
Alfred C. Haven,	"	Alexander D. Allen,	New York.
Charles S. Roberts,	"	Charles E. Bennett,	"

*Deceased.

The list on page 62 of the earliest graduates of the medical school at Syracuse University, published in the 1880 college catalog, shows how quickly the revived medical school established its reputation for academic excellence, innovative policies, and progressive social consciousness. A disproportionately large number of these graduates became prominent physicians, notably David Totman (top right), who taught physiology and materia medica at Syracuse University before becoming a surgeon, then chaired the Department of Surgery from 1913 until his death in 1920, bringing surgical pathology and other subspecialties into the curriculum; Nathan Jacobson (center right), who established his surgical practice in Syracuse in 1878 after a year of postgraduate study in Vienna, taught laryngology and clinical surgery at Syracuse University, and chaired the Department of Surgery from 1906 until his death in 1913; William Herbert Dunlap (bottom left), professor of materia medica and therapeutics, who studied the new science of dermatology in Germany and reintroduced it to Syracuse; A. Clifford Mercer (bottom center), who enjoyed a long career teaching pathology, histology, and clinical pediatrics at Syracuse University, chaired the Department of Pathology from 1886 to 1893, and was president of the American Microscopical Society in 1895; and Gaylord Parsons Clark (bottom right), who specialized in ear physiology, taught anatomy and physiology at Syracuse University from 1881 to 1904, and served as dean from 1905 until his sudden death in 1907.

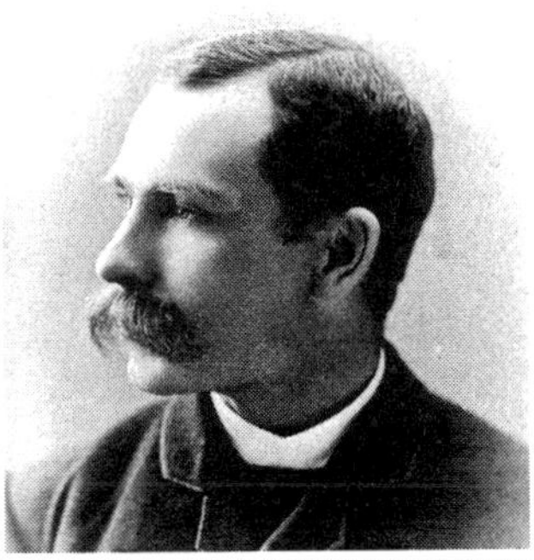

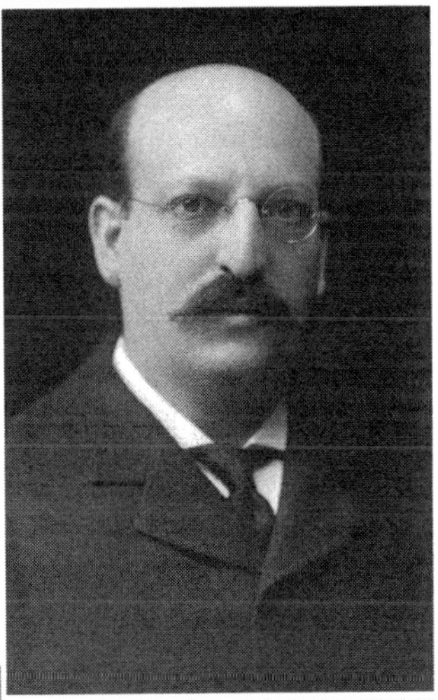

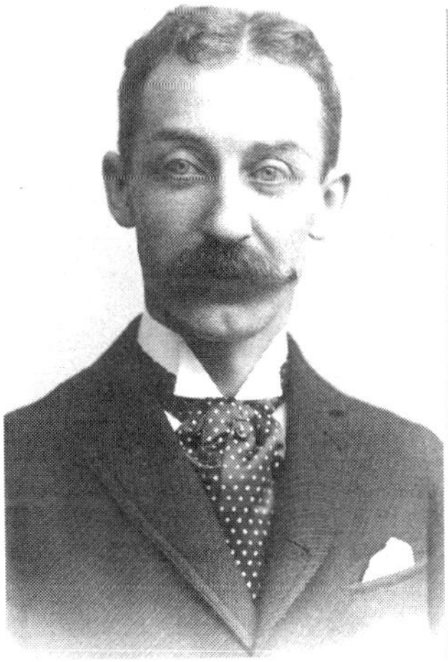

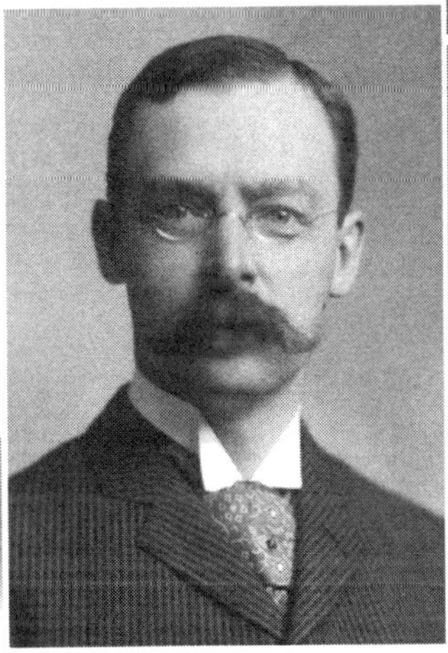

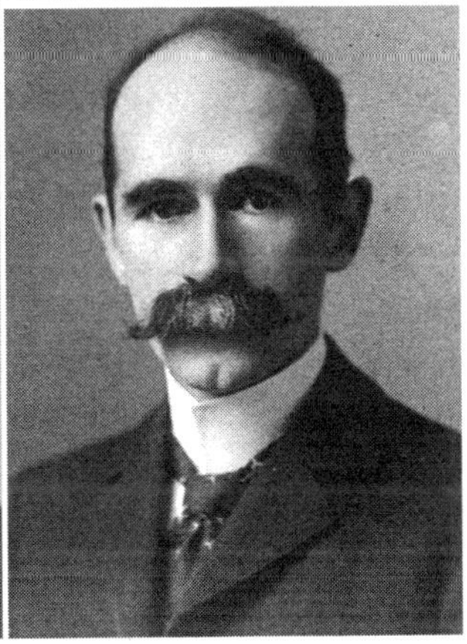

In the first six years of the Syracuse University College of Medicine, eleven of the 63 graduates, or 17 percent, were women. The percentage of women medical students in Syracuse fell after that, not to recover until the 1960s. Of these eleven — Sarah Van Tuyl, Laura Louise Nobles Woodin Graham, Harriet A. Woodward, Sarah Loguen Fraser, Margaret Stanton, Phebe Willett Dean, Caroline A. Hatch, Nettie E. Tripp Jenkins, Amelia E. Dann DeMott, Jennie Stevens Elder, and Mary Virginia Adams Glauner — one is truly outstanding: Sarah Loguen Fraser (shown painted by Susan Keeter).

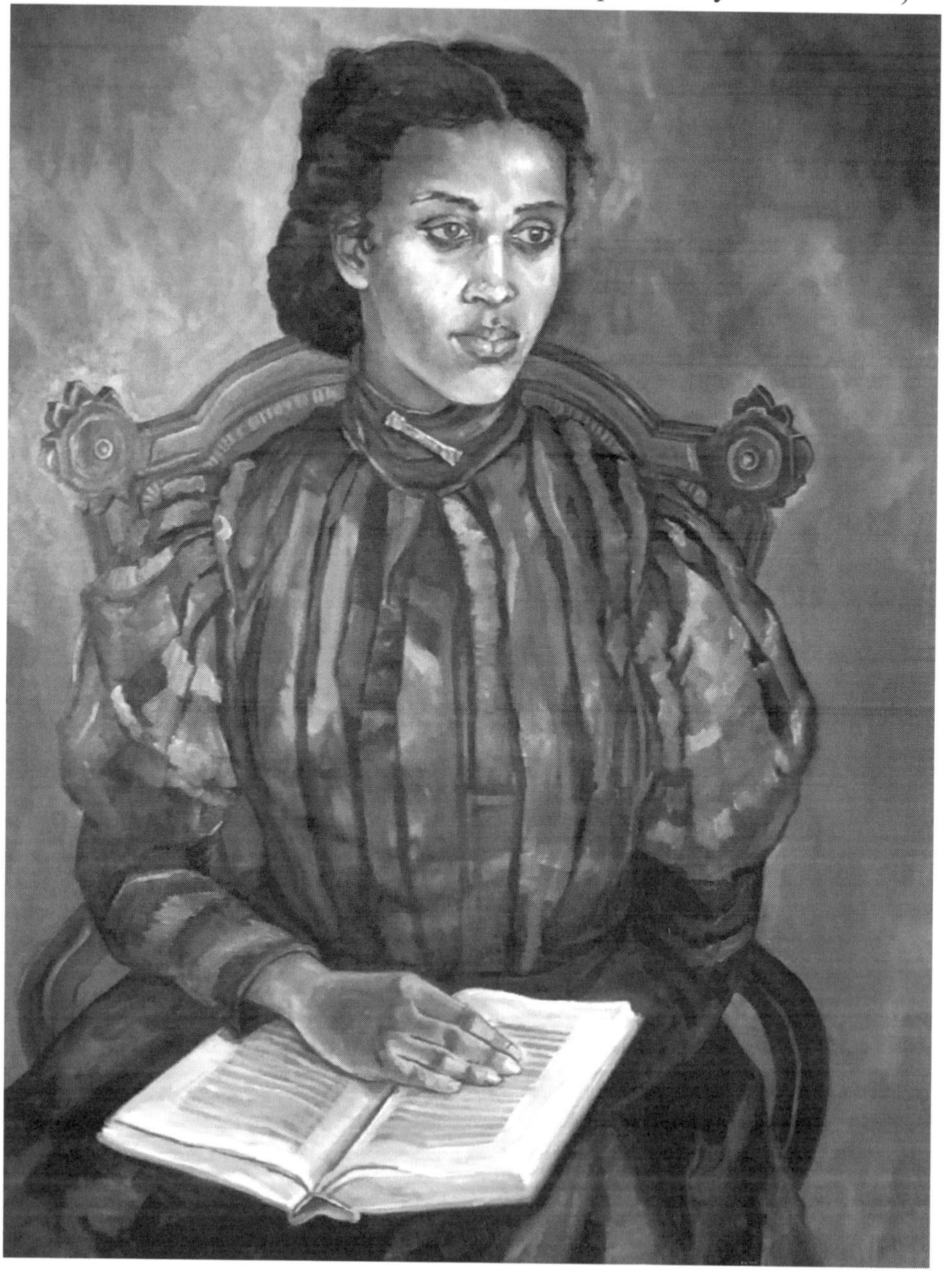

Around 1802 thugs kidnapped Jane McCoy, a seven-year-old free African-American girl, from her home in Ohio and sold her into slavery in Tennessee. She lost her name as well as her freedom. David Logue, her owner, called her only "Cherry." He raped her frequently from her teenage years on. Jermain Logue, their first child, was born around 1813. When he was about 21, he escaped to Ontario, learned to read, added "n" to his surname, chose "Wesley" as a middle name, and studied for the ministry, thus becoming the Rev. Jermain Wesley Loguen (pronounced "Logan"). In 1841 he settled in Syracuse, where he soon became a prominent citizen and a leading abolitionist. With a white Unitarian minister, Samuel May, he led the "Jerry Rescue" in 1851. Known locally as "The King of the Underground Railroad," he personally helped to liberate about 1500 fugitive slaves. His autobiography, *The Rev. J. W. Loguen as a Slave and as a Freeman*, appeared in Syracuse in 1859.

Sarah Marinda Loguen was born at the Loguen home in Syracuse on January 29, 1850, the fifth of eight children of Rev. Loguen and his wife, Caroline Storum. Sarah was always very close to her father. She finished high school in 1868, the same year he was consecrated a bishop in the African Methodist Episcopal Zion Church. Thereafter she rode his circuit with him, served as his secretary, and studied German in her spare time. Since her mother had died and since her older sister Amelia had married Lewis Douglass, son of Frederick Douglass, and moved to Washington, D.C., Sarah became head of the household when her father died unexpectedly in 1872. She was devastated, unemployed, and apparently without prospects.

At the railroad station in Washington, D.C. in the spring of 1873, about to begin her return to Syracuse after visiting Amelia's family and friends, Sarah heard a small boy scream in agony. A heavy wagon had just run over him and broken his leg. A crowd gathered to gawk but not to help. She was horrified that she was the only one present who seemed to show any compassion. Only she tried to find a doctor. Her frantic actions amazed the crowd, but still no one offered any comfort to the suffering boy. Finally someone took him away. She was so distressed by the crowd's indifference to the child's pain that she made this solemn vow: "I will never, never see a human being in need of aid again and not be able to help."

According to "Miss Doc," her daughter Gregoria's unpublished biography of her, deposited in the Moorland-Spingarn Research Center of Howard University, Loguen resolved on the train going home to become a physician. Emotionally drained, physically exhausted, half conscious, and with her eyes closed, she murmured, "I will, I will, I am going to be Doctor Sarah Marinda Loguen." Unknown to her, on the same train by sheer chance, was her family physician, an 1836 medical graduate of Yale University, a veteran of the Civil War, and in 1870 president of the Onondaga

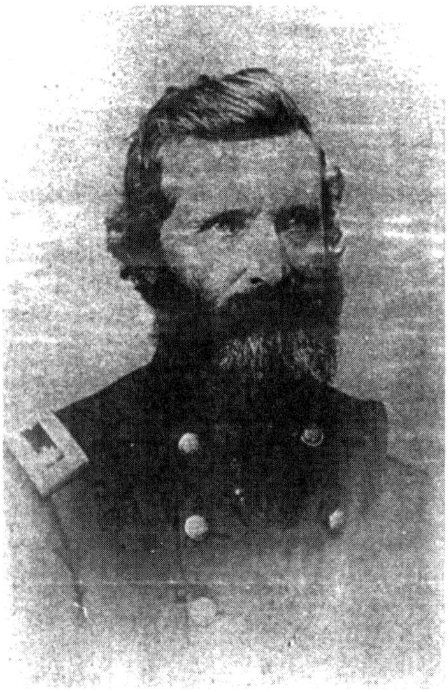

County Medical Society, Michael D. Benedict (left). As he overheard her reverie, his familiar voice startled her awake, "You are, are you?" For the rest of the trip the two discussed what being a physician means. He promised to help her all he could.

She studied with Benedict for the next five months. Through her hard work and his influence, she was admitted to the Syracuse University College of Medicine that fall. On October 4, 1873, the day after she matriculated, the Syracuse newspapers wrote: "We understand that Miss Sarah M. Loguen, daughter of the late Bishop J. W. Loguen, has commenced the study of medicine under the tuition of Doctor M. D. Benedict of this city. This is 'woman's rights' in the right direction, and we cordially wish the estimable young lady every success in the pursuit of the profession of her choice."

Even considering her race and gender, Loguen's medical school experience was quite normal for her time, including a graverobbing excursion in Oakwood Cemetery to try (and fail) to procure a cadaver for anatomical dissection. Such events were not unusual for medical students in the mid-nineteeth century.

The first African-American woman physician was Rebecca Lee Crumpler, who received her M.D. in Boston at Samuel Gregory's New England Female Medical College in 1864. The second was Rebecca J. Cole, with an 1867 M.D. from the Woman's Medical College of Pennsylvania; and the third was Susan Smith McKinney Steward, whose 1870 M.D. was from Clemence Sophia Lozier's New York Medical College for Women. When Loguen received her M.D. in the spring of 1876, she thus became probably the fourth African-American woman physician in the United States, the second in New York, and the first in the nation to earn her M.D. at a coeducational, regular medical school. Even if there were others before 1876 — the records are often hazy, with the race and sometimes even the gender of medical students difficult to determine — that would not diminish her status as a pioneer.

By 1890 about 115 African-American women had become doctors. By 1920 reaction from both the white community and African-American males had reduced that number to only 65 in active medical practice.

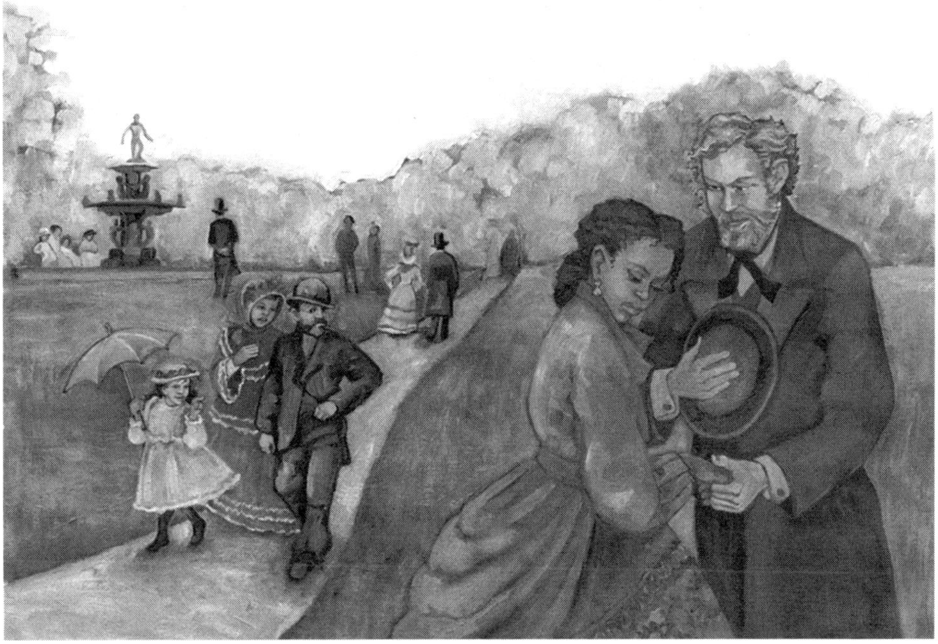

As depicted in Susan Keeter's painting, one of Sarah's classmates (we do not know which one) surprised her with a proposal of marriage shortly after their medical graduation. He claimed that his whiteness and her blackness did not matter and that a female physician of any color was such a social freak that she would need a male colleague to protect her. Rejecting his offer, she told him that whiteness and blackness did matter, that her job was to maintain the health of strong black bodies, that she was continuing her father's mission to improve African-American conditions, and that she would be abandoning all these ideals if she married a white man. He angrily went west and never contacted her again.

Loguen interned from September 1876 until the summer of 1878 at the Woman's Hospital of Philadelphia, which Ann Preston, who in 1866 became the first woman dean of the Woman's Medical College of Pennsylvania, had founded in 1861. Loguen was a favorite of the children in the wards, who called her "Miss Doc." She instituted a method to calm nervous patients by taking all bold or bright colors out of their environment and teaching them to knit with soft, pastel-colored yarn. In the twentieth century the psychology of color became well-established fact, but in the 1870s it was mostly trial and error, having barely reached the stage of theory.

In the fall of 1878 Loguen moved to Boston to fill a six-month vacancy in an internship at Marie Elizabeth Zakrzewska's New England Hospital for Women and Children. When she began private medical practice in Washington, D.C., in the summer of 1879, Frederick Douglass personally nailed up her shingle.

Douglass introduced Charles Fraser, a pharmacist from Puerto Plata, Santo Domingo (now the Dominican Republic), to the entire Loguen family and actively encouraged the courtship of Charles and Sarah from 1877 until he proposed to her in June 1881. Shortly after they were married in Syracuse on September 19, 1882, Douglass wrote to her: "Tell Mr. Fraser that while I would have been glad to have you here as long as I am in the land of the living, that I do not blame him a bit for taking you away."

Sarah Loguen Fraser was the first woman physician in Santo Domingo, licensed there in the spring of 1883, but by law only women and children could be her patients. Her practice prospered and she was well loved.

About to give birth on December 23, 1883, she was so frightened by the primitive midwifery procedures that were to be inflicted on her that she decided to manage her own labor. She did this until the pains became so harsh that she lost consciousness. At that point a traditional midwife took over. Sarah had a healthy daughter, Gregoria Alejandrina Fraser, but the midwife had damaged her reproductive system so much that she could never have another baby.

When Charles died of a stroke on September 30, 1894, Sarah gave up her medical practice in order to run the drugstore. Mostly for the sake of her daughter's education, she divided their time among Washington, Syracuse, and Paris from 1896 until finally settling in Washington in 1907. Thereafter she practiced medicine occasionally. As a private practitioner she was successful, but involvement with institutions sometimes made her the victim of racism. The Blue Plains (Maryland) Industrial School for Boys hired her in 1908 as Resident Physician with private quarters and an office, but as soon as she arrived she was housed in a cottage with fourteen boys and a girl. She and the girl were expected to be maids, cooks, and laundresses for the boys. Despite threat of a lawsuit, and with the help of Gregoria's intercession, she resigned. A few years later, while practicing two days a week at a women's clinic in Washington, she noticed that the white women physicians were taking credit for the black women physicians' work, and covering their backs by destroying case histories and charts that the black women physicians had written.

She retired from medicine gradually in the 1920s as she developed kidney disease and memory loss, probably Alzheimer's. She died quietly at home in Gregoria's arms on April 9, 1933, and was buried in Lincoln Cemetery in Washington. When news of her death reached Santo Domingo, its flags were ordered flown at half-mast for nine days.

Upstate Medical University dedicated its Black History Month celebrations to Sarah Loguen Fraser and erected a New York State historical marker in February 2000 in honor of her 150th birthday. A street on campus and an endowed medical student scholarship fund are named after her.

5

Surviving the Flexner Report

In 1877 a donation of $10,000 enabled the faculty to pay off the mortgage on the carriage factory campus. The university remained stingy toward the medical school, and the transfer of this real estate to the university, which was supposed to happen in exchange for better financial support, was delayed for ten years. After much wrangling, the final legal unification of the College of Medicine and Syracuse University was accomplished in 1887, with the university agreeing to contribute $500 a year to help maintain the medical school. But still the faculty was expected to cover the lion's share of operating expenses.

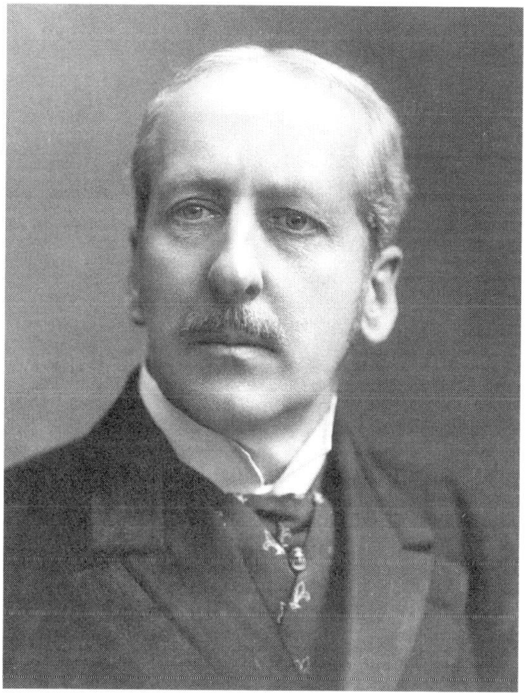

Also in 1877 William Pepper (right), gave an important speech that compared the Syracuse University College of Medicine favorably with the top medical schools in the country: the University of Pennsylvania, Harvard, Chicago Medical College, and the University of Michigan.* Pepper was at that time professor of clinical medicine at the University of Pennsylvania and shortly thereafter became university provost. In 1874, he had founded the Hospital of the University of Pennsylvania, thus creating the first academic medical center in America. So, coming from as eminent a physician as he, this praise was most valuable toward solidifying the reputation of the newly re-established medical school and enabling it to attract top-flight teachers and students.

---

* William Pepper, *Higher Medical Education, the True Interest of the Public and the Profession: Two Addresses Delivered Before the Medical Department of the University of Pennsylvania on October 1, 1877, and October 2, 1893* (Philadelphia: J.B. Lippincott, 1894), p. 41.

Despite this auspicious start, Syracuse University missed a golden opportunity to propel its new medical school into the absolute forefront of American medical education. When the College of Medicine established its three-year graded curriculum in 1872, only Harvard and Michigan had also already done so. Throughout the 1870s, 1880s, and 1890s, it continued with sometimes risky innovations to keep its curriculum among the best in the nation. It was among the first American medical schools to develop laboratory teaching methods, to improve bedside clinical protocols for students, to emulate the residency program designed by William Stewart Halsted at Johns Hopkins in the late 1880s, and to institute a four-year graded curriculum. But because Syracuse University failed to provide adequate financing, the quality of the medical school soon fell behind that of Hopkins, Harvard, Yale, the University of Pennsylvania, Jefferson, Michigan, Washington University of St. Louis, and a few others, all of which were blessed with generous and affluent administrations. Syracuse University College of Medicine faculty in the 1870s and 1880s were mostly voluntary, unsalaried, and had to provide their own utilities, pay their own overhead, conduct their own business, and solicit their own philanthropic contributions. Such philanthropy came mostly from the professors' friends and colleagues, because major donors could not be attracted when substantial support from the university coffers was absent. Since Syracuse University was more concerned to build its own general endowment, any separate endowment for the College of Medicine had to wait. Only in 1888 did the university begin to contribute its promised money to the the medical school's annual budget.

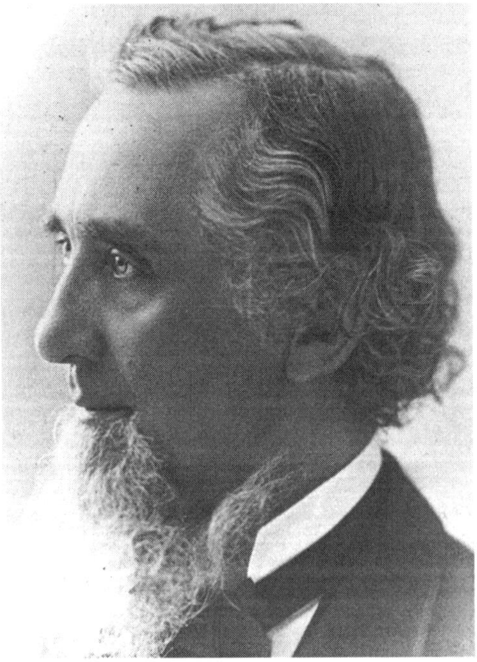

Professor of Medicine Henry Darwin Didama (right) became dean in 1887. In the 1870s he had led the movement to create three-year graded medical instruction, systematic medical research, and rigorous clinical training. In all his eighteen years as dean he fought for greater support from the university, for better teaching, and for national recognition of the medical school's achievements. In the latter two of these campaigns he was mostly successful.

Better teaching entailed less lecturing and more programmed "hands-on" instruction in laboratories and clinical settings. In this regard medical education in Syracuse under Didama was an unqualified success. The major reason that the transition from lecture to laboratory teaching worked so well was the influence of Henry Leopold Elsner (left).

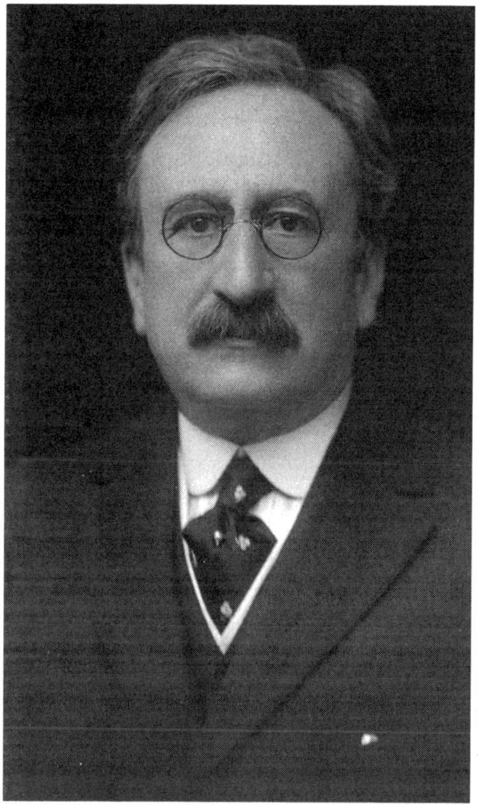

Born in Syracuse of German immigrant parents, his father also a physician, Elsner received his M.D. from Columbia in 1877 and took another year of medical study in Berlin and Vienna. Soon after his return to Syracuse in 1878, he built the most prosperous medical practice in Central New York. In 1882 he began teaching at the College of Medicine. His intimate familiarity with German methods of medical education enabled Syracuse to be one of the first medical schools in America after Johns Hopkins to build and upgrade laboratory facilities on the then state-of-the-art German model, a major improvement which many American medical schools did not accomplish until after the 1910 Flexner Report — if they survived that cull.

Elsner was promoted in 1886 to Professor of Clinical Medicine and in 1904 to Professor of Medicine. He was president of many professional organizations, including the Medical Society of the State of New York. In 1916, the year of his untimely death, appeared his life's work, *The Prognosis of Internal Diseases*, which Fielding H. Garrison praised in *An Introduction to the History of Medicine* as "almost the only important work on the subject" after Prosper Alpinus's 1601 *De praesagienda vita et morte aegrotantium*."

From 1905 to 1911 Good Shepherd substantially improved first its clinical diagnosis laboratory then its pathology laboratory, partially under Elsner's guidance. Urged by Elsner's relatives and the dean, his lifelong friend John Lorenzo Heffron, Class of 1881 (who himself had done graduate work in medicine at Vienna and Heidelberg in 1881-1882), Good Shepherd named these facilities the Elsner Research Laboratories shortly after his death. Heffron clearly recognized the great advantage that had accrued to the College of Medicine because of the European approaches that Elsner had taken. He wrote in his 1920 reminiscence, *Fifty Years of the College of Medicine of Syracuse University*, that the faculty in general and Elsner in particular "recognized the superiority of the laboratory method of teaching the sciences fundamental to medicine in the beginning, and, as rapidly as funds for equipment of material and men were available, they put each laboratory under a full-time, paid corps of teachers, so that all these sciences have been so taught from an early date. The laboratory method of instruction followed as a matter of course" (p. 13).

Improvements continued, even though still underfunded. The medical school built a new pathology laboratory in 1875, a new chemistry laboratory in 1876, and adopted the metric system in 1879. The new science of bacteriology became part of the pathology curriculum in 1894. The same year the faculty voted unanimously to extend the graded instruction to a mandatory four-year program, to begin in October 1896.

But by 1895 the carriage factory was crumbling. An emergency coalition of the faculty, the university, and alumni quickly raised $40,000 to design and construct a new medical school building at 309 South McBride Street. The carriage factory was razed, classes were held temporarily at St. Joseph's Hospital, and the new structure (below), finished within a year at a cost of $85,000, was occupied in the fall of 1896.

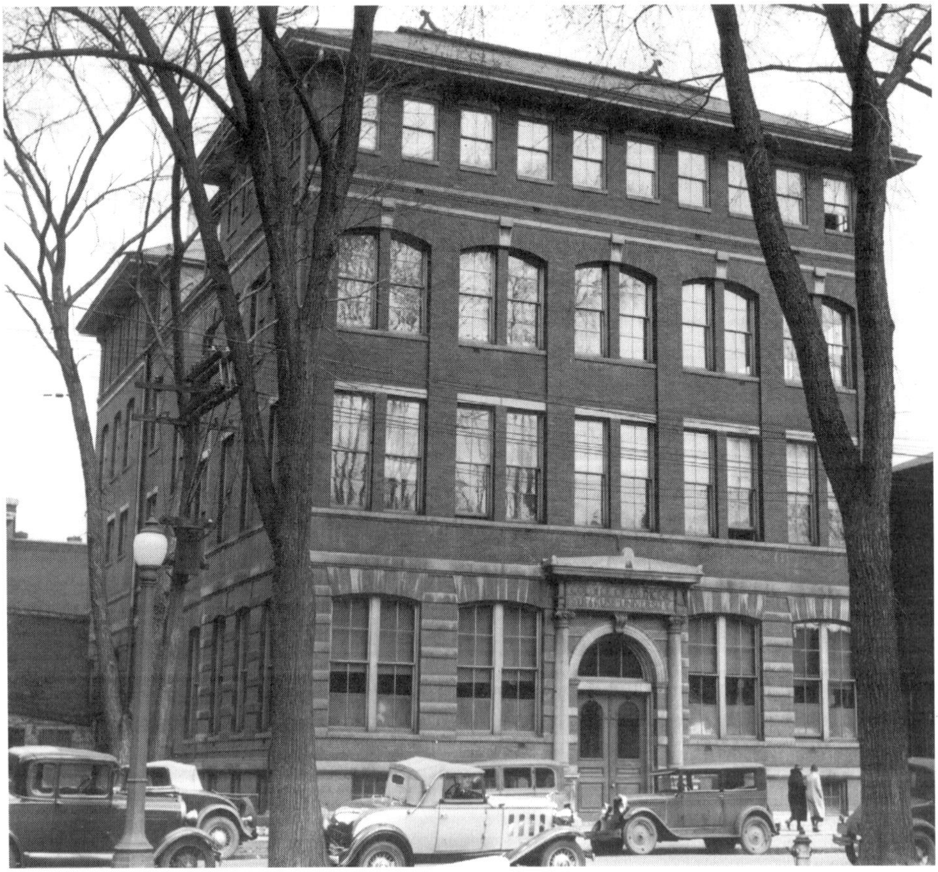

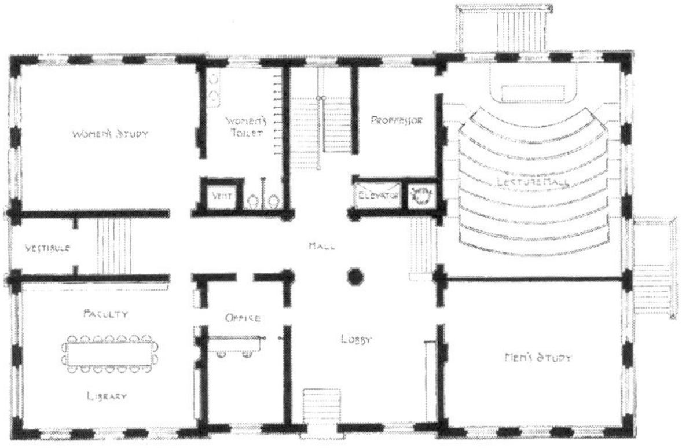

Plan of First Floor

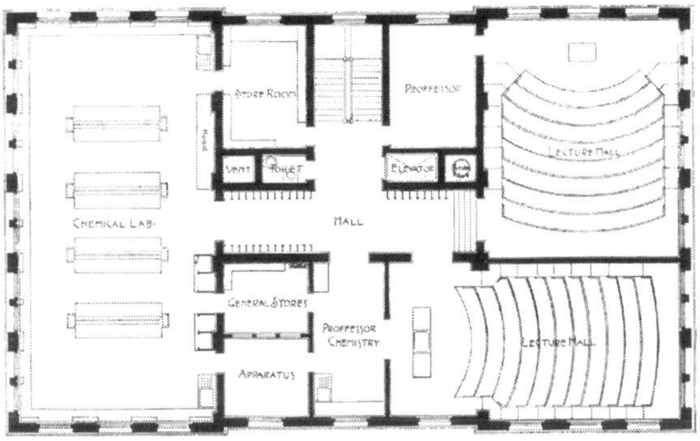

Plan of Second Floor

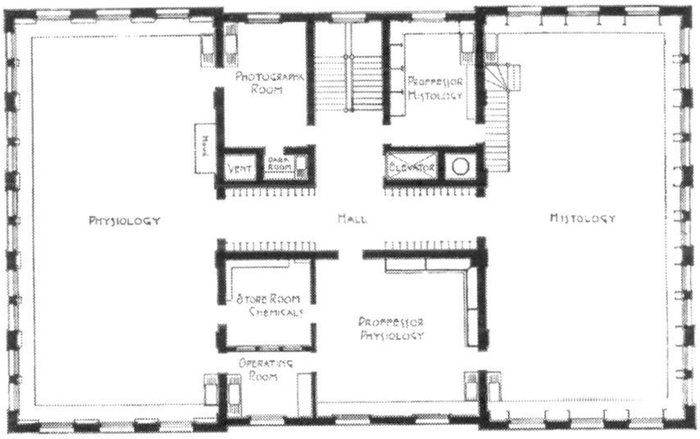

Plan of Third Floor

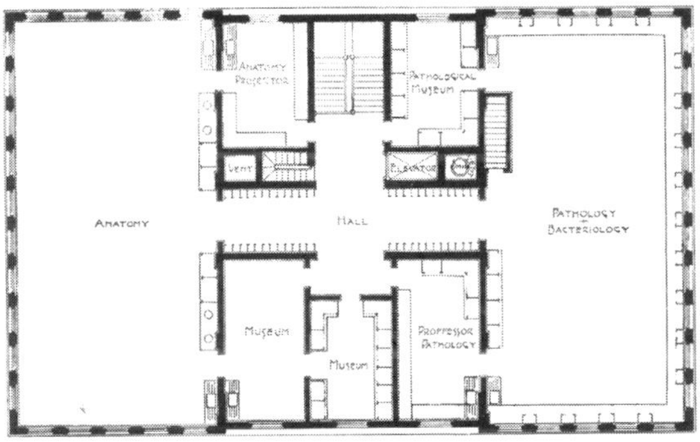

Plan of Fourth Floor

The faculty got nearly everything it wanted in the new building: three ample lecture halls, private offices, separate study areas for men and women students, a library that served as a faculty lounge, and up-to-date laboratories for anatomy, pathology, bacteriology, histology, physiology, and chemistry.

In Elizabeth Blackwell's time the library of Geneva Medical College was excellent, with not only current works but also older classics donated by Cutbush, Colman, and many others. But from 1872 to 1897 the collection was mostly in storage, unused, untended, and sometimes pilfered. Even though the Syracuse University College of Medicine from the beginning had designated a member of the clinical faculty as "Librarian," the title rotated and was just *pro forma*. The collection was regarded as a quaint curiosity from a bygone era. The 1875-1876 medical college catalog was the first in Syracuse to mention the library, and described it as comprising "the entire collection of the Geneva School, with some additions made by contribution and purchase. It is especially rich in the medical literature of an earlier day."

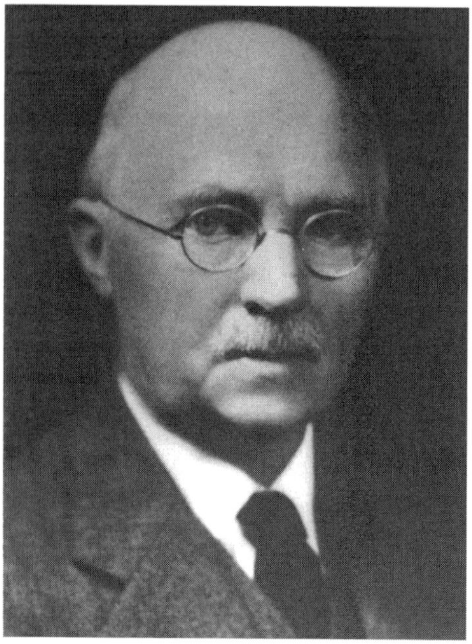

Professor of Ophthalmology Frank William Marlow, Class of 1885 (left), became librarian in 1890, remaining so until 1941, even after his retirement from medical teaching and practice. Marlow and Van Duyn seem to have been the first to discern the harm to the College of Medicine caused by neglecting the library. Marlow was especially disturbed that, apparently because there was neither a functional reading room nor a regular attendant, students were not using the library. In 1896 Marlow created a library committee consisting of himself, Clifford Mercer, and Lecturer on Hygiene and Public Health William H. Mills. He appointed the College of Medicine's secretary, Abby M. Bond, and assistant secretary, Mary A. Barker, to serve as assistant librarians. The minutes of the earliest library committee meetings are in Bond's hand.

Marlow managed to build the collection even though library funding remained inadequate for respectable acquisitions. He negotiated an impressive gift of about 1100 titles from Stephen Smith, a bargain purchase of about 2500 volumes for $300 from Philadelphia ophthalmologist and "Medical Library Movement" founder George Milbry Gould, a substantial bequest from the estate of Syracuse Professor of Anatomy Scott Owen, Class of 1883 (left); and ongoing gifts from such faculty members as Van Duyn, Clifford Mercer, and Didama.

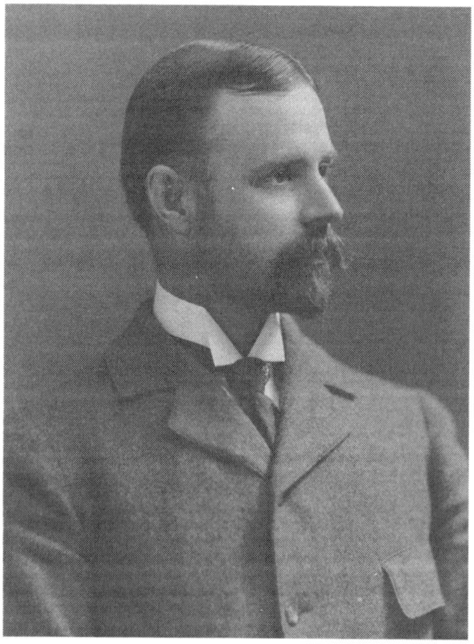

But the situation did not really begin to improve until the fall of 1897 when Marlow hired a first-year medical student, Elizabeth Latimer Shrimpton, at 12½ cents an hour to reorganize the library in its new quarters and to serve as the medical school's first regular library attendant.

Shrimpton was born on July 1, 1875, in Fayetteville, New York. She received her B.S. from Knox College in 1896 and her M.D. in 1901. Her medical career was entirely in Syracuse, in general practice until she retired in 1951. She never married, but at the age of 44 adopted a son, David MacDill Shrimpton. She died at home in Syracuse on June 6, 1955.

Little of Marlow's dream for the library could have been actualized without Shrimpton's tireless and careful work. She was the first "real" medical librarian in Syracuse. Her four years in charge of daily activities marked the turning point for the library's utility and relevance to modern medical education. Most of the thousands of accession entries from 1897 (the year accessions started) to 1901 are in her hand, with many in Bond's and some in a third, perhaps Barker's.

At least 811 and probably over a thousand volumes were in the original Geneva Medical College Library, but when Shrimpton completed the accession process for the Geneva books in 1898, only 406 of these volumes remained in the collection. What happened to the rest is unknown. Because of Marlow's collection development ability and Shrimpton's management skill and initiative, the library by 1901 had officially recorded 5072 volumes. That total would have been far fewer without her. Her effort and dedication brought the library into the twentieth century with efficient methods of cataloging, inventory control, and reader services. She can be credited with originating the policies and practices which continue to make

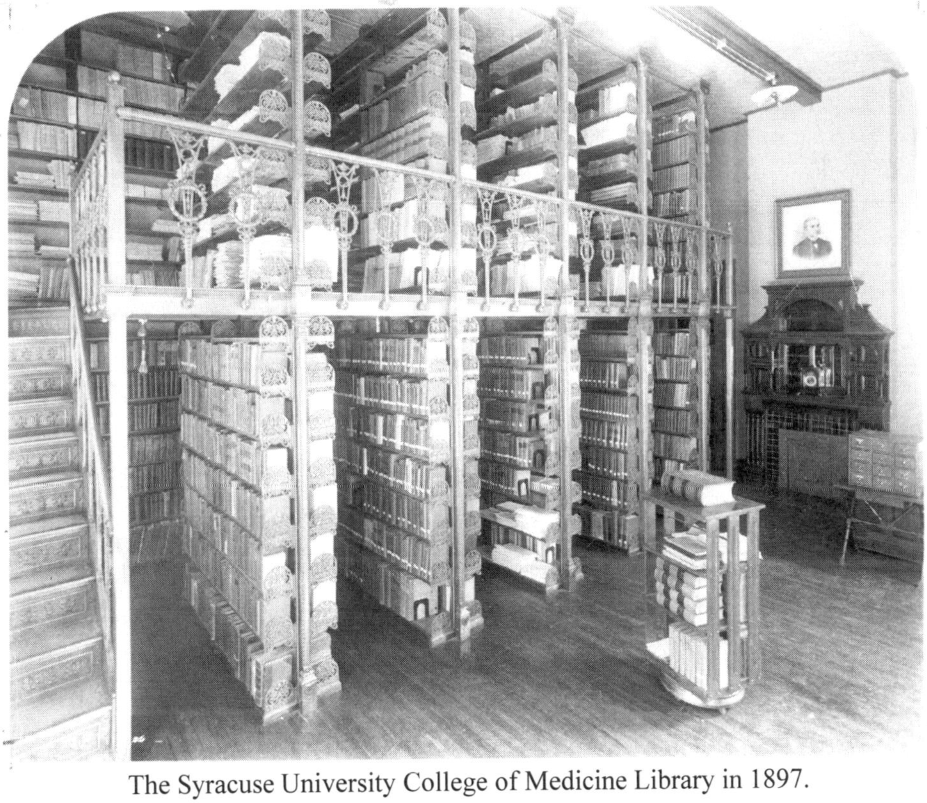

The Syracuse University College of Medicine Library in 1897.

the resources of the Health Sciences Library accessible to its main group of users, the medical community of Central New York.

The Flexner Report strongly underscored the necessity of medical libraries for the whole process of educating doctors. Despite Flexner's admonition and the medical deans' protests, Syracuse University continued to underfund, understaff, and undersupport its medical library. From 11,503 volumes in 1922, it grew to only 23,262 by 1949, and did not reach Dean Weiskotten's 1940 goal of 100,000 volumes until the early 1970s.

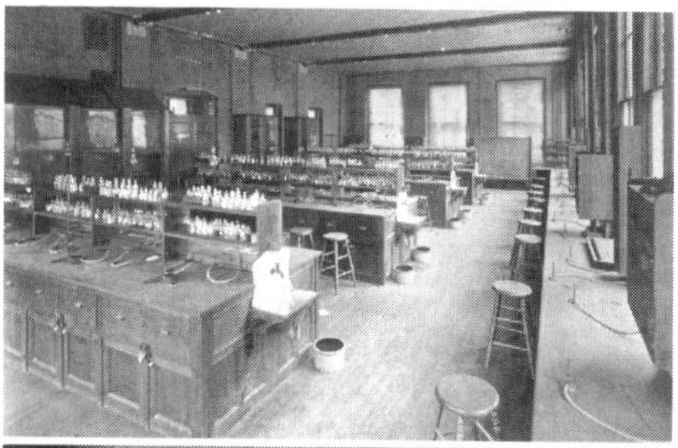
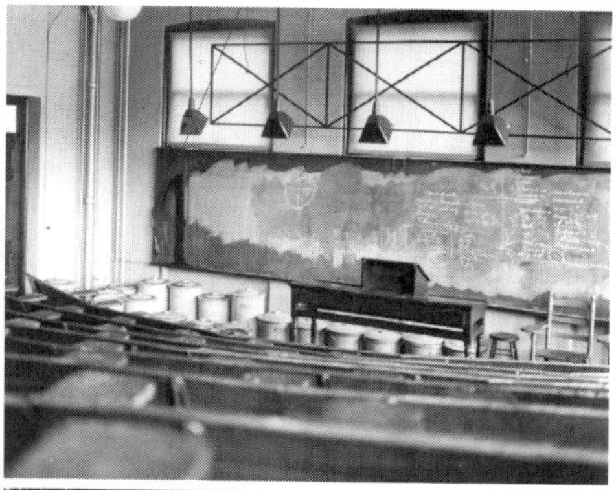
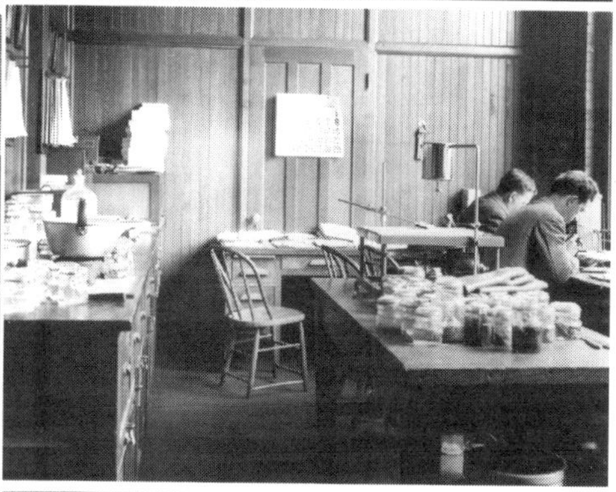
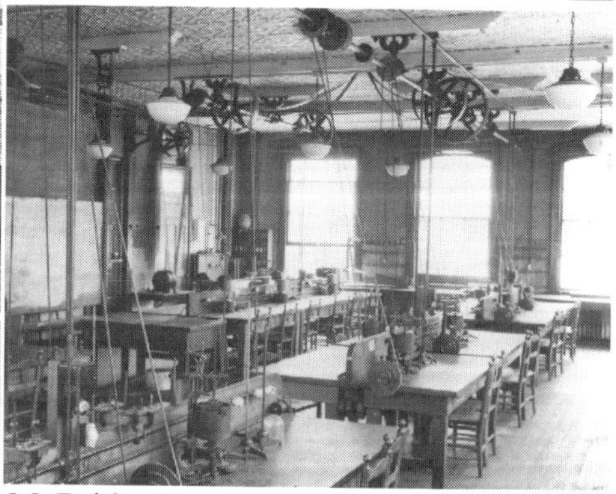
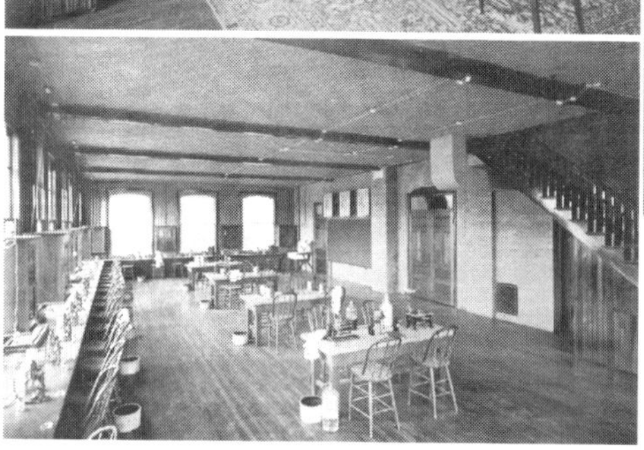
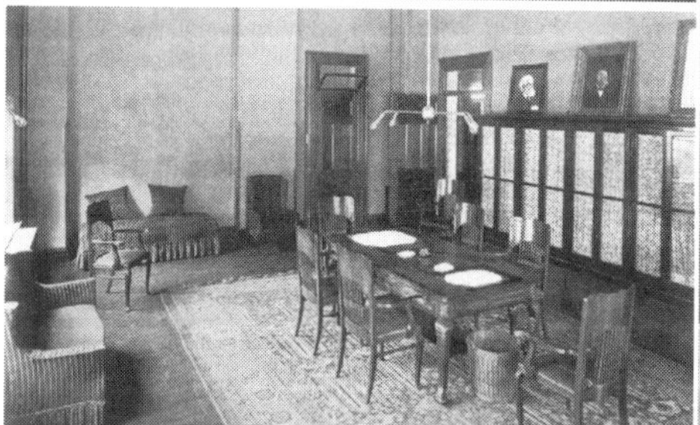
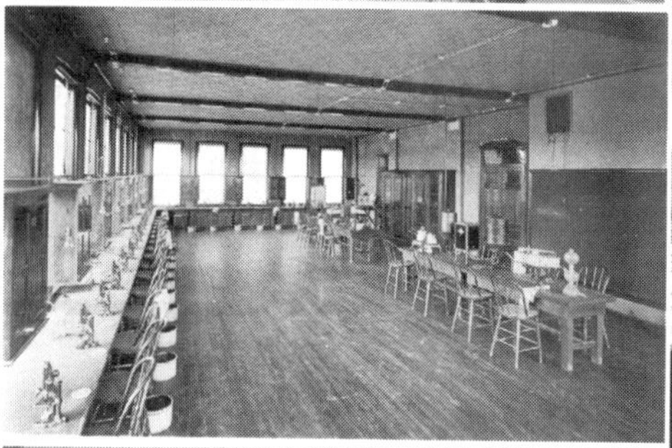

McBride Street campus in 1897, clockwise from top left: chemistry lab, pathology lecture hall, pathology office, physiology lab, histology lab, women's study, pathology lab.

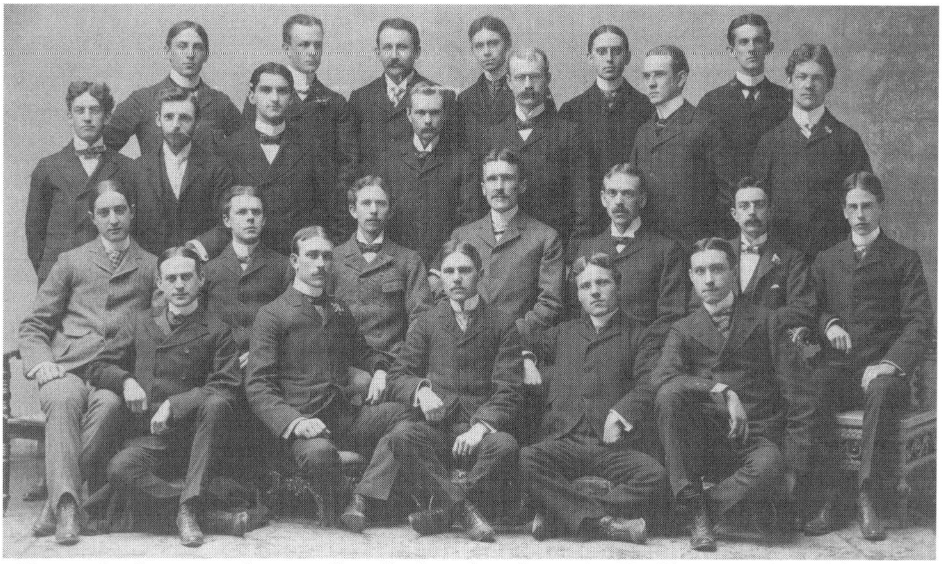

Above, the Syracuse chapter of medical student fraternity Nu Sigma Nu (NΣN) in 1898. Below, roommates George Clayton Feigel (left) and Charles Wesley Lanning (right) of the Class of 1898. Note the half pelvis on the wall and the femur and hangman's noose on the bookcase. Such macabre humor was typical of nineteenth-century medical students.

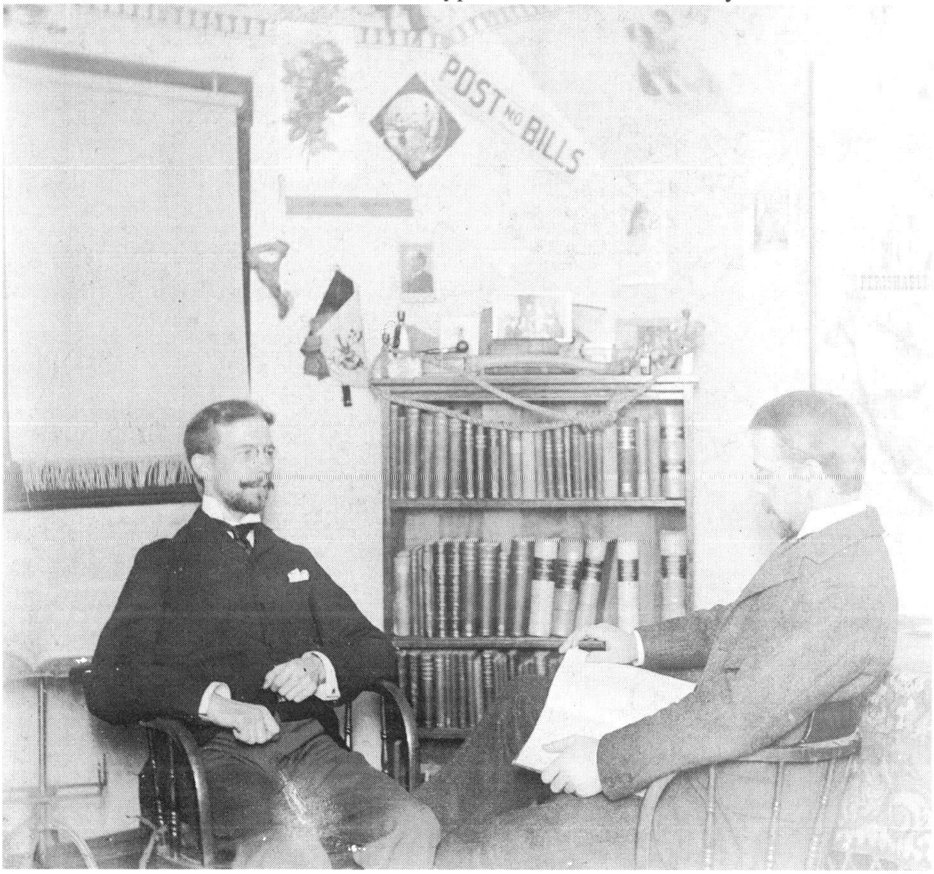

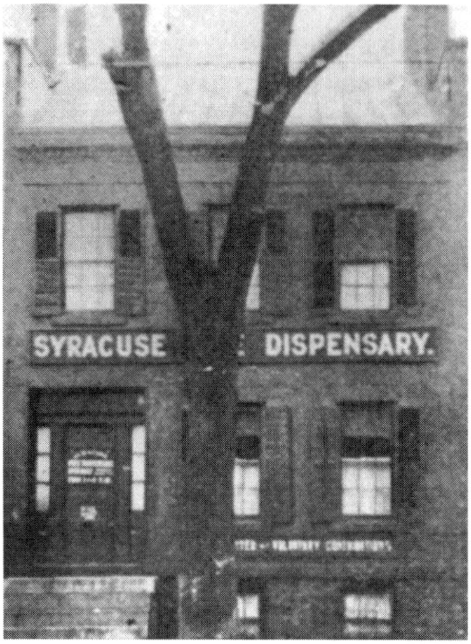

On January 1, 1876, the College of Medicine's earliest public dispensary opened in a small room on the carriage factory campus. In its first year it served about 900 patients and its staff filled about 250 prescriptions. In 1885 the faculty began to see advantages in moving the dispensary off-campus to a location nearer the center of the city, but they took no action until 1897, when it reopened at 407 South Warren Street, just south of East Jefferson Street, as the Syracuse Free Dispensary (right). This building had facilities for most of the then common diagnostic outpatient procedures, including ophthalmological examination (page 79 top). It moved in 1904 to slightly larger quarters at 506 South Warren, on the corner of East Onondaga Street (below), where it remained until 1914. Both of the Warren Street buildings proved inadequate, and in 1912 the cornerstone was laid for a new dispensary adjacent to the medical school at 610 East Fayette Street (page 79 bottom). Also in 1912 the Department of Bacteriology separated from the Department of Pathology. When the Syracuse Free Dispensary and City Health Department

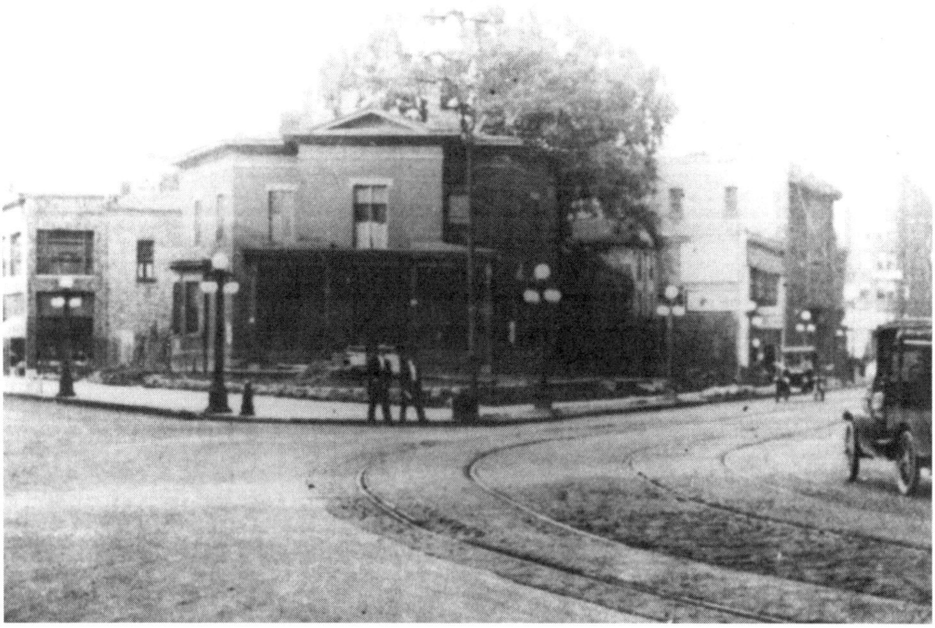

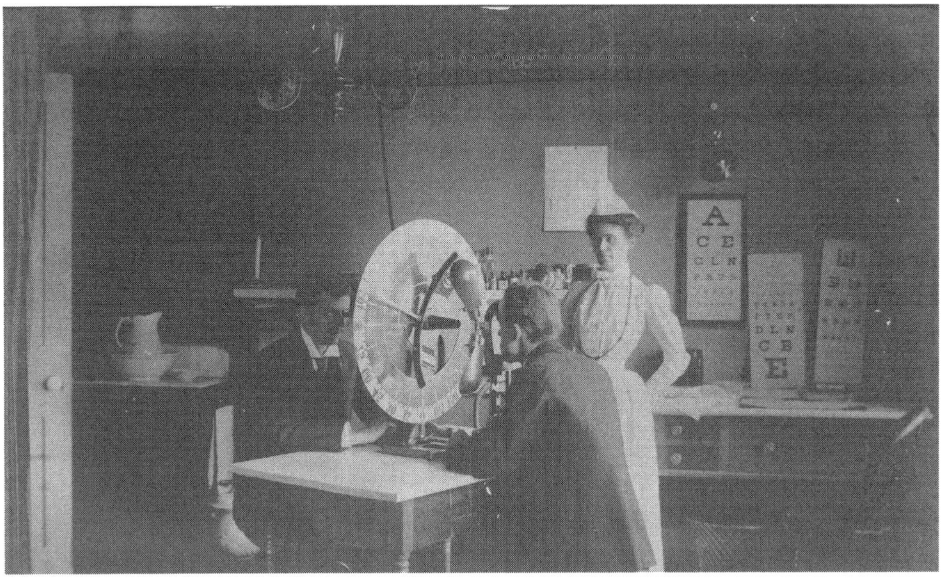

Clinic reopened on Fayette Street in 1914, Bacteriology occupied the third floor under the directorship of Oliver Wendell Holmes Mitchell, who became professor and chair in 1917. The faculty had strongly recommended since the beginning of bacteriological instruction in 1894 that each student own a microscope, but in 1912 this recommendation became a requirement. Reuben C. Hanchett, Class of 1884, ran the Dispensary sporadically from

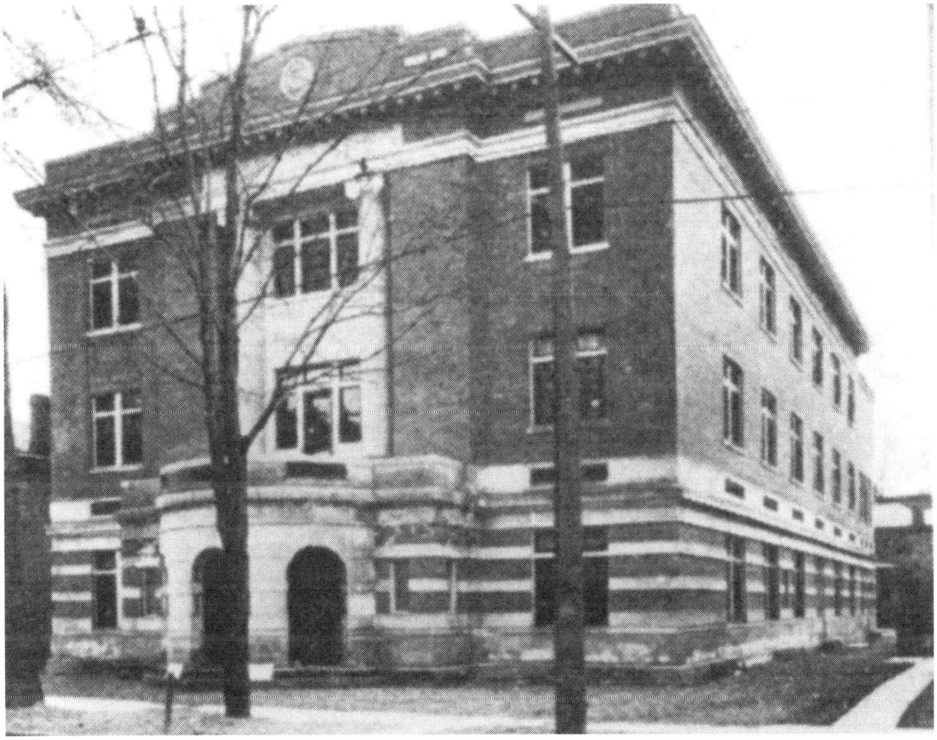

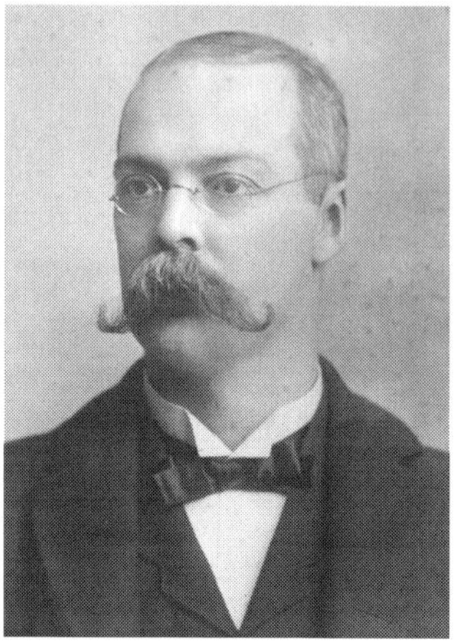

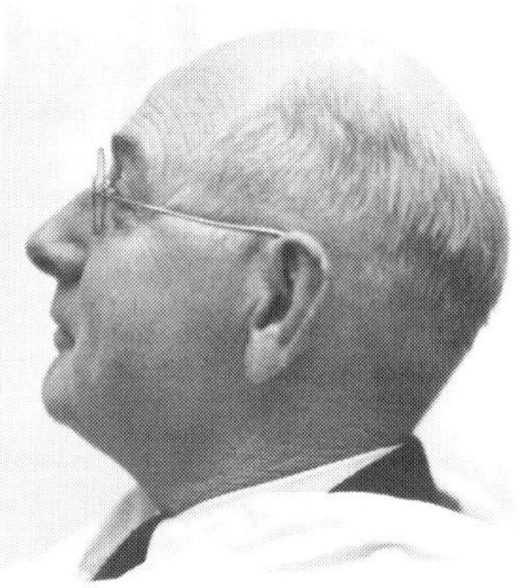

1893 to 1898. After interning for a year at St. Thomas' Hospital in London, Hanchett (top right) returned to Syracuse, taught physiology at the College of Medicine from 1885 until 1889, then switched to teaching materia medica. He resigned from the faculty for unknown reasons in 1908, but kept the appointment he had held at Good Shepherd since 1902. Mitchell (bottom right) taught hygiene, sanitation, and public health, as well as bacteriology, all with dry wit, good humor, and sometimes shocking presentations. His interests gradually drifted more toward public health. When the Department of Bacteriology divided into the Department of Bacteriology and Parasitology and the Department of Public Health in 1943, Orren D. Chapman, Class of 1924, became chair of the former while Mitchell became the first chair of the latter. In the 1950s Bacteriology and Parasitology evolved into the Department of Microbiology under Chapman and Public Health into the Department of Preventive Medicine under Harry A. Feldman.

William H. May, Class of 1890 (left), became Syracuse City Bacteriologist in 1892, part-time lecturer in pathology and bacteriology in 1892,

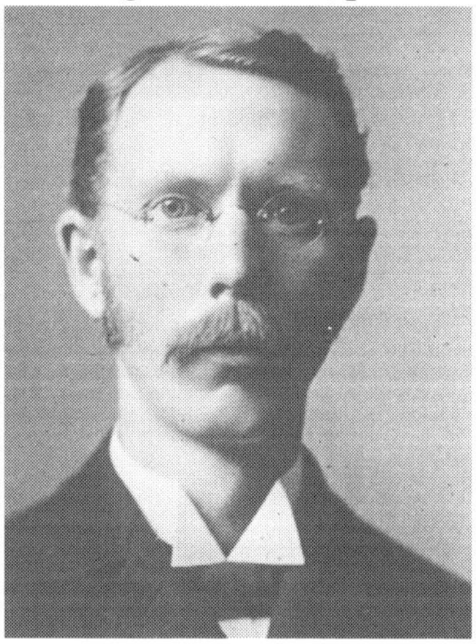

staff pathologist at both Good Shepherd and St. Joseph's in 1893, and — upon Clifford Mercer's resignation from the Department of Pathology to become a pediatrician in 1893 — chair of that department. May continued part-time as a teacher, and when the faculty decided in 1900 to hire a full-time professor of pathology, he preferred to resign from the College of Medicine rather than from his other posts. Halbert S. Steensland, an odd person but a very fine scientist, was brought in as the full-time pathologist to replace May. Steensland was chiefly responsible for inculcating the rigorous scientific methods in the Department of Pathology that became its watchword under Weiskotten in the 1920s. He arranged in 1901 for students to participate in microscopic analysis of morbid laboratory specimens at Good Shepherd.

Several other departments also gained from reforms instituted in the last decade of the nineteenth century and the first decade of the twentieth.

For example, the strong legacy that Plant had left in pediatrics was soon built upon. Clifford Mercer chaired and improved that department from 1895 until 1926, but he was really a pathologist and histologist, not a pediatrician, and the students judged him a poor teacher. They requested several times beginning in 1907 that Edward Judson Wynkoop, Class of 1892, assume Mercer's pediatric teaching duties, but all these requests were denied. Wynkoop finally became chair in 1926 and served until 1933.

In 1892 the College of Medicine adopted Halsted's residency plan and, with one graduate selected as a house officer at St. Joseph's, began participating in the program that would soon become the national norm for postgraduate medical education. The following year two graduates were selected for residencies. Good Shepherd entered the residency program in 1897, thus providing a ready outlet for new graduates of the College of Medicine.

Also in 1892 Gaylord Clark became the first College of Medicine professor to earn a regular salary, rather than rely on the vicissitudes of whatever money might come his way through tuition and fees. He then earned $500 a year to teach physiology, but by 1896 — the year he oversaw the design and construction of the first modern physiology laboratory in the United States, on the third floor at McBride Street — his salary had grown to $1500 a year. When, for reasons of health, Didama resigned the deanship four months before his death in 1905, the faculty unanimously voted Clark to succeed him.

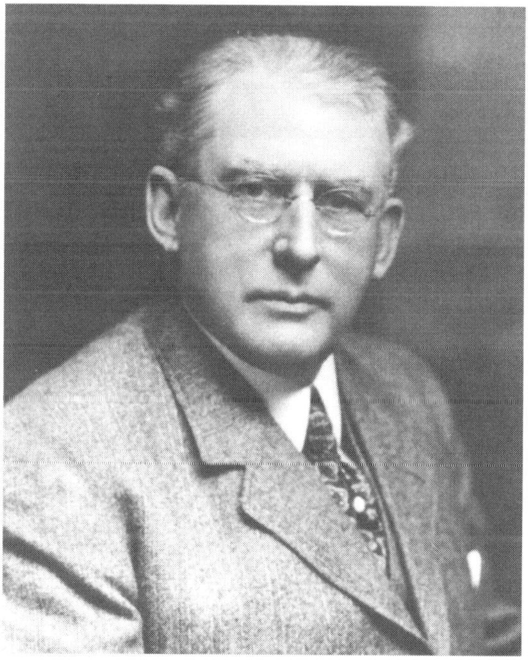

Clark had little time to realize his goals for the College of Medicine. When he died at the age of only fifty on September 1, 1907, just two years into his term as dean, the faculty immediately named John Heffron (left) as acting dean, and the Syracuse University Board of Trustees confirmed his appointment as permanent dean in January 1908.

Heffron, an internist, began at the College in 1882 as an instructor in histology, and since then had taught microscopy, materia medica, and therapeutics before being named Professor of Clinical Medicine in 1894. He was an administrator of uncommon vision as well as a superb clinician and a popular teacher. Ferguson wrote of Heffron in § I.2. of his "Chronological Calendar":

> He came to the deanship at a time when medical education was undergoing radical changes brought about by the studies resulting in the Flexner Report. Requirements for admission were being broadened, continuation courses established. Much more intensive bedside teaching, and consequently closer hospital relationships, became a necessity. In several thoughtful and scholarly reports to the Board of Trustees he outlined the changes necessary if this Institution was to continue to hold its place in medical education. He was the first to conceive of this College as a medical center, and his programs and support led to the building of the new Dispensary in 1912, the absorption of the Hospital of the Good Shepherd by the University in 1915, the planning for a medical center on the downtown site, and the ultimate establishment of the Yates Castle grounds as the site for the future development of the Medical Center. He deeply felt the need of a financial sponsor for the College, so that his plans for development could be fulfilled and the school hold its previous rank in the top few in the country. The inability of Syracuse University to provide the funds and the lack of an "angel" made it necessary to accept a "good school," but did not permit the desired level of expansion.

Heffron was not satisfied with a "good school." He wanted a "great school." He consistently increased his annual budget requests for the sake of improving and maintaining quality in the medical school, but the university chancellor almost as consistently denied or reduced these requests, citing university deficits. Thus Heffron's term as dean was marked by conflict and discouragement.

The downtown medical center never materialized, and the Uniersity Hill medical center did not materialize during Heffron's lifetime, but with the new buildings in 1896 and 1914 came additional innovations, including bedside teaching on rounds, mostly at Good Shepherd and St. Joseph's and mostly designed to enhance the students' clinical experience. Despite the chronic lack of financial support from Syracuse University, Heffron could take comfort in two facts: first, that he had an excellent faculty, committed to modernization and growth; and second, that much construction and renovation of hospitals was then occurring in Syracuse.

A group of public-spirited women founded Syracuse Women's Hospital and Training School for Nurses in 1887 as a facility to treat sick or injured women and children. It began accepting residents in 1897, but at first only women. Sometimes known at first as Syracuse Children's Hospital, it changed its name in 1902 to Syracuse Hospital for Women and Children and by 1908 it was also admitting men. For about its first two decades it had little contact with the College of Medicine, but, after existing in

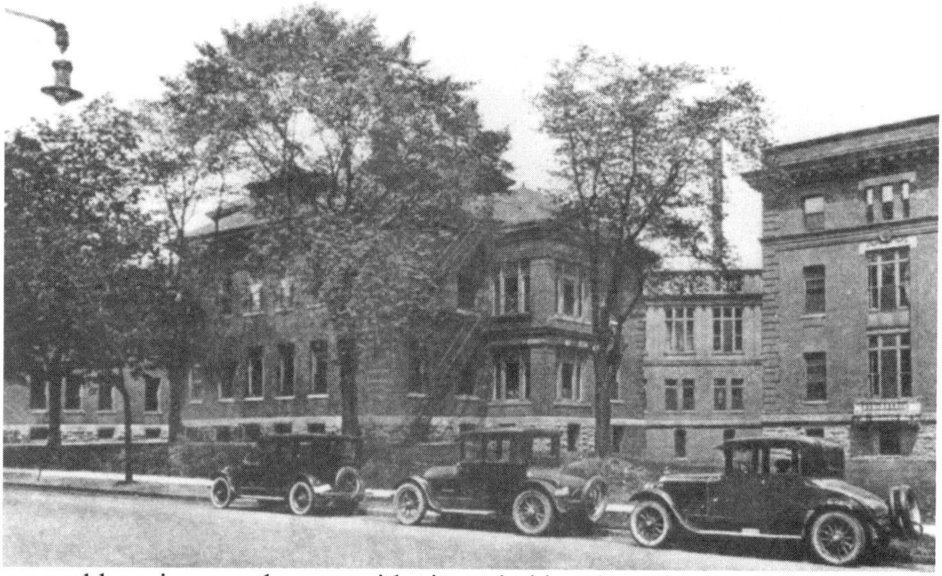

several locations on the west side, it settled in a large building at 1214 West Genesee Street (above), where several faculty members received appointments as attending physicians.

William L. Wallace, Class of 1897, led the group of physicians and investors that founded Crouse Irving Hospital in 1910 and opened it in 1912 at 720 South Crouse Avenue. Supported entirely by private funding and intended to treat everything except contagious diseases on a for-profit basis, it started its nursing school in 1913. From the beginning, many College of Medicine faculty and students were affiliated with it.

The Dispensary, Good Shepherd (which was remodeled in 1902), St. Joseph's, and these two new hospitals gave Syracuse medical students stellar opportunities for clinical training.

William Dunlap had become professor of dermatology in 1887, but after his untimely death in 1895, dermatology again lapsed into a ten-year hiatus. Henry Clay Baum (left) revived the study at the College of Medicine in 1906. Baum was an 1883 University of Michigan M.D., the staff dermatolologist at Syracuse Women's Hospital since 1898, and the younger brother of the author of *The Wizard of Oz*. As his course topics included syphilis and other sexually transmitted (then called "venereal") diseases, he was promoted to Professor of Dermatology and Syphilis in 1911. Henry A. McGruer, Baum's colleague since 1914, took over the chair in 1917, following Baum's early death in 1916. Baum and McGruer did most of their teaching in outpatient clinics at the Dispensary.

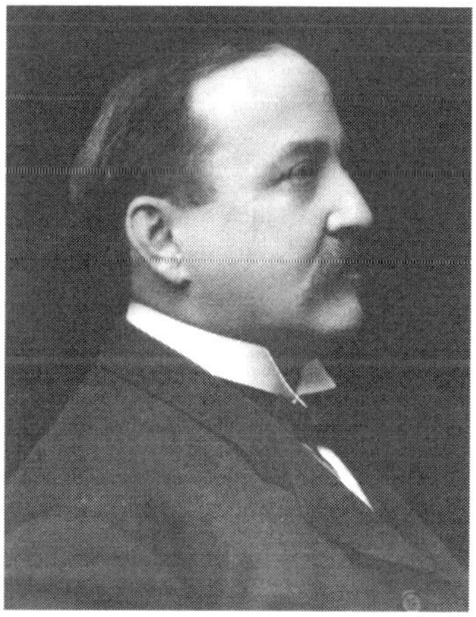

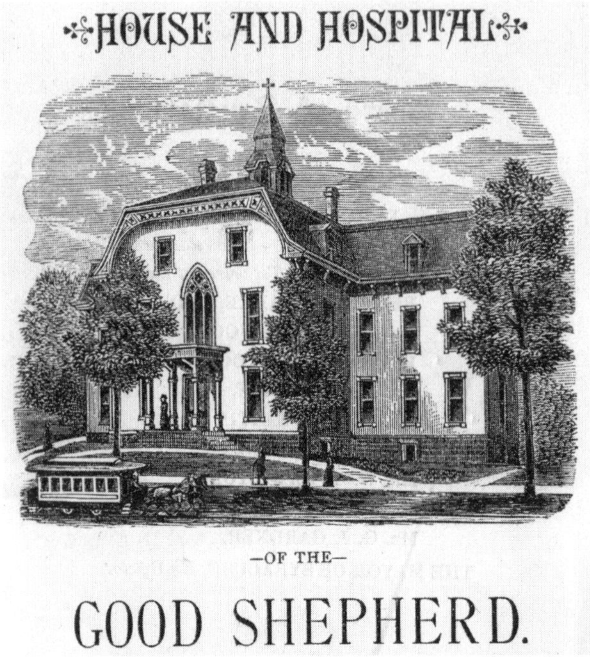

Good Shepherd (shown at left as it looked in 1880) prospered after it moved to Marshall Street in 1875. Even though it was a long walk up the hill from the medical campus on McBride (then Orange) Street to the hospital, medical students almost immediately began using its facilities. By 1902 there was significant overlap between the attending staff of Good Shepherd (below) and the faculty of the Syracuse University College of Medicine.

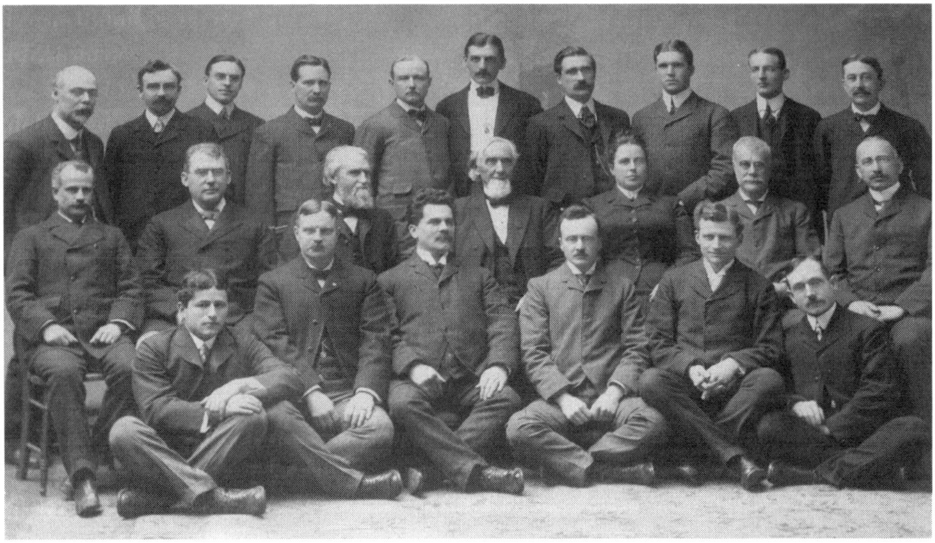

Top row: Reuben C. Hanchett (materia medica), Sargent Francis Snow (otolaryngology), Francis Roe Benham (obstetrics), Frank L. Harter (medicine), Eugene W. Belknap (obstetrics), Porter R. McMaster (surgery), J. Roberts Johnson (pediatrics), Julius H. Kevand (ophthalmology), Halbert Severin Steensland (pathology), Leonard A. Saxer (medicine); *middle row:* William Graham Hinsdale (obstetrics), John Lorenzo Heffron (medicine), Alfred Mercer (medicine), Henry Darwin Didama (medicine), Juliet E. Hanchett (gynecology), John Van Duyn (surgery), Edward L. Mooney (otolaryngology); *seated:* I. Harris Levy (medicine), George Griffin Lewis (ophthalmology), Antoine F. Vadeboncoeur (neurology), Robert Burns (surgery), George M. Price (surgery), William L. Wallace (surgery).

Syracuse University bought Good Shepherd in 1915 from the Episcopal Diocese for $76,000, thus acquiring its own teaching hospital. *De facto*, however, Good Shepherd had already been the College of Medicine's main teaching hospital since at least the 1890s and, along with the Dispensary, its main clinical facility.

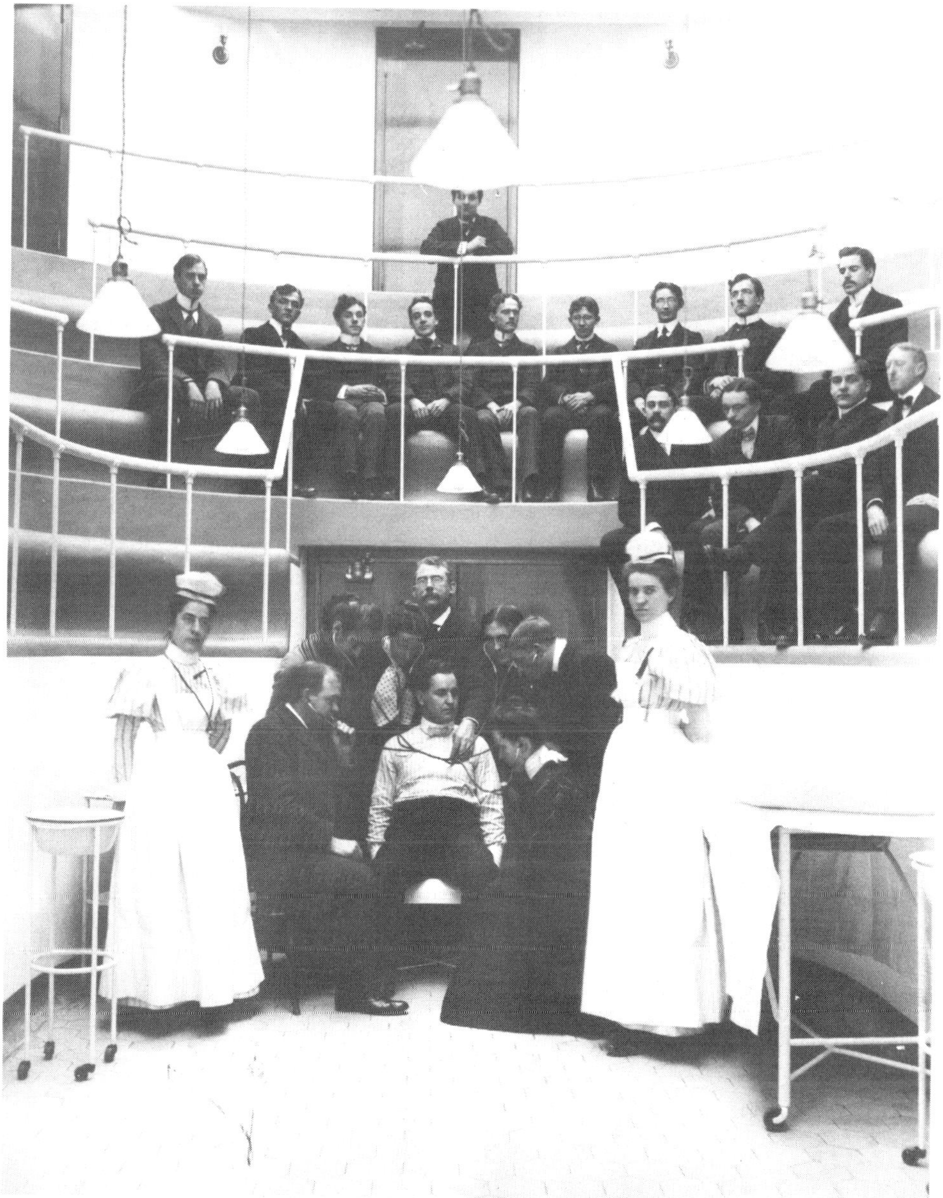

The Class of 1902 is shown at Good Shepherd on February 1, 1901, learning stethoscopy from Dean Heffron (center, behind the patient). Albert George Swift, who would chair the Department of Surgery from 1933 to 1946, is second from the left in the long row at the top. Swift did a four-year

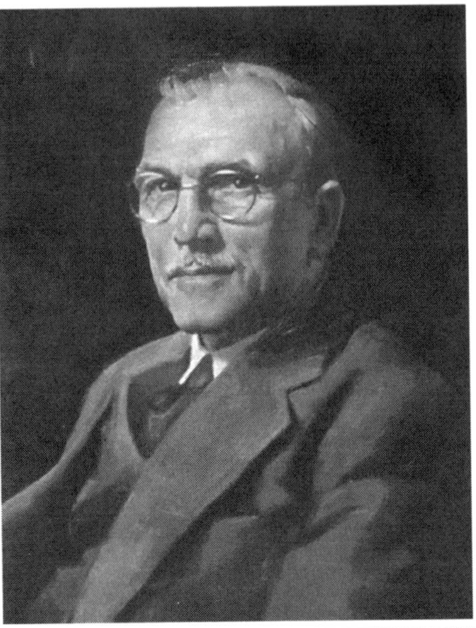

surgical residency at Mt. Sinai Hospital and practiced surgery for six years in New York City before returning to Syracuse to become a member of the surgery faculty in 1912. Despite his quick temper, Swift (shown at right in Joseph Kozlowski's painting), was popular with colleagues and students alike because of his surgical expertise, his excellence as a teacher, and his consummate loyalty to the College of Medicine. He operated mainly at St. Joseph's after taking over Jacobson's practice in 1913, but after succeeding Edward Van Duyn as chair, most of his work was at Good Shepherd.

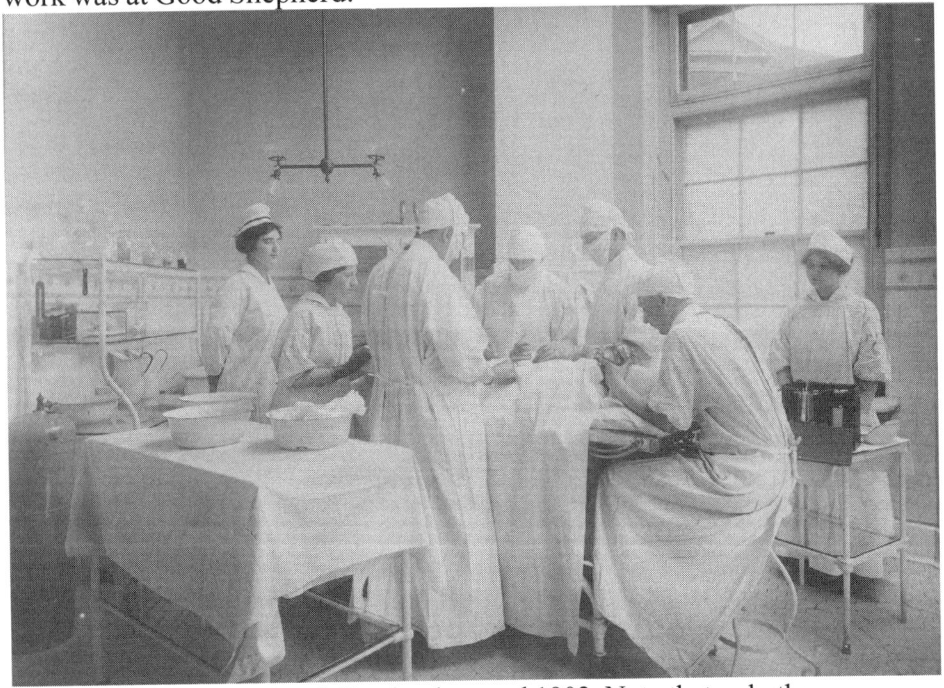

Surgery at Good Shepherd around 1902. Note that only the surgeons wear masks and that gloves seem to be optional.

Along with nurse Laura Mills Marlow and Bishop Huntington's daughter Aria, Juliet Hanchett co-founded the Visiting Nurse Association of Central New York in 1890. All three women were members of the "In As Much Circle" of the King's Daughters, a national charitable organization. Hanchett was one of the earliest women physicians to succeed in Syracuse. She received her M.D. from the Woman's Medical College of Pennsylvania in 1885, was licensed in New York and began to practice in Syracuse in 1887, and was admitted to the Onondaga County Medical Society in 1892. The gender barrier had not been much of an issue at the Society since Margaret Stanton became its first woman member on April 9, 1878.

Despite the accomplishments of Elizabeth Blackwell, Mary Walker, Sarah Loguen Fraser, Sarah Dolley, Juliet Hanchett, and many other early women physicians with ties to Central New York — most of whom were alumnae of coeducational medical schools — including women in the medical educational process remained controversial locally as well as nationally. This controversy particularly surrounded coeducational medical schools, where morality and natural modesty were thought to be compromised. The general population was beginning to believe that women could be educated to professional callings, but many writers of both genders still wanted to restrict higher education to single-sex institutions. In 1874 Dean George Fisk Comfort of the Syracuse University College of Fine Arts, and his wife, Anna Manning Comfort, published *Woman's Education and Woman's Health*, their rebuttal to Harvard Medical School Professor of Materia Medica Edward Hammond Clarke's inflammatory and misogynistic 1873 diatribe, *Sex in Education*. Among its other rebutters were Julia Ward Howe, lyricist of *The Battle Hymn of the Republic*, and Anna C. Brackett, the first woman principal of an American secondary school. In 1903 Grafton Press in New York City published *Woman's Unfitness for Higher Coeducation* by Ely Van de Warker, a gynecologist practicing in Syracuse. Van de Warker did not dispute that women were capable of great intellectual success, but argued only against coeducation, mainly on the grounds that men and women have sufficiently different physical needs, moral characters, and social expectations to preclude their commingling in classrooms.

In 1908 the Carnegie Foundation for the Advancement of Teaching, the AMA, and the Association of American Medical Colleges (AAMC), for the sake of supporting and and promoting high quality regular medical education throughout the United States and Canada, appointed Abraham Flexner, a former secondary school principal with no medical training, to evaluate all American and Canadian medical schools directly. From January 1909 to April 1910 Flexner made 175 site visits to 167 medical schools, comparing each summarily with Johns Hopkins, which he upheld as a paragon. His data, conclusions, and recommendations were published in 1910 as *Medical Education in the United States and Canada*, better known as the "Flexner Report." As a direct result of this report, the number of schools immediately dropped to 126 and was around 80 just ten years later. Only because of the foresight of Didama, Van Duyn, Elsner, Clark, Heffron, the Mercers, and a few others, and because of the Dispensary and the various Syracuse hospitals available for clinical instruction, the Syracuse University College of Medicine just managed to squeak by. Flexner wrote on page 276:

> Of the eleven medical schools now existing in the state, only the bona-fide university departments can then expect to survive; outside of New York city, Syracuse University alone has just now a chance. The schools of Buffalo, Albany, and Brooklyn belong to the past. None of the three has even yet entirely emerged from the fee-dividing stage. Syracuse, with a smaller total fee income than any of them, devotes every dollar to the development of the fundamental branches and has fairly earned support from outside.

Of course, the University of Buffalo Department of Medicine, Albany Medical College, and the Long Island College Hospital (now SUNY Downstate Medical Center) all survived, but in the short run in 1910 they had much more desperate catching up to do than the Syracuse University College of Medicine did.

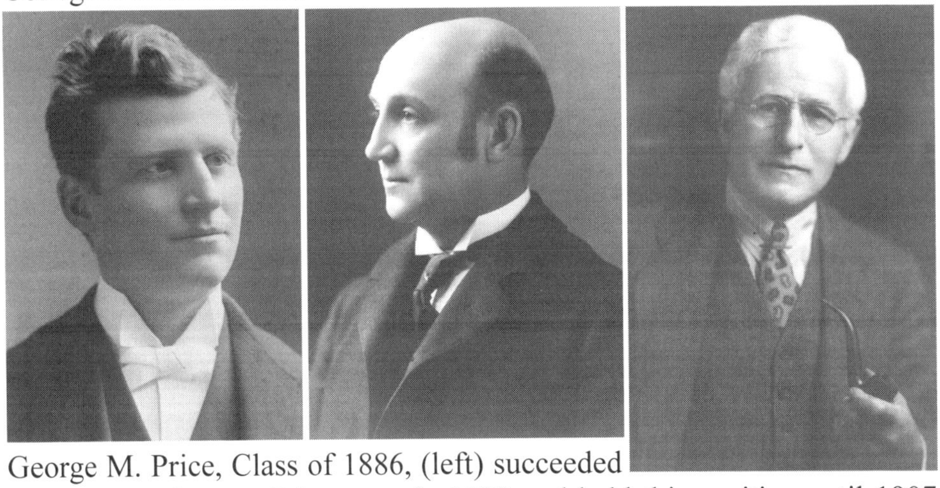

George M. Price, Class of 1886, (left) succeeded Owen as Professor of Anatomy in 1899 and held this position until 1907 when he became Professor of Clinical Surgery. Aaron B. Miller (center) taught gynecology from 1884 to 1925 and was chiefly responsible for separating it from obstetrics. In 1903 I. Harris Levy, Class of 1893 (right), co-taught with William Dewey Alsever, Class of 1900, the College of Medicine's first full course in physical diagnosis. Like many teachers of internal medicine in Syracuse, Levy began by teaching histology. In 1906 he was promoted to Associate Professor of Clinical Medicine and to full professor in 1916. His intensity in the study of cases and his determination to find always the right answer made him a star of clinical-pathological conferences. He chaired the Department of Medicine from 1916 to 1932.

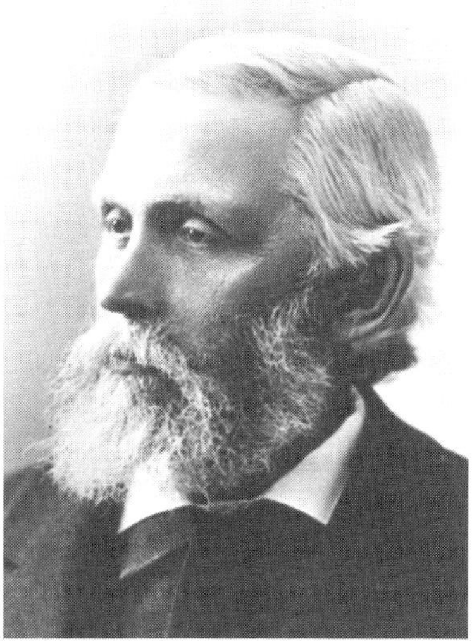

Towler continued to teach chemistry after the medical school moved to Syracuse, but between 1877 and 1880 gradually relinquished these duties to William Manlius Smith (right). Under Smith, who had been president of the Onondaga County Medical Society in 1865 and who held the chair of chemistry until 1899, the department's name changed from just "Chemistry" to "Medical Chemistry."

From 1900 until 1908 chemistry at the Syracuse University College of Medicine was taught by various instructors, lecturers, and junior faculty. From 1908 until 1917 the offerings in chemistry at the medical school were directed by the chair of the Syracuse University Chemistry Department, Ernest Noble Pattee, who apparently had little interest in biochemistry. Dean Heffron saw the situation as critical for the medical curriculum and acted quickly. In 1909 he hired a 23-year-old chemist who had just received his M.A. from the University of Wisconsin. This new instructor, Robert Kemp Brewer (below), earned his M.D. at Syracuse over the next four years, all the while teaching chemistry. He was promoted to assistant professor in 1914, associate professor in 1915, and full professor in 1917. Brewer essentially reinvented the department, bringing its research and teaching into the modern era.

Throughout the nineteenth century neither Geneva Medical College nor the Syracuse University College of Medicine demanded any specific prerequisites for the study of medical chemistry. Only in 1902 was a college undergraduate course in inorganic chemistry first required for admission to the medical school. Brewer wanted his entering students to have more advanced analytic experience with both qualitative and quantitative methods. Gradually he stiffened the requirements so that by 1920 undergraduate organic chemistry was required for admission. Thereafter freed from the obligation to teach remedial organic chemistry to first-year medical students, Brewer could concentrate instead on teaching aspects of chemistry that have more immediate clinical importance. Using mainly laboratory sessions rather than lectures, he covered, according to the 1921-

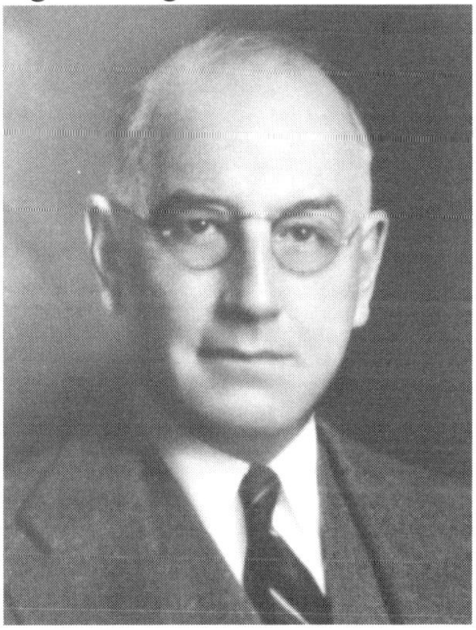

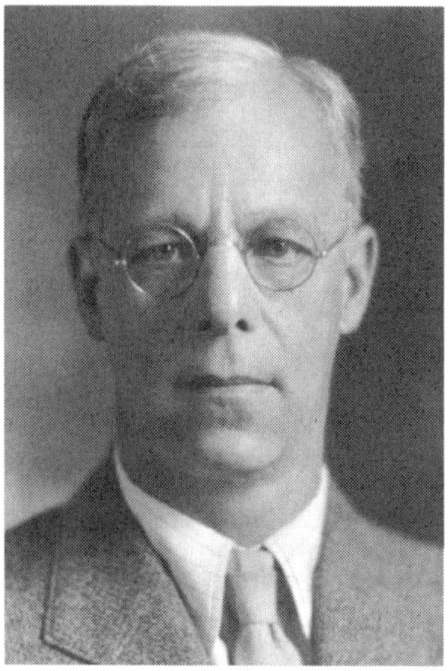

1922 *Bulletin of the Syracuse University College of Medicine*, "foodstuffs, connective, muscular and nervous tissues, the digestive fluids and their enzymes; the bile, milk, blood, and urine ... [and] clinical methods of the qualitative and quantitative study of the constitutents of the body fluids which are of especial diagnostic importance."

Van Duyn, Brewer, and Swift all had sons who became prominent physicians in Syracuse. Edward Seguin Van Duyn, Class of 1897 (left), chaired the Department of Surgery from 1920 to 1933. David Wyman Brewer, Class of 1941, became the protégé of otolaryngologist Gordon D. Hoople, Class of 1919, specialized in voice research, and eventually had several professional singers among his patients. Surgeon Edward Swift and his pediatrician wife Miriam, both of the Class of March 1943, had a nephew, Peter, Class of 1977. But the most prolific ancestor of a Syracuse medical family, even more so than Alfred Mercer, was Alfred Green Doust, Class of 1887. His brother, Henry Burton Doust, Class of 1900, a specialist in tuberculosis and public health, founded Central New York's first tuberculosis clinic in 1908. Their nephew, Brewster Clark Doust, Class of 1914 (right), joined the Department of Pediatrics in 1916 and succeeded Wynkoop to chair the department until 1947. A.G. Doust's son, Alfred Webb Doust, Class of 1935 (left), practiced and taught otolaryngology in Syracuse; and his grandnephew, William Charles Doust, Class of 1945, did postgraduate work at the Mayo Clinic under Benjamin Spock then practiced child psychiatry in Los Angeles. A.W. Doust's grandson, Matthew Webb Doust, Class of 1998, completed an anesthesiology fellowship at the Mayo Clinic in 2003. Two other Dousts, Brewster Jr. and his wife Victoria, earned their medical degrees respectively at the University of Rochester and Johns Hopkins, but practiced internal medicine in Syracuse.*

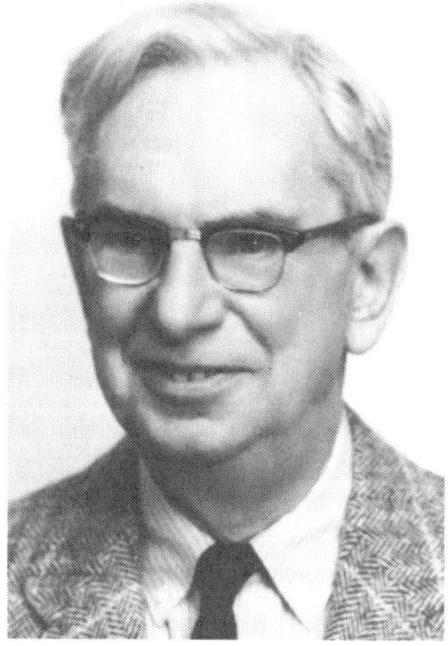

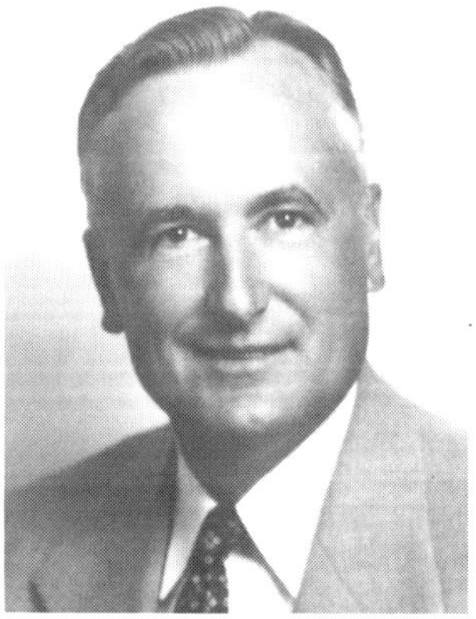

* In 2002, substantial gifts from both the Swift and the Doust families created the Swift Foyer and the Doust Boardroom on the ninth floor of Weiskotten Hall.

THE SYRACUSE HERALD: SUNDAY MORNING, OCTOBER 6, 1918.

Epidemic Reaches Alarming Proportions, With Estimate of Ten Thousand Cases of Influenza Among Civilians

10,000 CASES OF INFLUENZA NOW THREATEN CITY

Epidemic Assumes More Serious Proportions in Civilian Life.

Number of Cases Takes Drop at Cantonment in the Last 24 Hours.

(Continued From Page 17.)

in the grip of the epidemic are: East Syracuse, Cicero, North Syracuse, Marcellus, Camillus, Navarino, Marietta, Amber and Minoa.

The epidemic among the Camp Syracuse recruits is regarded by Maj. Arthur F. Thompson, camp surgeon, as well on the way to being stamped out.

Only twenty new cases were found among the soldiers while discharges from hospitals here and on the camp grounds totalled more than 100.

Recruits from the camp in local hospitals numbered 555. In addition to these there were fifty from the Syracuse university training detachment undergoing treatment.

Major Thompson said the cases discovered on Saturday were of a much milder character than those of a week ago.

Close Sunday Schools.

At least two Sunday schools will be closed to-day on account of the epidemic. They are those of the First Methodist church and the Good Will Congregational church.

There will be no Sunday school at the Furman Street Methodist church, on account of the annual session of the conference.

The Rev. William H. Powers, pastor of the James Street Methodist church, was taken home from the session of the New York Central Methodist conference yesterday morning, suffering with what was believed to be Spanish influenza.

The Rev. Dr. Arthur Copeland, ... Genesee Street Methodist church this morning, has notified the pastor, the Rev. S. S. Pratt, that he might not be able to keep the appointment, as he had contracted a hard cold. He is in attendance upon the session of the conference.

Commissioner of Public Safety Nicholson has ordered all physicians to report all cases of the plague to Dr. Totman, health officer. Upon these reports will depend whether or not public meetings and assemblies will be forbidden.

All the Rochester & Syracuse, Auburn & Syracuse and the Syracuse & Northern electric railway cars will be disinfected every night as a precaution against the epidemic.

Toll of Deaths.

The toll of deaths in the influenza epidemic among civilians in this city and immediate vicinity during the week, follows:

Sunday—Harold F. Davin, 33, No. 505 Second street, Liverpool; Mrs. Anna Rooney, 62, East Syracuse; Frank Race, North Syracuse; Frank Nitschke, 28, No. 212 Ash street; Martin H. Murphy, No. 507 Tully street; Madd Madsen, 32, No. 515 Lodi street; Miss Myrtle Carpenter, R. N., Crouse-Irving hospital; Miss M. Pauline Curtin, student nurse, Skaneateles.

Monday—Miss Dorothy Shapley, student nurse, Hospital of the Good Shepherd; Miss Emma J. Hooper, R. N., Hospital of the Good Shepherd; Mrs. Lydia Waibel, No. 1110 South Crouse avenue; Miss Jane Piddick, 25, R. N., Hospital of the Good Shepherd; Miss Fannie Claxton, student nurse, Homeopathic hospital; Leland Thayer, 33, No. 721 South Salina street.

Tuesday—Miss Hazel I. Dodd, No. 202 West Corning avenue; Mrs. Ada Leroy, No. 226 West Brighton avenue; Mrs. May Peterson, No. 4313 South Salina street; Homer E. Jackson, Solvay; Merritt McQuinn, 23, South Warren street; Mrs. Celia F. Wentworth, 32, Amboy; Mrs. An-

Soldier Patients in Local Hospitals

Figures announced at local hospitals concerning the soldier epidemic victims follow:

	Total Cases	New Cases	Discharged	Deaths
Crouse-Irving	220	0	3	[illegible]
Good Shepherd	196	3	21	1
St. Josephs	94	6	6	0
Homeopathic	96	1	5	1
Memorial	39	4	7	0
Totals	605	14	44	4

East Adams street; Anthony Palgino, 29, Solvay; Jarred Thorpe, 69, Cicero road; Lucia Romana, Camillus; Mrs. Elizabeth P. Maher, 34, No. 130 Coolidge avenue; George Hill, 46, No. 501 Bryant avenue; William H. Merrill, 50, No. 109 Brewster avenue; Joseph V. Flanagan, 31, East Syracuse; Mrs. Alma T. Putnam, Hazelton, Pa.

Thursday—Ludwik Wesolowski, 25, No. 122 Lakeview avenue; John De Marchi, 30, No. 215 Lamont avenue, Solvay; Mrs. Jessie F. Bixby, No. 883 South Beech street; Mrs. Florence D. Sniffin, No. 1240 South State street; Joseph Sanford, 32, No. 744 South avenue; Miss Grace Bird, 16, No. 500 Park street; Edward P. Meyer, No. 451 Wilkinson street; Fred L. Grover, No. 120 Parkside avenue; Charles H. Brown, 63, No. 719 South Clinton street.

Friday—Edward Burns, 34, No. 309 Harrison street; Miss Florence F. Carrigan, 19, No. 724 Otisco street; Ermina Heppeler, 12, No. 203 Herbert street; Jessie McEvitt, 36, No. 122 Parkside avenue; John J. O'Boyle, No. 204 North Geddes street; Dallas C. Mark, 21, No. 400 West Willow street; Mrs. Francis Flach, 41, No. 402 Craig street; Mrs. Florence Hennessey, 30, No. 110 Grace street; Frank Lang, 86, No. 709 Irving avenue; Charles W. Garlock, 45, No. 305 Cedar street; James E. Chapman, No. 4 West Towpath; Miss Ethel Merrill, student nurse, Hospital of the Good Shepherd.

Saturday—Miss Ruth Markert, 24, No. 709 Danforth street; Charles Foster, 24, Psychopathic hospital; Roberta C. Austin, 10, No. 213 Gifford street; Patrolman Michael W. White, No. 703 West Belden avenue; Miss Agnes J. Post, 17, No. 244 ... No. 204 Van Buren street; Mrs. Rose Pettenuk, 25, No. 940 South State street; Mrs. Francis Koziol, 35, Solvay; George Williamson No. 217 Erie street; Miss Olive Lewis, No. 517 Turtle street; James Coogan, No. 1201 Burnet avenue.

Wife of Lieutenant O'Brien Succumbs

Mrs. Regina C. North O'Brien, wife of Lieut. Charles V. O'Brien, M. R. C., died Saturday morning at her home in Brooklyn. Lieutenant O'Brien is a former resident of Solvay and is well known here. Besides her husband she is survived by her son, Charles V. O'Brien, jr., and her parents, Mr. and Mrs. F. T. North of Brooklyn, and one sister, Miss Genevieve North, also of Brooklyn. The news of Mrs. O'Brien's death was received here by Mrs. Mary O'BBrien, mother of Lieutenant O'Brien. Miss Margaret and Miss Alice O'Brien, his sisters, of Solvay and Michael and Robert E. O'Brien of Detroit will attend the funeral at Brooklyn. Mrs. O'Brien was an influenza victim whose illness lasted but a few days.

MISS POWER, SCHOOL TEACHER, IS VICTIM

Miss M. Bernadine Power, a public school teacher, died at her home, No. 1602 South Geddes street, late Saturday night, a victim of pneumonia which developed from influenza. Death followed a brief illness.

Miss Power leaves three brothers, Frank J., John A. of this city, and Thomas P. Power, stationed at the Artillery Officers Training camp,

Mrs. H. Burton Doust Dies on the Anniversary of Her Wedding Day

Wife of Physician in Service Had Just Learned of Promotion.

Husband Made Major, She Lives Only to Learn of Honor.

Three hours after she had received a cablegram from her husband, Dr. H. Burton Doust, somewhere in France, bearing a tender message in commemoration of their seventh wedding anniversary and telling her that he had been promoted to the rank of major, Mrs. Jane Munro Doust died of double pneumonia at her home, No. 309 Summit avenue, at 1:30 o'clock yesterday afternoon.

Mrs. Doust was taken ill with influenza on Monday and pneumonia developed a few days later. On Friday her condition became critical, but she did not lose consciousness and when the cablegram from her husband arrived, she had it read to her and held it in her hand.

Happy Marriage.

Mrs. Doust was the daughter of the late Mr. and Mrs. Thomas Munro of Camillus and her marriage to Dr. Doust, which took place on October 5th, 1911, was an ideally happy one. When the Van Duyn unit was organized and her husband, who was physician in charge of the Municipal Tuberculosis clinic and one of the most prominent specialists in lung diseases in the city, expressed a desire to join and report for duty overseas, Mrs. Doust gave her consent and her blessing, her only regret being that she could not accompany him.

While the unit was in training quarters at Atlanta, Ga., waiting for foreign orders Mrs. Doust, with the wives of some of the other physicians of the unit, formed a "Syracuse colony" there in order to give the husbands a taste of home as long as possible. She returned home in May and has since devoted herself to Red Cross work and other war time enterprises.

Major Notified.

Mrs. Doust, while socially a favorite, was very much interested in charities of the kind that are not advertised. Her purse was always opened for the aid of those in need and her sympathy and attention were ready to respond at any time to the call of suffering.

Besides her husband, Major Doust of the Van Duyn unit, Mrs. Doust is survived by her brother, Thomas Munro of Camillus, and a sister, Mrs. William Wilson Nichols of Rochester. Arrangements for the funeral have not yet been completed. A cablegram was sent to Dr. Doust last evening notifying him of his bereavement.

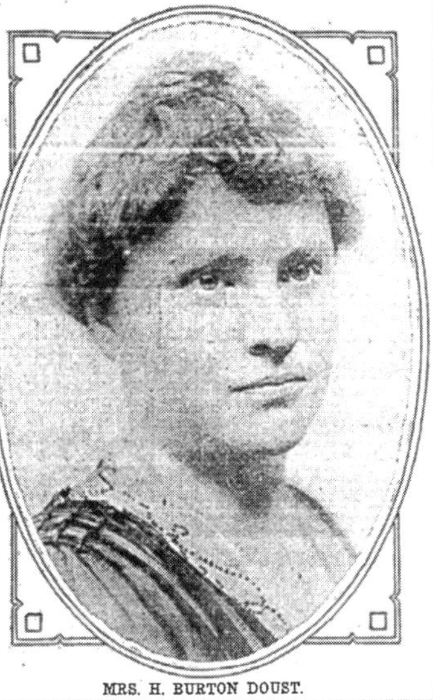

MRS. H. BURTON DOUST.

MANY OLD-TIME LIQUOR DEALERS QUIT BUSINESS

Deputy State Excise Commissioner Rubin up to last evening had received $417,110 from the issuing of 352 licenses in the city and towns. This year 299 certificates were issued for the city as against 363 last year. Three wholesale dealers, The Cushing company, John J. Lowery and Hubbard & Sons did not renew their licenses.

Among the well known dealers who did not take out licenses were August Birchler in Butternut street; Michael Walsh, No. 1919 W. Fayette street; John H. Schmidt, No. 456 N. Salina

Military Measures Have Kept Down Epidemic at Princeton, Says Dr. Luby

Syracuse Man Home for Week-end Declares Work of Health Board Has Resulted in Minimizing Spread of Influenza.

Dr. Daniel F. Luby, medical officer for the Princeton Officers Material Schools Pay corps of the United States navy, who arrived in town last night to spend Sunday with his family here, says that the keeping down of influenza at Princeton is due in his opinion in great part to the Military Board of Health.

The board has closed all schools, churches, motion picture houses, bowling alleys, billiard and pool rooms and all other places where the public gather. This action was taken as a precautionary measure rather than because there is any unusual amount of sickness at this time.

The new military board consists of the local health officer, T. W. Margerum, Dr. J. M. Carnochan, Lieutenant Lub- and Capt. F. E. E. Priestly. The body has been given unlimited authority to enforce all federal and State sanitary codes and to regulate conditions throughout the town.

"Every morning the navy boys are inspected by Admiral Goodrich and the medical officers look for influenza symptoms. If any are found, the boys are sent to the temporary isolation hospital, which was formerly the old athletic house on the Princeton athletic field. After a few days there they are returned to their classes, the disease never being given a chance to develop.

Preventive Methods.

"Recently 200 petty officers arrived at the school from the infected districts around Boston, Newport and the Great Lakes stations. Every boy had his clothes fumigated, took a hot bath, had his nose and throat sprayed with a chlorozine solution and afterwards with dichloromen T solution. Eight hours afterwards they were given back their clothes and all contacts were isolated. As a result of these precautionary measures the incidents of influenza remain very low.

Henry Burton Doust's wife was a victim of the worst public health crisis ever to hit Syracuse, the swine influenza pandemic that sickened two billion people and killed forty million worldwide in 1918 and 1919. Ironically, her nephew-in-law, Brewster Sr., began research in 1917 that led to developing the facial masks that are now commonly used against airborne infections.

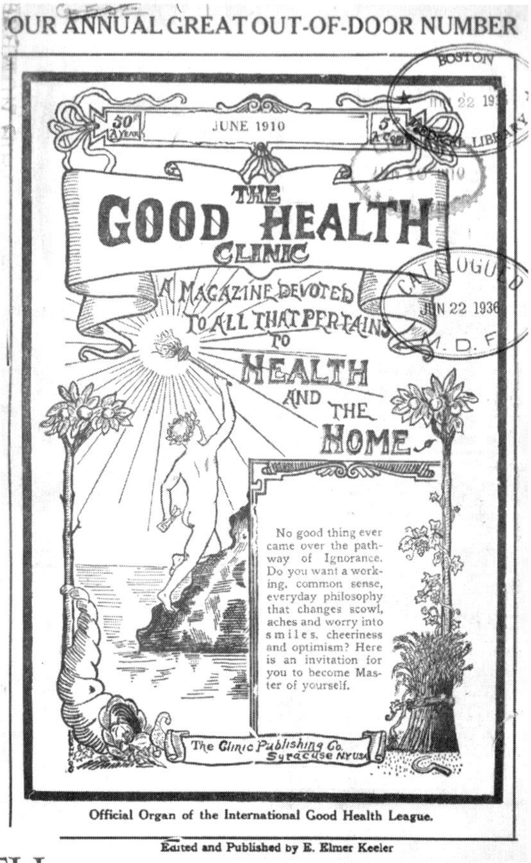

Questionable medical business persisted even after the so-called "Golden Age of Quackery" that began in the 1860s ended with the passage of the federal Pure Food and Drug Act in 1906. Some alternative practitioners managed to stay just on the edge of the new law. Edward Elmer Keeler, a homeopathic physician practicing ophthalmology and otolaryngology in Syracuse, published twenty-nine volumes of a popular medical journal from 1898 to 1925. Calling it first *The Syracuse Clinic* then either *The Good Health Clinic* or just *The Clinic*, he touted it as the "Official Organ of the Medico-Chirurgical Society of Central New York and the International Health League." These organizations were not really medical societies, but just clubs for Keeler's supporters. He promoted hypnotic and hydropathic cures, offered hints for exercise and good vegetarian nutrition, and advertised patent medicines, natural remedies, and astrological services, all in a folksy, lighthearted style. His publication went out of business when the Department of Health of the City of Syracuse became his competitor, bringing out six volumes of its own popular medical journal from 1924 to 1931, *Better Health*, which, in a similar format aimed at the same audience, offered authoritative and practical advice buttressed with statistics.

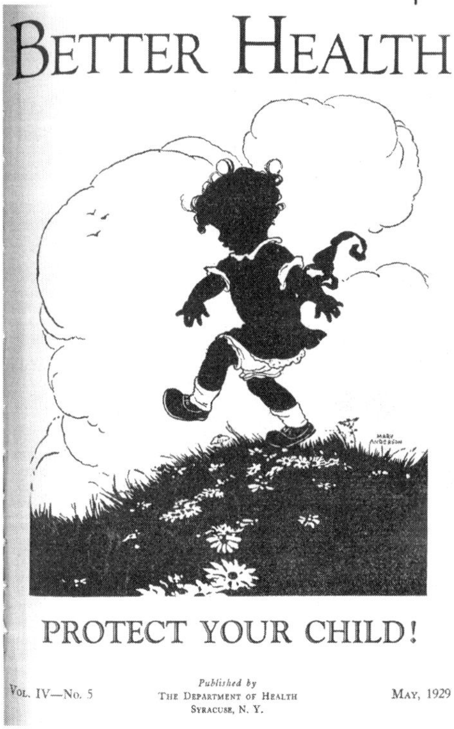

6

The Weiskotten Years

When Heffron retired as dean in 1922, outgoing Syracuse University Chancellor James Roscoe Day offered the deanship to Weiskotten, who declined on the grounds that Day was a lame duck. He served instead as acting dean. Three years later, Day's successor, Charles W. Flint, made him the permanent dean. Weiskotten remained until 1951, bringing the school successfully through the difficult years of the Great Depression and World War II into the modern medical world.

Trends toward greater specialization gained momentum in higher education in general and medical education in particular during his long tenure. These and other rapid changes proved difficult to manage as they demanded larger numbers of better trained people for professional employment in an industrial society and transformed the public persona of the medical profession from the individual doctor to the corporate entity. He complained in the *Journal of the American Medical Association* in 1937 that too many preclinical courses were "merely a mimicry of nonmedical university courses inflicted on the medical students by teachers whose sole experience has been a graduate course in a single subject which has been almost devoid of any of its medical implications." Thus one of his main goals — and achievements — was to reform preclinical training so that it would more naturally and logically proceed into real clinical education.

At the critical juncture of the early 1930s, with the country and its institutions in deep economic trouble and no one quite sufficiently aware of the problems facing medicine, Syracuse University was fortunate that its medical school was led by someone who not only influenced the local trajectory but also determined some of the reforms that affected the national future of medical education. These reforms began in earnest when the AAMC created its Commission on Medical Education (CME) in 1925. About the same time the AMA revamped its Council on Medical Education and Hospitals (CMEH), which had not fully inspected American medical schools since the Flexner Report. In 1927 concerned citizens formed the Committee on the Costs of Medical Care (CCMC), chaired by Ray Lyman Wilbur, the physician president of Stanford University. In 1934 the CMEH, also chaired by Wilbur, undertook a new medical school survey, which Weiskotten would design and direct. Weiskotten was away from Syracuse for much of 1934 to 1936 making this survey, personally examining all medical schools in the United States and Canada, except schools of osteopathy and a few unapproved schools that refused to be inspected. His report was published in 1940 as *Medical Education in the United States, 1934-1939*, by Herman G. Weiskotten, Alphonse M. Schwitalla, William D. Cutter and Hamilton H. Anderson. This team found about twenty of the 89 American and Canadian schools below accepted standards, placed some of these on probation, and required others to make specific adjustments. At the time, only 66 of the 79 American schools had full four-year programs.

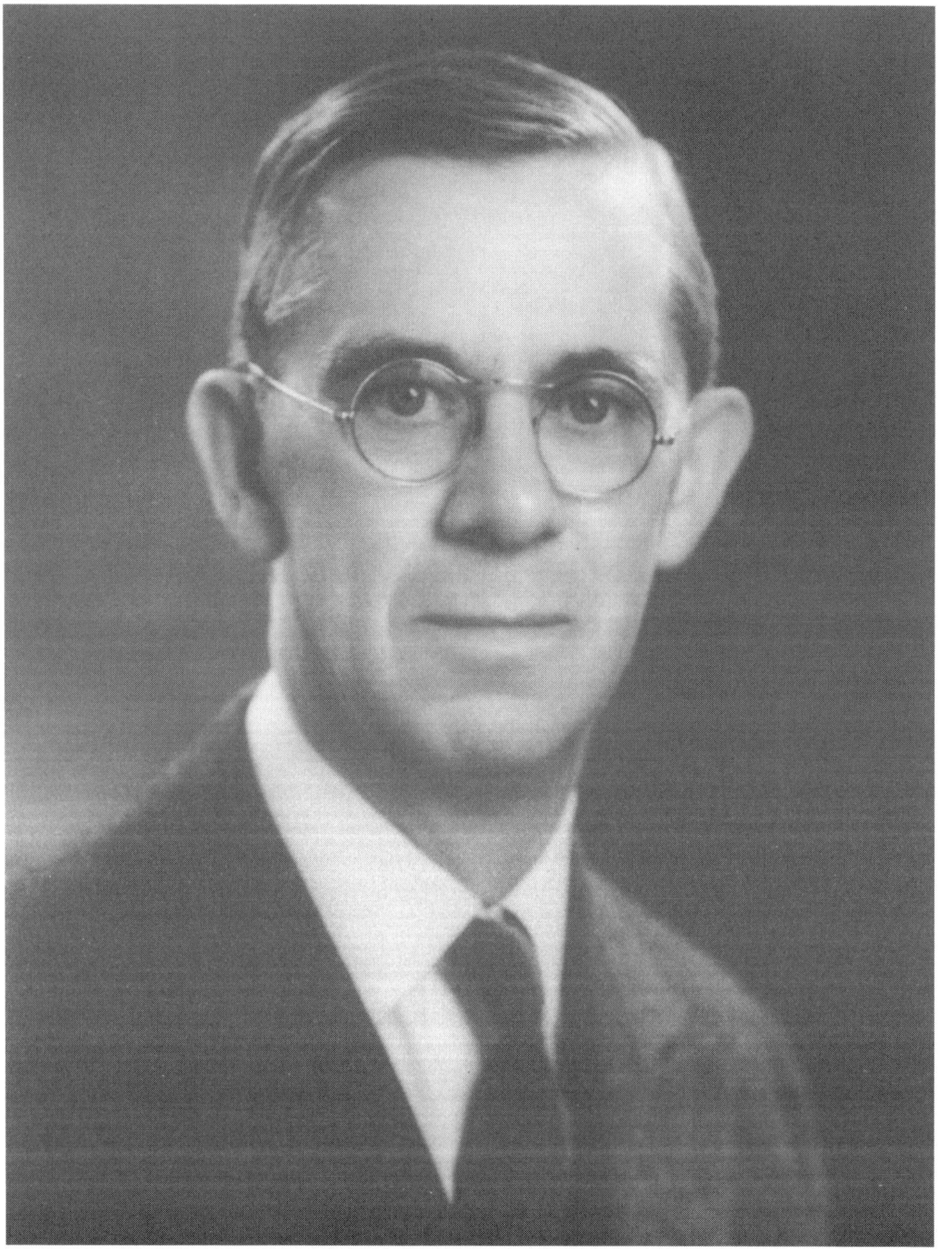

The Weiskotten Report established the standard model of American medical education as:

1. Four years to earn a bachelors' degree, achieving high grades and a solid background in science.
2. Four years in medical school, the first two years for basic science, the last two for clinical training.
3. One year of general internship in a hospital or clinic.
4. Three to seven years of hospital residency to learn a specialty; the length of the residency being determined by the complexity of each particular specialty.

This model persists even in view of the trend, initiated by students in the 1990s, away from lecture teaching in large halls to hands-on learning in small groups. To a large extent it was Weiskotten's personal influence that sparked the positive changes at the College of Medicine, especially in the 1930s. Whatever he either commended or condemned when he discovered it at other schools naturally soon emerged in better form at his own institution. His forceful personality ensured that it did.

After graduating from Syracuse High School on West Genesee Street in 1901, Weiskotten had entered Syracuse University in 1901, earning his Ph.B. in 1906 and his M.D. in 1909. His first mentor was Steensland, who had trained in pathology at Johns Hopkins and Harvard. When Good Shepherd opened its pathology laboratory in 1909 under Steensland's direction, Weiskotten became its first pathology resident. He was promoted to instructor in 1910, assistant professor in 1912, associate professor in 1913, and full professor in 1916. He chaired the department from Steensland's suicide in 1924 until J. Howard Ferguson (right) of the Class of 1926 was appointed to that post in 1942. Weiskotten remained active in pathology throughout his administrative career. His major research concerned the actions of benzene, about which he published a nine-part series of articles from 1915 to 1930. He refined Steensland's teaching methods, emphasizing the anatomical study of pathology, and took additional postgraduate pathological training in Vienna in 1924.

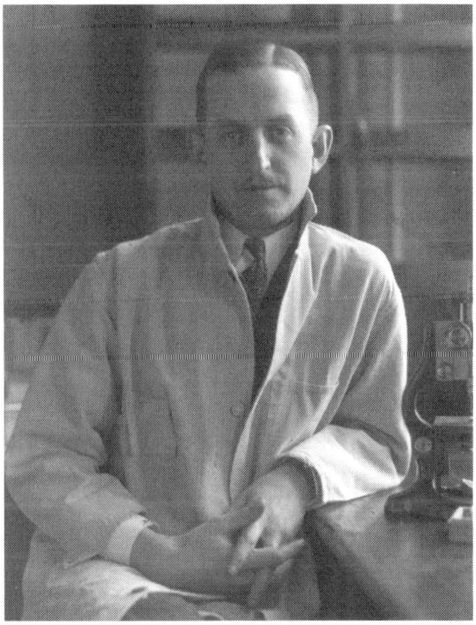

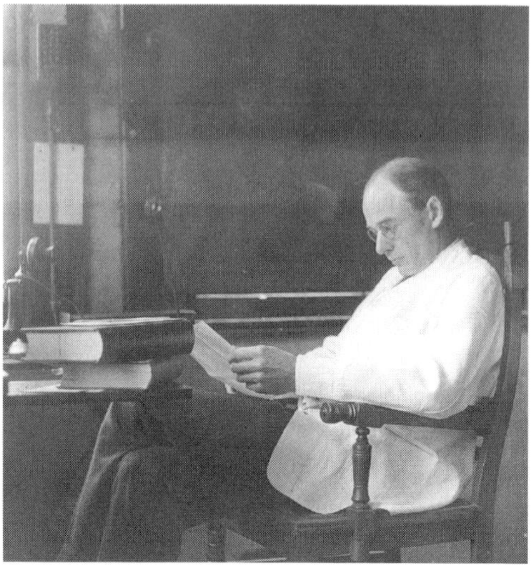

In 1929 Syracuse University set the pace for first-year postgraduate medical study nationwide by publishing *Interns Handbook: A Guide to Rational Drug Therapy, Clinical Procedures and Diets*. The authors were most of the College of Medicine faculty, chaired by pharmacologist Marion S. Dooley (right) of the Class of 1914. "The young doctor entering his internship [who] soon learns that the hard-won knowledge behind his diploma is not correlated for bedside use" was the intended reader of this book — and there were thousands of such doctors. Dooley's work was well received. The second edition appeared in 1938 and the third in 1944, both with a new subtitle, *A Guide, Especially in Emergencies, for the Intern and the Physician in General Practice*. All

1930 staff of the University Hospital of the Good Shepherd: *top row:* Alexander Mason (urology), Leon E. Sutton (surgery), Frederick James O'Connor (otolaryngology), Philip Rosenberg (pediatrics), Jacob Joshua Levy (radiology), Raymond Burns (obstetrics), George Clifford Goewey (allergy), Edward Charles Hughes (obstetrics/gynecology), Ed-

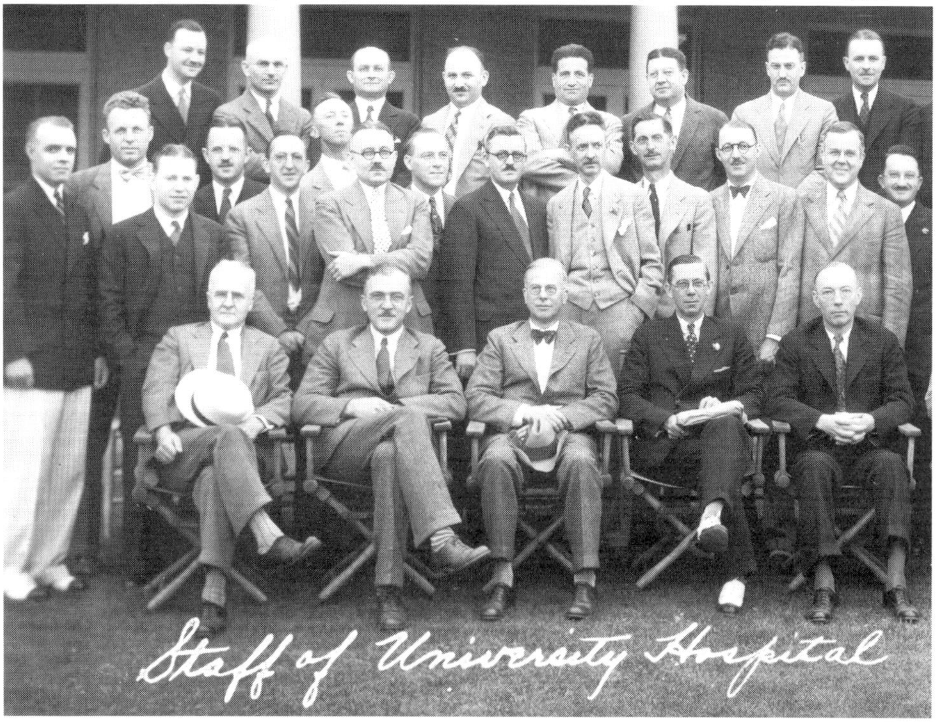

three editions were dedicated to the memory of Dean Heffron "as an expression of appreciation of his culture, ideals and especially his devotion to the better teaching and practice of rational therapy."

Weiskotten was not satisfied with the McBride Street campus. He envisioned a grand medical center on University Hill, closer to the heart of the Syracuse University campus. It would consist of not just a medical school, but a medical school endowed with excellent basic science facilities and surrounded by a variety of hospitals within easy walking distance. For these purposes he set his eye on the grounds of Yates Castle, a rambling estate on Irving Avenue.

In 1852 Colonel Cornelius Tyler Longstreet, a wealthy local clothing merchant, began construction of his 24-room mansion in the shape of a Norman castle. Its architect, James Renwick, also designed St. Patrick's Cathedral in New York City and several buildings at Vassar College. The castle was completed in 1855 at a cost of $200,000. First known as "Longstreet's Folly," it acquired its more familiar name, Yates Castle, from its second owner, Alonzo Chester Yates Sr., who bought it in 1867 and spent thousands of dollars to transform it into an elegant palace of high society.

ward G. Schweinberger (surgery), Morris A. Schoenwald (gynecology), Louis George Fournier (obstetrics/gynecology), Aaron Harry Kallet (medicine), Arnold Burnet Kauffman (otolaryngology); *middle row:* Noble Russell Chambers (psychiatry), Richard Sumner Farr (orthopedics), Abraham S. Lavine (surgery), Paul Hubbard Lowry (surgery), Benedict William Reifenstein (medicine), Murray Allen Cain (surgery), Maynard Edward Holmes (medicine), Herbert Carl Yeckel (medicine), Arthur Dubois Meyers (medicine), Clyde Orrin Barney (surgery), Harry Ethan Burdick (gynecology), John Charles Frey (anesthesiology), Charles Joseph Wells (anesthesiology), Lopo de Mello (dermatology), Thomas Forrest Laurie (urology), Thomas P. Farmer (gynecology), Robert J. McGuire (gynecology), Leo Eaton Gibson (urology), Roscoe D. Severance (orthopedics), Tracy L. Bryant (surgery); *seated:* Robert Burns (surgery), Albert George Swift (surgery), Henry Burton Doust (pulmonology), Herman Gates Weiskotten (pathology), William John McNerney (medicine), Frederick H. Knoff (anesthesiology), I. Harris Levy (medicine), George Sidney Britten (otolaryngology).

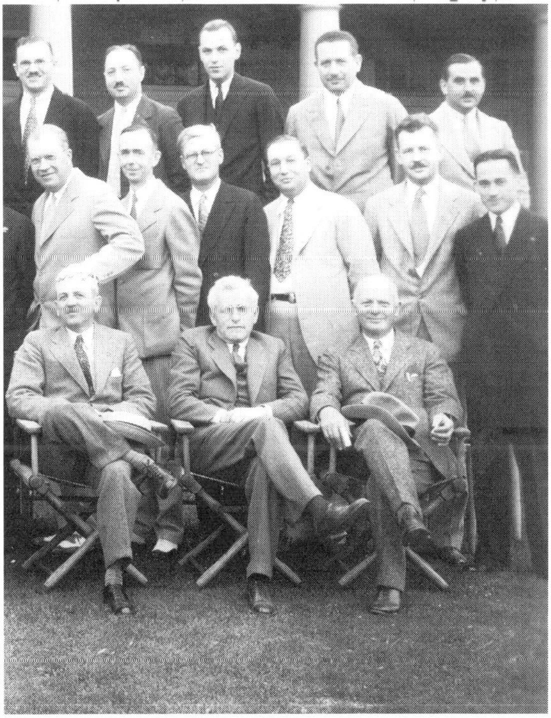

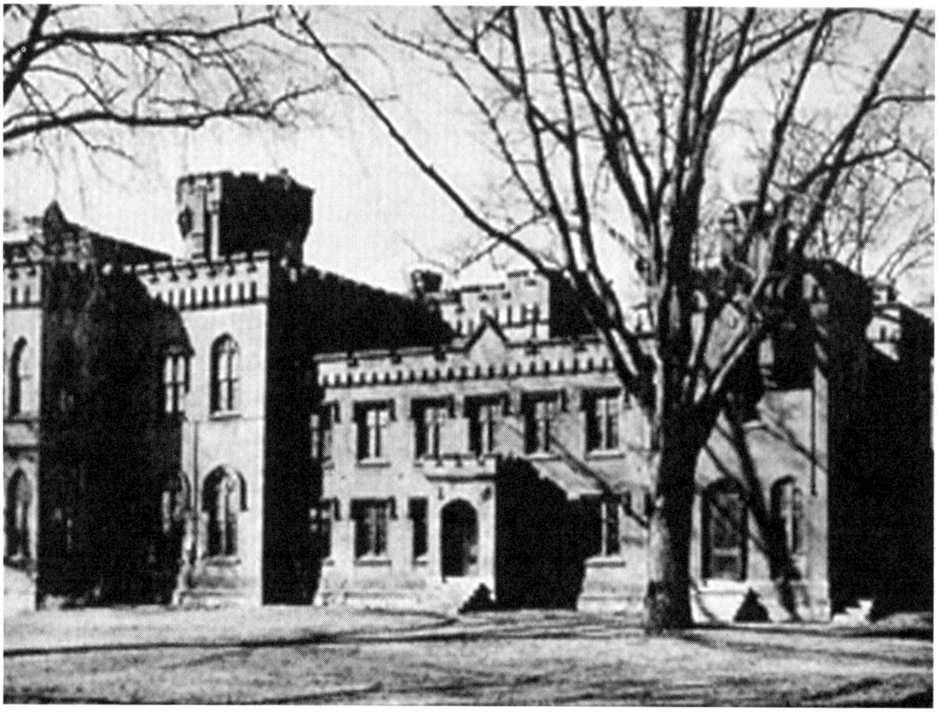

The profligate heir, Alonzo Jr. ("Lonnie"), allowed the property to fall into ruin, and most of its furnishings and art treasures were sold at public auction in 1898. The Yates family rented it in 1900 to Hudson River Institute Professor of English and History Abraham Lincoln Travis, who used it for the Syracuse Classical School, a preparatory school, until 1905. Syracuse University bought the 14-acre site in 1906 and used it from 1907 to 1934 for its School of Education and from 1934 to 1953 for its School of Journalism.

The focus of Weiskotten's new medical campus would be a Georgian style basic science building to be erected just northwest of Yates Castle, just northeast of the City Hospital for Communicable Diseases, just south of Syracuse Memorial Hospital, just southwest of Crouse Irving Hospital, one block south of the Syracuse State Psychopathic Hospital, and two blocks west of Good Shepherd. This building was commissioned in 1934 with a federal loan of $825,000. President Franklin Delano Roosevelt (shown flanked by Syracuse University Chancellor William Pratt Graham [left] and Weiskotten [right]) laid its cornerstone on September 29, 1936. It opened on November 14, 1937 and was dedicated on November 22 with speeches by Henry Asbury Christian of Harvard Medical School, New York State Commissioner of Health Edward Settle Godfrey, and Weiskotten's friend and mentor, Ray Lyman Wilbur. The building did not really have a name, but was called either the College of Medicine Building or, later, the Basic Science Building. On December 8, 1972, celebrating 100 years of regular medical education in Syracuse, it was renamed Weiskotten Hall.

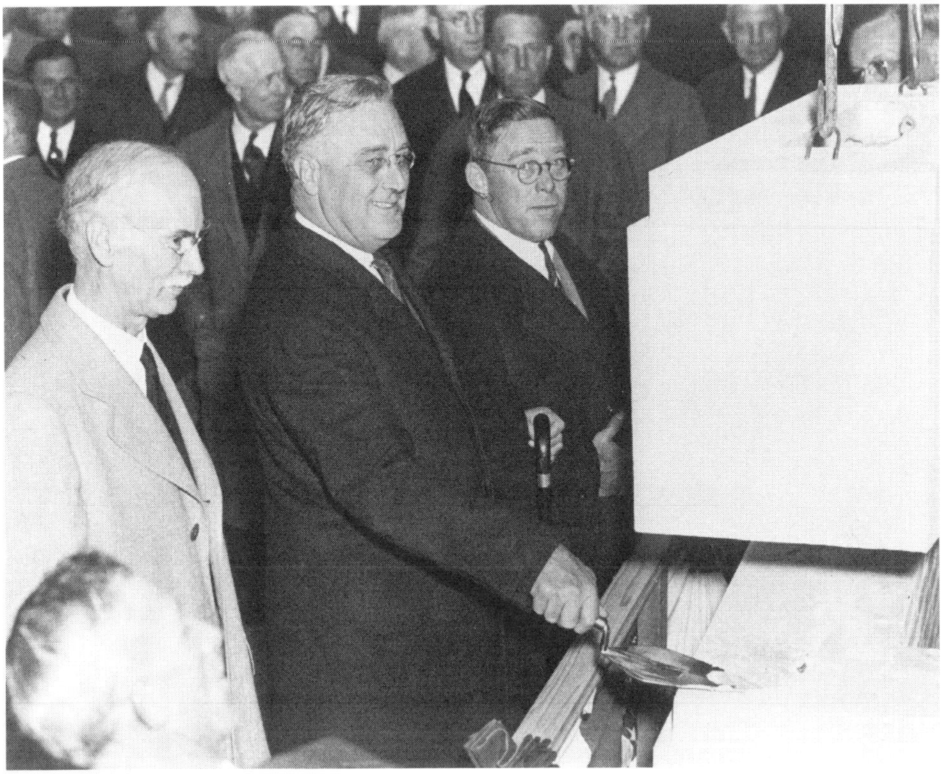

The main medical school building completed Weiskotten's vision of a medical center. He had already successively persuaded the City Hospital for Communicable Diseases, Syracuse Memorial Hospital, and the Syracuse State Psychopathic Hospital, and would later persuade the new Veterans Adminstration Hospital, all to locate or relocate near Crouse Irving Hospital and Good Shepherd, adjacent to the new College of Medicine campus. These four hospitals opened respectively in 1928, 1929, 1930, and 1953.

Pediatrician, epidemiologist, and public health administrator A. Clement Silverman, Class of 1915, was the motivating force behind the revitalization of City Hospital. The separate psychiatric hospital in Syracuse was Weiskotten's own idea. Through his efforts, the New York State Legislature in 1926 authorized creating the Psychopathic Hospital at the southwest corner of Irving Avenue and Adams Street. In the mid-1920s the City Hospital, to succeed the mid-nineteenth century "Pest House" on Teall Avenue, and the Psychopathic Hospital each began construction according to Weiskotten's specifications on land that Syracuse University provided.

In 1918, the Syracuse Hospital for Women and Children became Syracuse Memorial Hospital to reflect its broader new range of services. In 1925, its trustees approved moving from West Genesee Street to construct a new 340-bed facility, and that same year it also started construction where Weiskotten wanted it. Dwight James Baum, the architect who designed this hospital, also designed the 1936 College of Medicine building, Hendricks Chapel, and the Maxwell School of Citizenship. In 1929 Memorial Hospital moved to its present location on Irving Avenue. After establishing a co-operative arrangement with the Syracuse University School of Nursing in 1946, it dissolved its School of Nursing, but reacquired a nursing school when it merged with Crouse Irving Hospital in 1968.

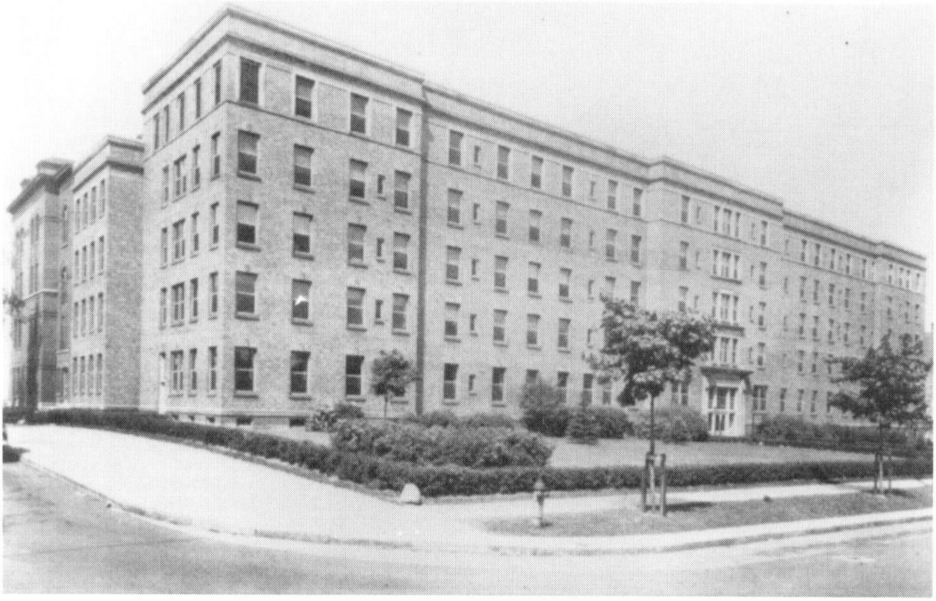

Thus by 1930 three new hospitals were grouped about the site proposed for the medical center campus. St. Joseph's (above at its Prospect Avenue site in 1927) was the only major hospital in Syracuse that did not locate or relocate on University Hill during Weiskotten's administration.

The Syracuse Veterans Administration Medical Center was conceived as a thousand-bed neuropsychiatric hospital, and was so approved by President Harry Truman in December 1945. By the time ground was broken in December 1949 the federal government had decided on a 500-bed general hospital instead. Its doors opened in June 1953 with Ralph Matheny as its first manager, John Duggan, Class of 1943, as its first chief of medicine, and Lloyd S. Rogers as its first chief of surgery. In 1959 the VA became the site for the first artificial kidney machine in Syracuse.

Of the nine medical colleges in New York in the 1930s, Syracuse was seventh in size followed by Rochester and Albany. Using data from the late 1930s, Weiskotten reported in 1940 that the city had 992 general hospital beds and 86 medical students, or 11.5 hospital beds per student (the average of all the schools surveyed was 14.2 beds per student); but Boston, home of Harvard, had only 8.2 beds per student, and Philadelphia, home of five medical schools including the nation's oldest, had only 10.5.

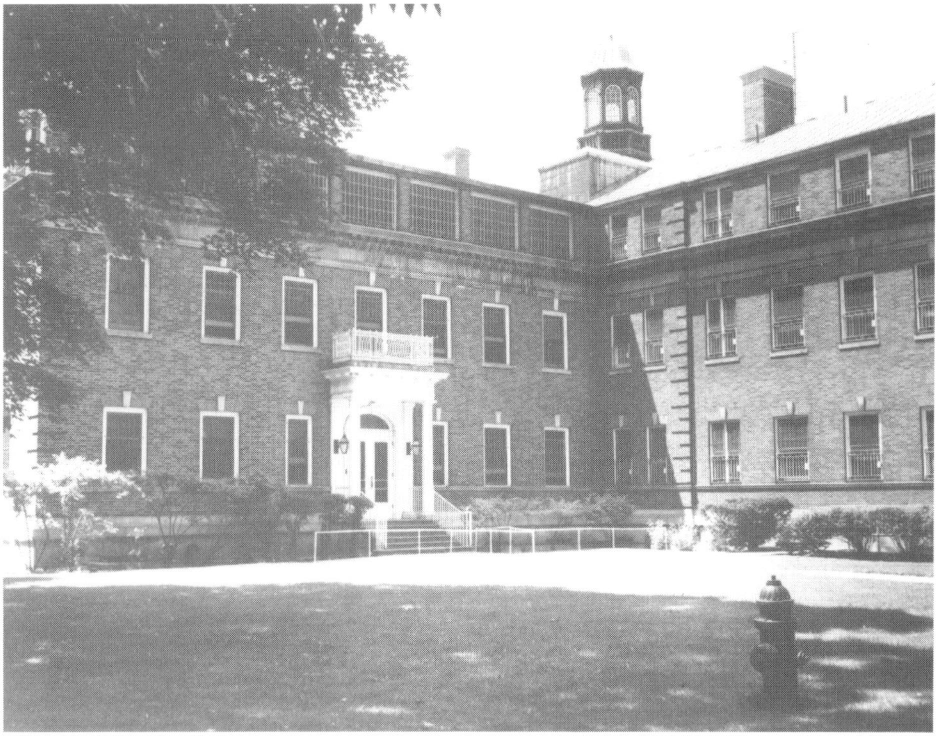

Syracuse State Psychopathic Hospital, renamed Syracuse Psychiatric Hospital in 1956, was razed in September 1990 to build the East Wing of University Hospital.

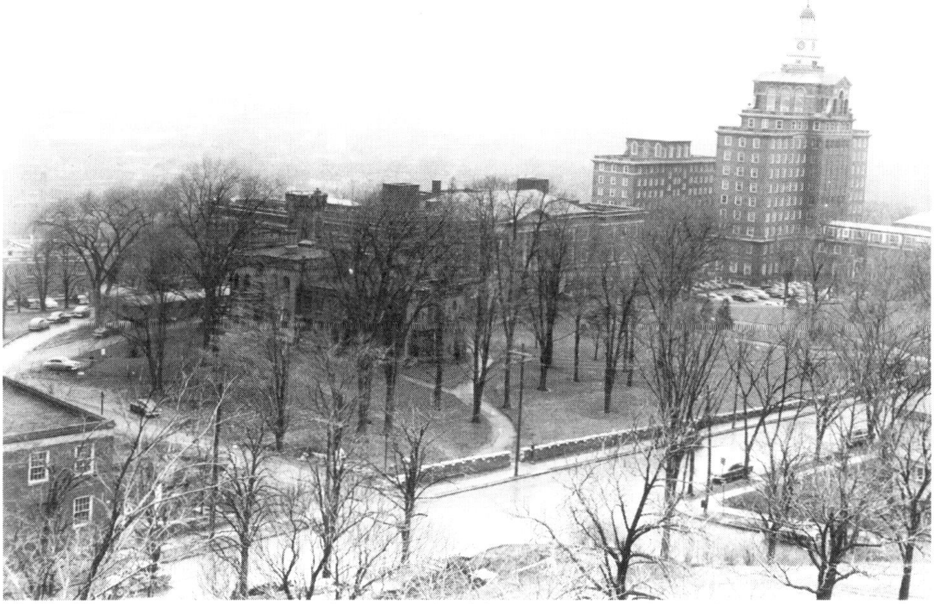

The Irving Avenue campus in 1945, looking northwest from the Crouse College hill: The nursing school in the lower left, Yates Castle behind the trees, the main building of the College of Medicine behind the castle, and Syracuse Memorial Hospital with its familiar clock tower in the upper right.

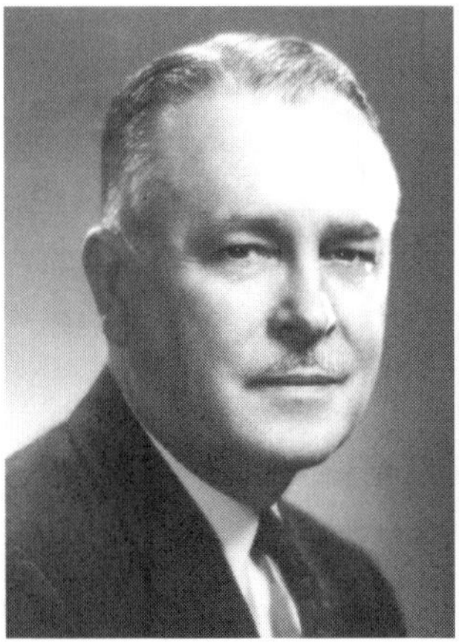 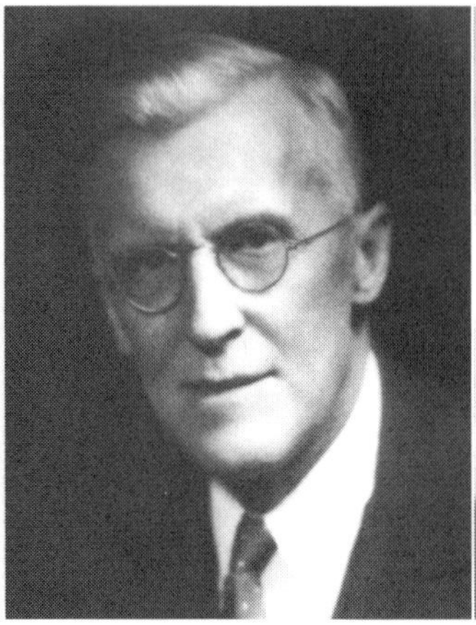 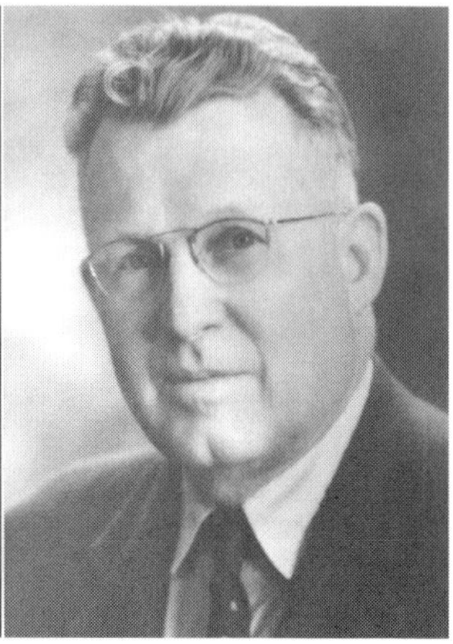

Edward C. Hughes, Class of 1924 (top left), began teaching obstetrics at the College of Medicine in 1923 and served as chair of the Department of Obstetrics from 1943 until it merged with the Department of Gynecology in 1961. Clarence E. Coon, Class of 1898 (top center), from 1919 to 1931 and Richard S. Farr (top right) from 1931 to 1954 taught orthopedic surgery within the Department of Surgery. Orthopedics did not become its own department at the College of Medicine until 1966. Coon formerly taught anatomy, general surgery, and radiology (then called roentgenology) and was attending orthopedist at St. Joseph's and attending radiologist at both the Dispensary and the Syracuse Hospital for Women and Children. Farr came to Syracuse from Vermont after World War I to establish private orthopedic practice. Edward C. Reifenstein, Class of 1904 (bottom left), taught internal medicine from 1915 to 1946, chaired the department from 1932 to 1946, and founded Syracuse's first cardiology clinic in 1932. Alfred M. Wose from 1908 to 1940, Thomas F. Laurie (bottom center) from 1918 to 1946, and Leo E. Gibson, Class of 1920 (bottom right), from 1928 to 1954 were the College of Medicine's earliest teachers of urology. The Department of Urology was semi-independent until 1941, then part of Surgery until 1966.

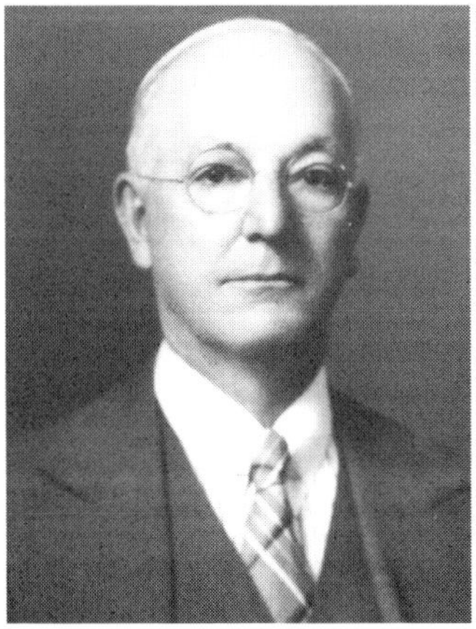 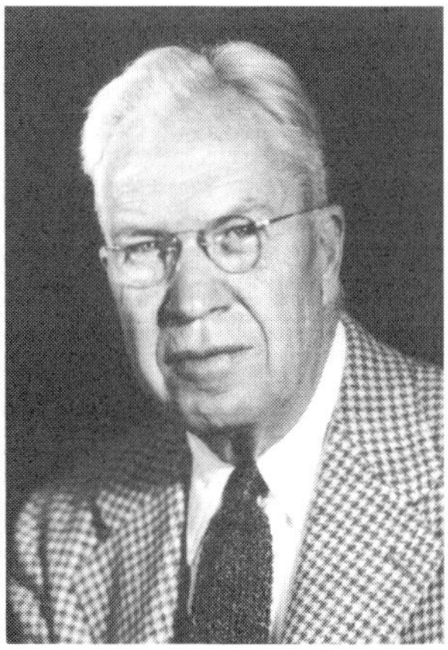 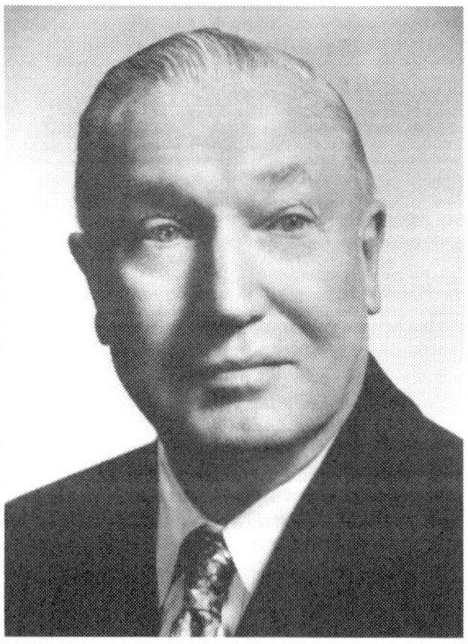

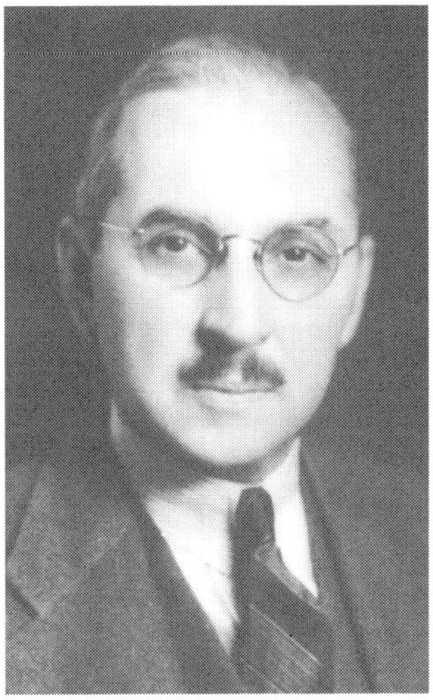
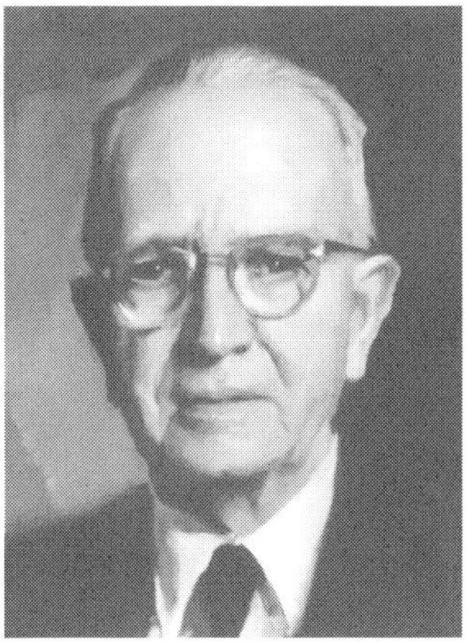
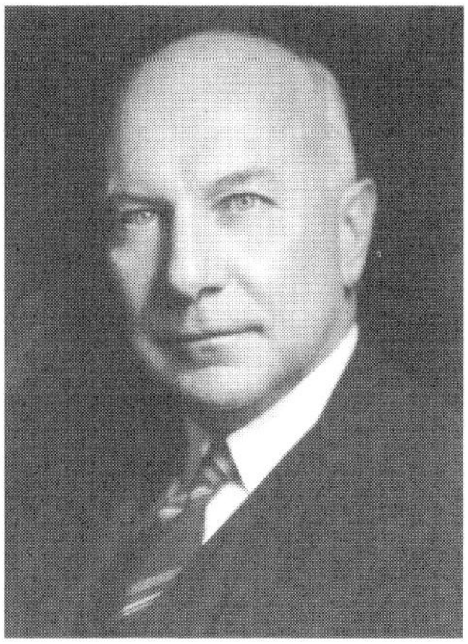

Much progress in psychiatry, psychology, and the neurosciences occurred during the Weiskotten era. Wardner Ayer (top left) joined the faculty in 1915 as an instructor in histology and embryology. In 1919 he moved from the Department of Anatomy — chaired from 1910 to 1938 by the colorful and flamboyant Henry W. Stiles (bottom left) — to the Department of Medicine, where he taught neuropathology, neurology, and neuropsychiatry until 1948, always emphasizing the clinical importance of the neurosciences. Another pioneer in psychiatry at the College of Medicine was Eugene N. Boudreau, Class of 1912 (top center in a detail from Everett Raymond Kinstler's 1961 painting), who concentrated on neuroanatomy and epilepsy while on the faculty from 1920 to 1946. Richard H. Hutchings (bottom right), after whom the Hutchings Psychiatric Center at 620 Madison Street in Syracuse is named, taught psychiatry from 1908 to 1933 and administered the psychiatric hospital in Utica. Harry A. Steckel (top right) came to Syracuse in 1931 to direct the new State Psychopathic Hospital. Under him, Psychiatry became a separate department from Medicine in 1933. He retired in 1948.

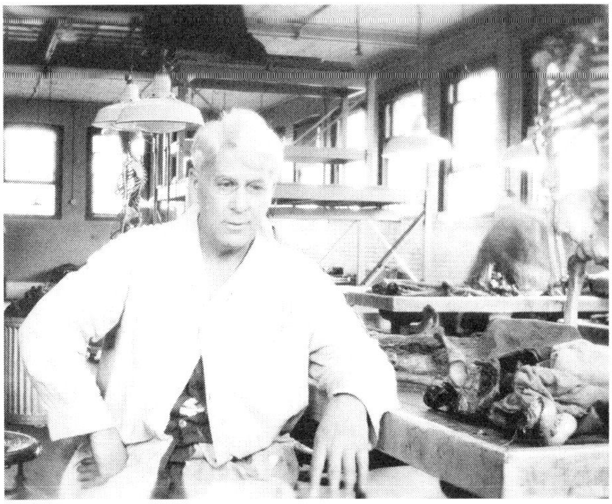
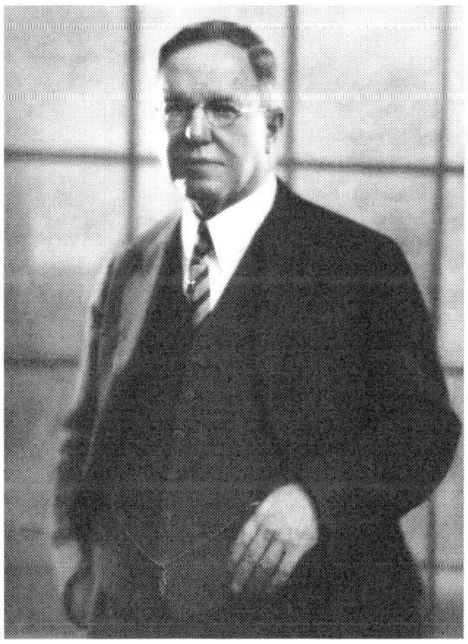

Weiskotten's first love was pathology. As an expert in pathological anatomy, he served Onondaga County as the coroner's necrotomist from 1913 to 1926. He was president of the Onondaga County Medical Society in 1923 and director of Good Shepherd from 1925 to 1941. As Syracuse City Commissioner of Health from 1926 to 1928, he modernized the program of the Visiting Nurse Association. He was absolutely tireless, but nevertheless complained in the mid-1920s that his three simultaneous full-time jobs of college dean, hospital director, and county health official left him little time to be also a professor of pathology. He called this part of his life "hectic but interesting."

He aimed to surround himself with physicians who were as dedicated to medical science and education as he was and — asymptotically — who would work as hard as he did. During his frequent absences from Syracuse, Brewer acted as dean, running the medical school with ample assistance from Weiskotten's secretary, Lucy Pelton Faigle, Swift, and Ayer.

Weiskotten's twenty-nine year administration must be seen as a remarkable benefit to both his own medical institution and medical education in general. Syracuse medical alumni over the years have recalled his fatherly concern with their financial plights as students. He personally enabled many financially troubled students to stay in medical school. Yet he was aloof, unfriendly, monomaniacal, and not well-rounded. Though perhaps not as eccentric as Steensland, his personality, demeanor, and dedication to medical science reflected Steensland's. Hoople wrote in his eulogy of Weiskotten in the *Bulletin of the Onondaga County Medical Society*, "he was not lovable and warm ... he was a scientist through and through." This extreme devotion to his life's mission and his detachment from the non-scientific world often appeared as hostility, intolerance, or ruthlessness.

The two keynote speakers at the centennial celebration on June 4, 1934 were Harvey Cushing, the world's foremost neurosurgeon, and George M.B. Hawley, a lawyer representing Hobart and William Smith Colleges. Cushing acknowledged the value of what he and many others believed was Syracuse University's greatest contribution to the general development of American medical education in the nineteenth century:

> What is historically important is that your school here at Syracuse was the first in New York State and the second in the country [behind only Harvard] to replace the traditional but outworn order of things by progressive exercises for nine months in the year over a period of three years — a programme to which other schools quickly followed suit.

Weiskotten's main significance was in furthering this legacy.

The Department of Medical Chemistry was renamed Physiological Chemistry in 1939 and Biochemistry in 1946. Brewer's successor, Wilfred Westerfeld, wrote in his 1989 typescript memoir, *The Making of a Medical Center: A Personal History of the Background*, that when he arrived in July 1945, "Syracuse was not known as a research-oriented medical college," but that Weiskotten "was quite supportive of the idea" of making it one. The Syracuse University Department of Chemistry wanted to make any expansion of the physiological chemistry or biochemistry program part of the graduate program in chemistry. Westerfeld persuaded Chancellor William Pearson Tolley that the Department of Chemistry was incompetent to manage a graduate program in biochemistry on its own. Thus, through the efforts of both Brewer and Westerfeld, the independent Department of Biochemistry was created at Syracuse University under the control of the College of Medicine. Brewer, unfortunately, did not live to see it.

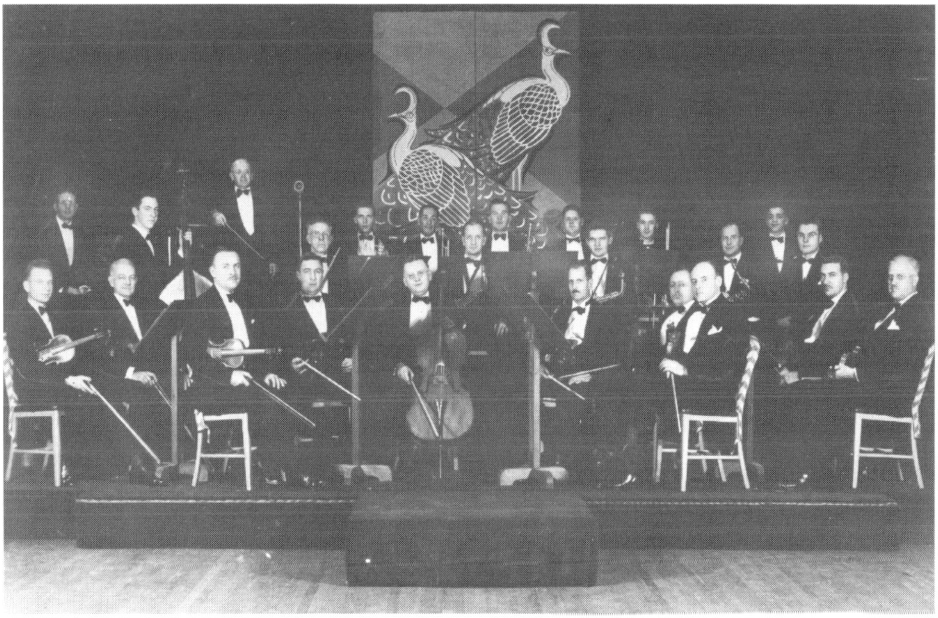

In 1938 the Alumni Association assembled an orchestra consisting of five professional musicians and nineteen alumni, medical students, faculty, local physicians, and amateur musicians: *front row:* Mr. Moses; Carlton Frasier Potter, Class of 1910; Edward C. Hughes, Class of 1924; Vilas George Van Ornam, M.D.; professional cellist; Charles M. Greene, Class of 1918; Nicholas Warner Van Lengen, Class of 1909; Ellery G. Allen, M.D.; professional musician; Frederick Stephen Wetherell, Class of 1913; *back row:* Foster C. Rulison, Class of 1918; professional bassist; professional conductor; Peter Campbell Ten Eyck, Class of 1897; professional musician; Herbert R. Diaso, Class of 1934; Mr. Lipes; C. Eugene Erway, Class of 1939; Frederic R. Fenno, Class of 1938; Gordon H. Bobbett, Class of 1940; Arthur E. Harris, Class of 1935; Jesse Overton, Class of 1935; Joseph J. Frank, Class of 1939; David W. Brewer, Class of 1941.

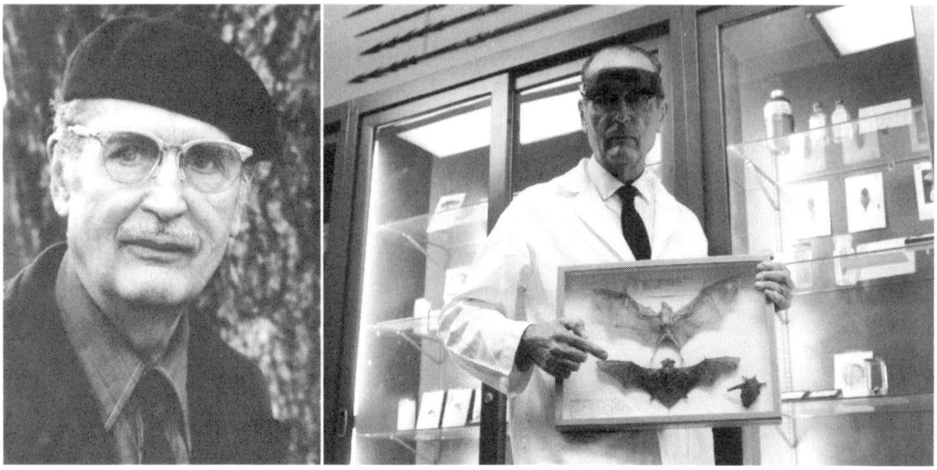

One of the most gifted, unconventional, and admired professors ever to teach in the College of Medicine was Justus F. Mueller (above), who began as an adjunct lecturer on parasitology, medical entomology, and microbiology in the Department of Bacteriology in 1930. To better describe its scope, much of which Mueller had shaped, this department was renamed Bacteriology and Parasitology in 1943 and Microbiology in 1954.

As an undergraduate, Mueller studied zoology at Johns Hopkins and drawing at the Corcoran School of Art and the Maryland Institute College of Art. He received his Ph.D. in parasitology in 1928 at the University of Illinois as the protégé of the leading American parasitologist of his time, Henry Baldwin Ward. That experience further toughened Mueller's already tough character. As he recalled in a speech to the American Society of Parasitologists (ASP) in 1973, "If you took Ward's guff, you could stand anything." Eager to leave Illinois, he took a job in 1928 teaching zoology at the New York State College of Forestry (now the SUNY College of Environmental Science and Forestry). He stayed there until 1943, when he was promoted to associate professor at the College of Medicine.

In the late 1930s he made the first of his many scientific expeditions into the rainforests of Central and South America, including a perilous trip from Huánuco, Peru, to the mouth of the Amazon in 1941. These adventures earned him election to the Explorers Club in 1980.

Mueller was an extraordinary scientist, making basic discoveries about the life cycle of *Spirometra mansonoides* and *in vitro* laboratory methods, but he was as much an artist as a scientist. In 1935 he published *A Manual of Drawing for Science Students*, a practical set of lessons that emphasized and clearly described theoretical principles of observation. He also designed the emblem of the ASP, several prize medals, and 118 three-dimensional zoological instructional models. His main advice in his 1961 Upstate commencement speech was: "It's no good unless you sweat!"

7

The U.S. Army 52nd General Hospital

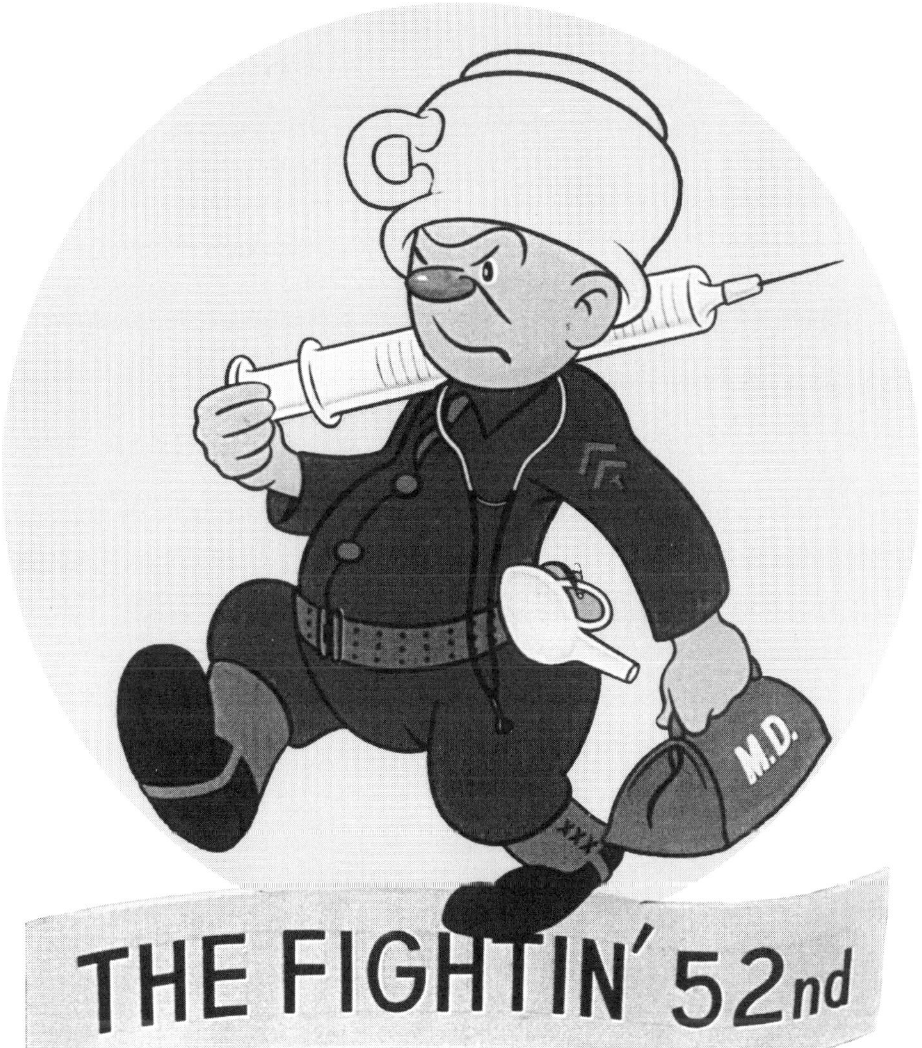

As World War II began, many American institutions of higher learning, including Syracuse University, organized local hospital units to serve medical and surgical needs overseas. The Department of War authorized the creation of these mobile hospitals in 1940 — before the United States

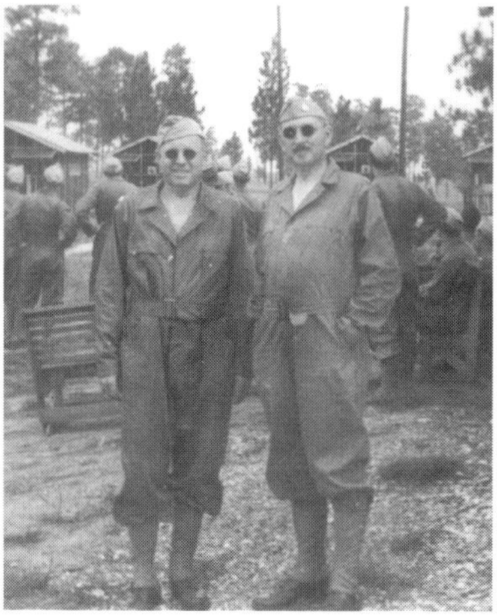

entered the war. The first recruitment meeting for the unit affiliated with the Syracuse University College of Medicine, the U.S. Army 52nd General Hospital, occurred early in 1941, many months before Pearl Harbor. The five members of the original committee, internist Wardner D. Ayer, surgeon Clyde O. Barney, orthopedist Richard S. Farr, psychiatrist Harry A. Steckel, and Dean Weiskotten, chose Farr (left) as senior officer and Ayer (right) as his aide.

The Army commissioned the 52nd on September 1, 1942. After basic training at Camp Livingston, Louisiana (above), and additional training at Camp Kilmer, New Jersey, it sailed for Britain on January 6, 1943 aboard the Cunard liner *Queen Elizabeth*, which had been converted into a troop ship. Her swimming pool had been drained and equipped with five levels of bunks. Staterooms intended for two held six. She had no naval escort because she was too fast for destroyers to keep up. To avoid U-boats she zigzagged at full speed all the way, making people fall, furniture slide, and food spill every seven minutes. She also carried the "black box," one of the first sonar devices. When it alerted her to the presence of a wolfpack near the Azores, she had time to hightail it toward Iceland before any danger arose. The Royal Air Force provided an escort when she reached Irish waters.

After a harrowing week at sea, the 52nd debarked in Scotland, travelled by train to cold, wet, coke-heated temporary quarters in Somerset, then moved gradually that spring into its permanent quarters in Wolverley (aerial view below), near Kidderminster, Worcestershire, with Spartan facilities for 600 staff and 1700 patients.

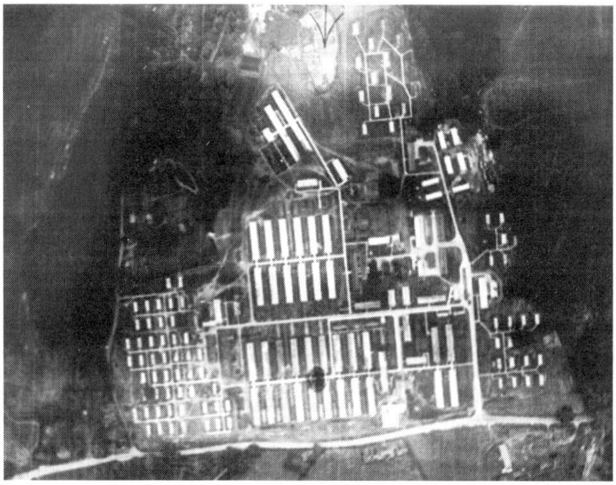

The views of the Wolverley camp on page 109 are, clockwise from top left: officers' quarters, officers' mess, headquarters parade ground, officers' barracks, ambulance and patients, main gate, Thursday afternoon retreat, nurses on Thursday afternoon retreat, post-D-Day expansion of tents behind every hospital building, nurses' quarters.

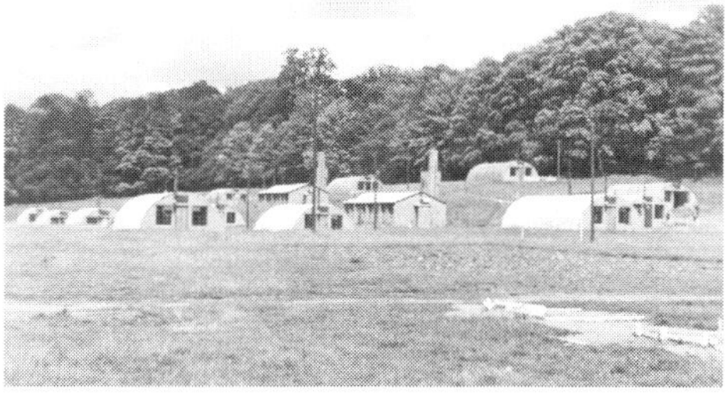

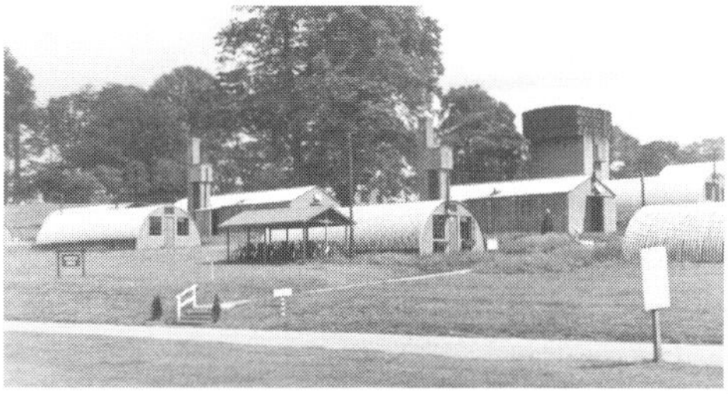

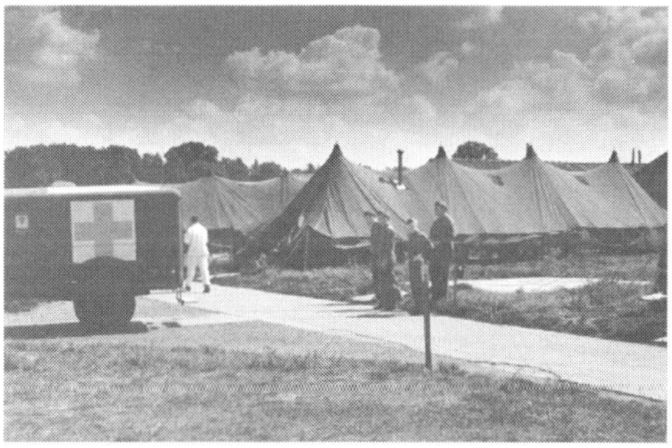

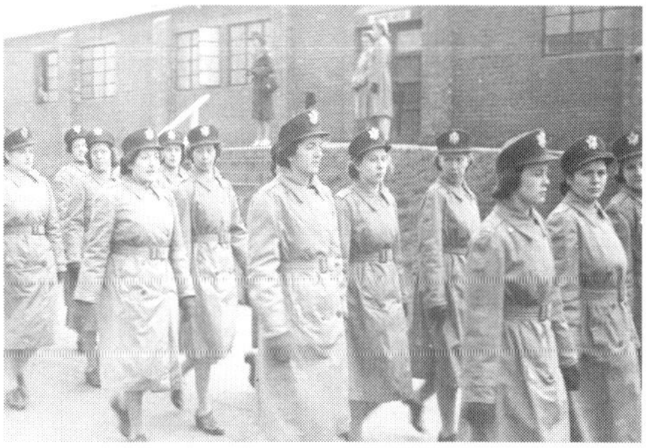

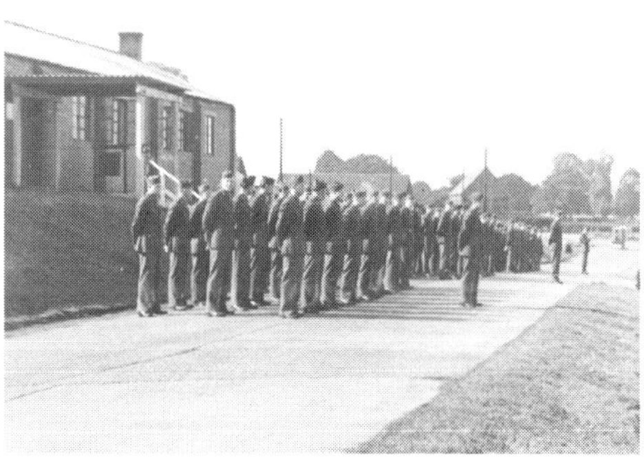

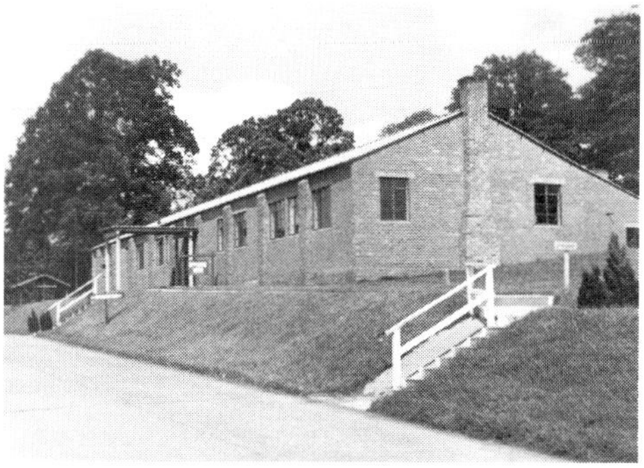

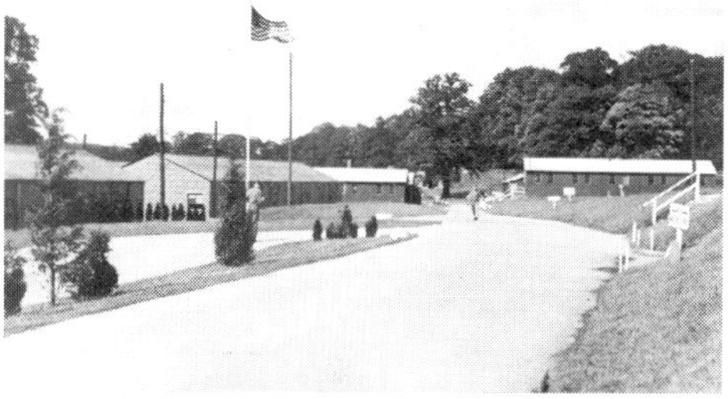

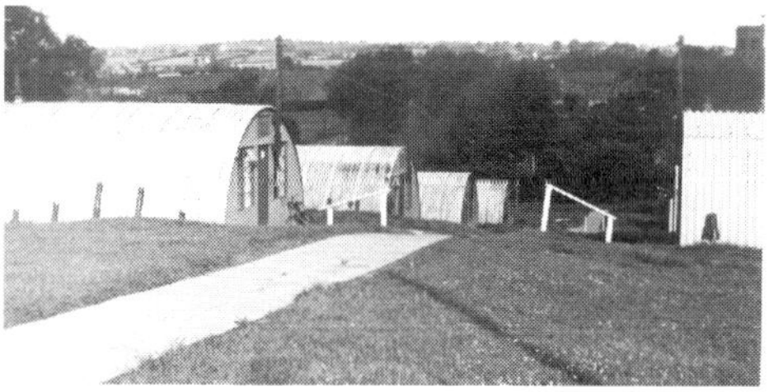

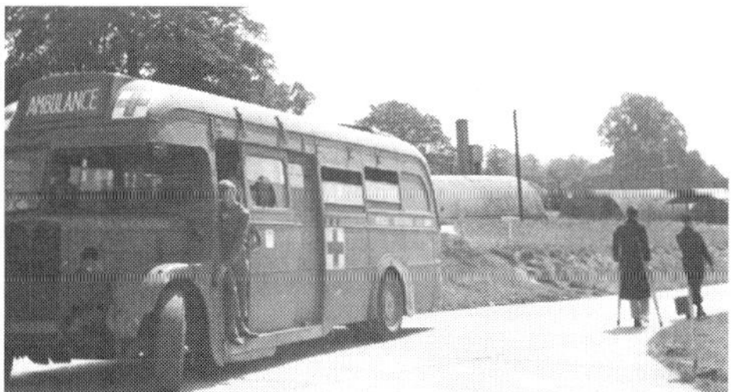
AMBULANCE

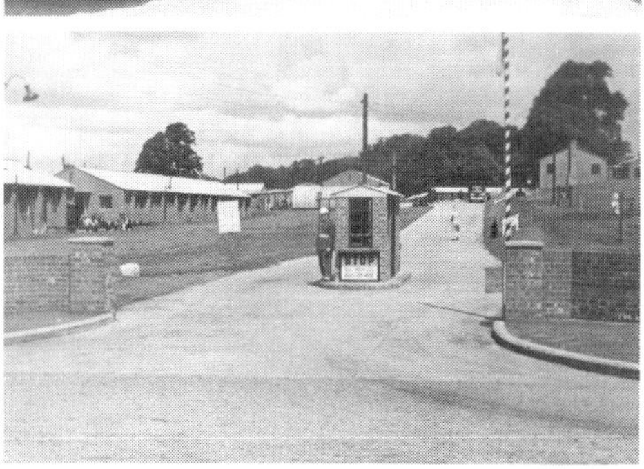

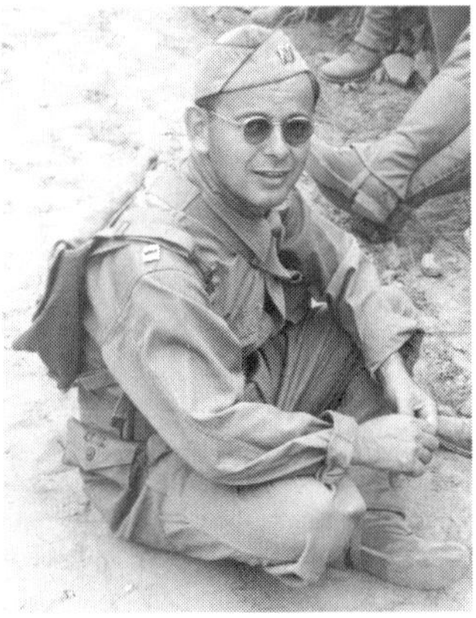

There was not much to do for the nearly seventeen months that the 52nd was in England before D-Day. Keeping the enlisted men occupied and out of trouble was a problem. Colonel Farr appointed Captain Max Kutzer (left) as the morale officer and ordered him to build a recreational sports program. Kutzer took this mission seriously and decided on a baseball team. He understood baseball as well as anyone, having played shortshop as an undergraduate at Harvard and with the semi-professional Dorchester Club while a student at Harvard Medical School in the 1930s.

In the spring of 1943 Kutzer arranged with the farmer whose land abutted the hospital for the use of a suitable field. He advertised for any patients, officers, or enlisted men to try out. He chose twelve good players for hardball, four officers and eight enlisted men, and organized the rest for intramural softball. His starting pitcher was Captain Ted Kleinhans, a Syracuse University athlete who had also pitched for the Philadelphia Phillies, Cincinnati Reds, New York Yankees, and Syracuse Chiefs. Every day Kutzer would scan the incoming patient and duty rosters, looking for more men who might make good ball players.

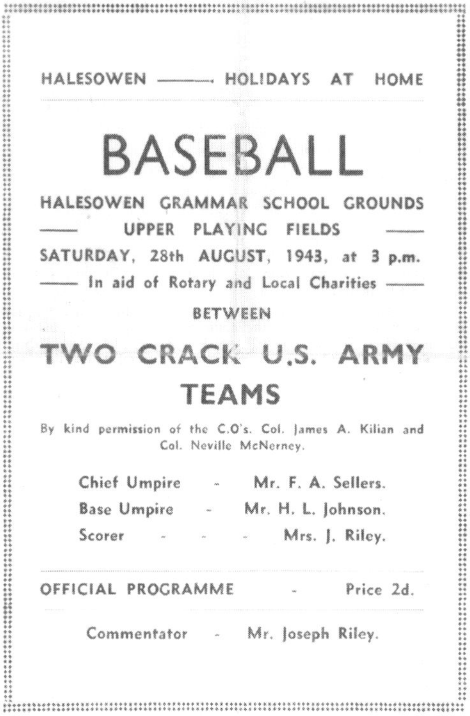

HALESOWEN —— HOLIDAYS AT HOME

BASEBALL

HALESOWEN GRAMMAR SCHOOL GROUNDS

—— UPPER PLAYING FIELDS ——

SATURDAY, 28th AUGUST, 1943, at 3 p.m.

—— In aid of Rotary and Local Charities ——

BETWEEN

TWO CRACK U.S. ARMY TEAMS

By kind permission of the C.O's. Col. James A. Kilian and Col. Neville McNerney.

Chief Umpire - Mr. F. A. Sellers.
Base Umpire - Mr. H. L. Johnson.
Scorer - - - Mrs. J. Riley.

OFFICIAL PROGRAMME - Price 2d.

Commentator - Mr. Joseph Riley.

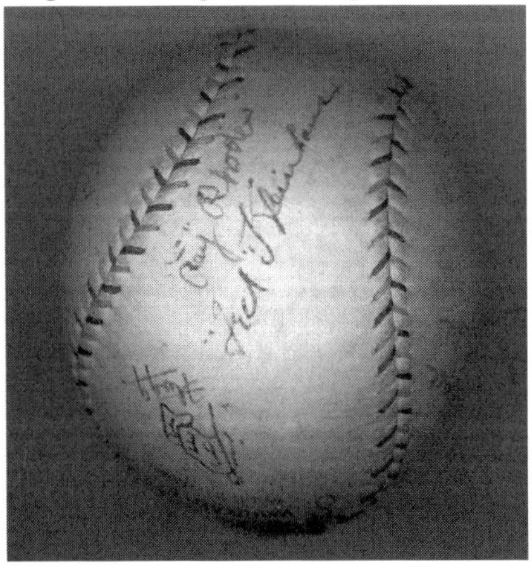

Russell Lee Bauers, a six-foot-three-inch right-hander, pitched for the Pittsburgh Pirates from 1936 to 1941, then for the Chicago Cubs in 1946 and the St. Louis Browns in 1950, ending his career with a 31-30 record and a 3.53 lifetime earned run average. His best year was 13-6 in 1937, when he helped the Pirates to third place in the eight-team National League. One day Kutzer

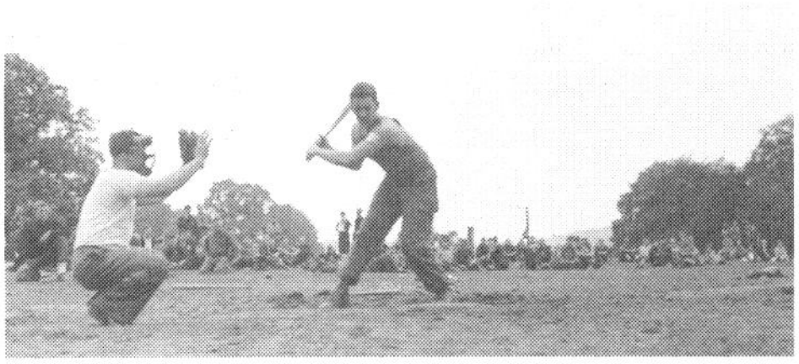

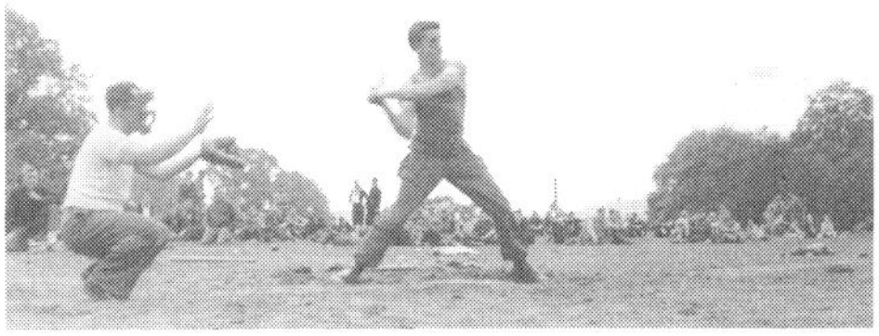

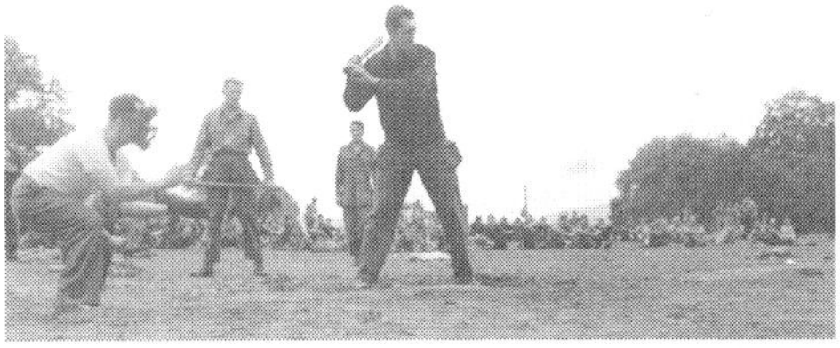

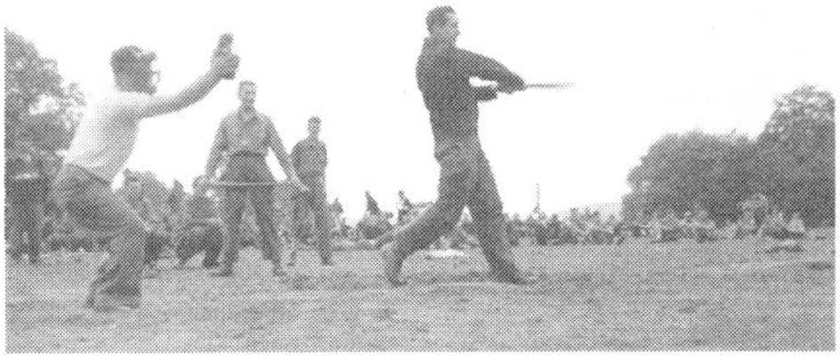

recognized his name among the new psychiatric patients. Private Bauers had suffered a nervous breakdown and was afraid to return to combat. Kutzer offered to get him transferred out of his battle unit and into Klein-hans's rehabilitation unit if he would agree to pitch. Bauers jumped at the chance and the 52nd then had two major league pitchers on its team.

Calling its team the "Chiefs," the 52nd played against other American units throughout England and won most of its games. The only team with a better record was the 10th Replacement Depot, which could put together an entire team of major leaguers from a pool of over ten thousand men.

Kutzer also organized intramural basketball for enlisted men, swimming lessons, and dances with the WACs and nurses.

PLAYERS

	AMERICANS.	CHIEFS.
Pitcher	Sgt. Collins.	Capt. Kleinhans.
Catcher	Pte. Hughes.	Pte. Joyce.
1st Base	Pte. Mattivello.	Master Sgt. Flagg.
2nd Base	Sgt. Kocur.	Pte. Costa.
3rd Base	Pte. Garratt.	Pte. Monaco.
Short Stop	Pte. Daily.	Capt. Kutzer.
Right Field	Pte. Pearsall.	Cpl. Todd.
Centre Field	Sgt. Capinos.	Lieut. Rhodes.
Left Field	Pte. Tranter.	Cpl. Towers.
Substitutes	Cpl. Davis, Pte. Phillips, and Pte. Romano.	S. Sgt. Bercume, T. Sgt. Lerner and Pte. Sweet.
By kind permission of the C.O's.	Col James A. Kilian	Col. Neville McNerney.

BOX SCORE

Innings	1	2	3	4	5	6	7	8	9	Total
Americans										
Chiefs										

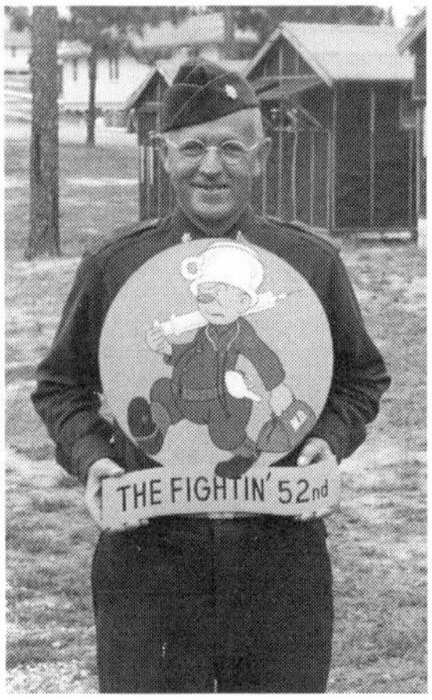

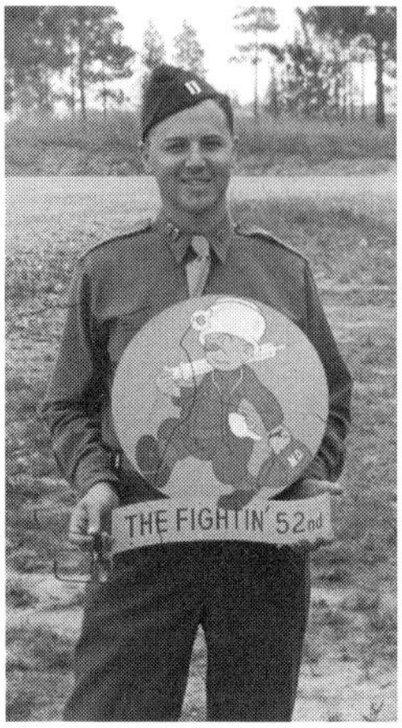

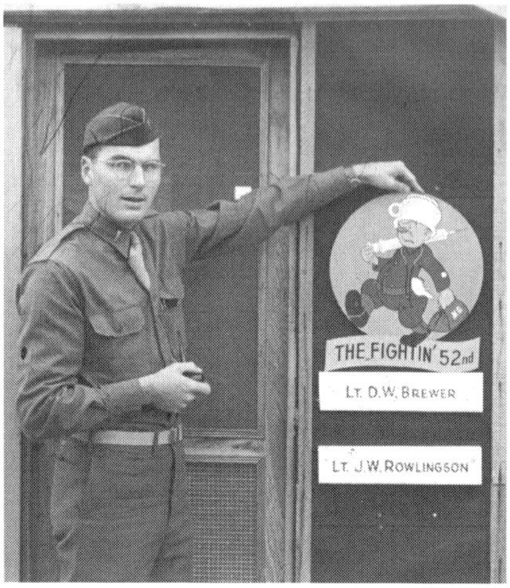

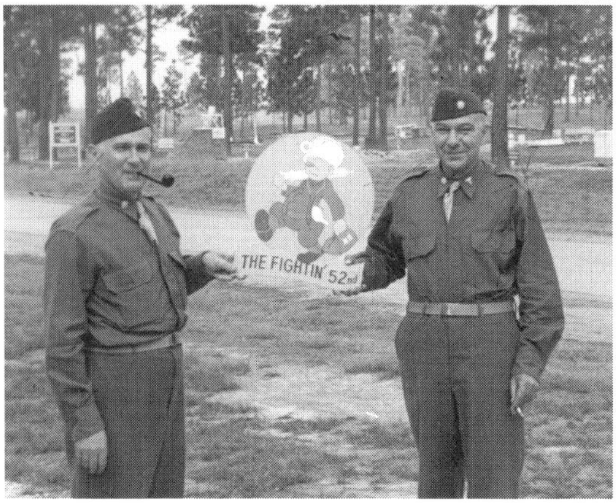

Besides Kutzer, another morale booster in the 52nd was a Corporal Fitzgerald, whom everyone knew as just "Fitz." A natural artist and satirist, Fitz created the unit's ubiquitous mascot, the stubby corporal with a chamber pot for a helmet, a syringe for a rifle, and a bedpan for a kit. Fitz modelled the face on the features of the commanding officer, Colonel Neville McNerney. Displaying the mascot at Camp Livingston are, clockwise from top left: Paul H. Lowry, Class of 1922; neurosurgeon Arthur David Ecker; David W. Brewer, Class of 1941; Wendell V. Brown, Class of 1928; and Tyree C. Wyatt, Class of 1922.

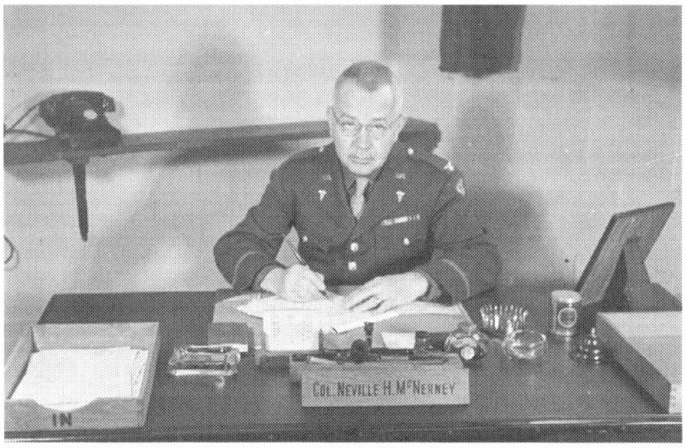

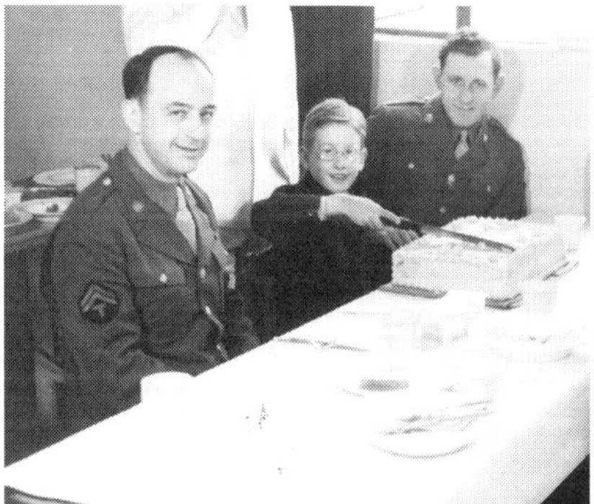

The 52nd enjoyed a friendly relationship with the British people. Throughout the war, British families living near likely bomb targets would send their children north to be safe from the Nazis. The 52nd welcomed these children, entertained them and the local kids, played sports and games with them, and sometimes even gave them birthday parties.

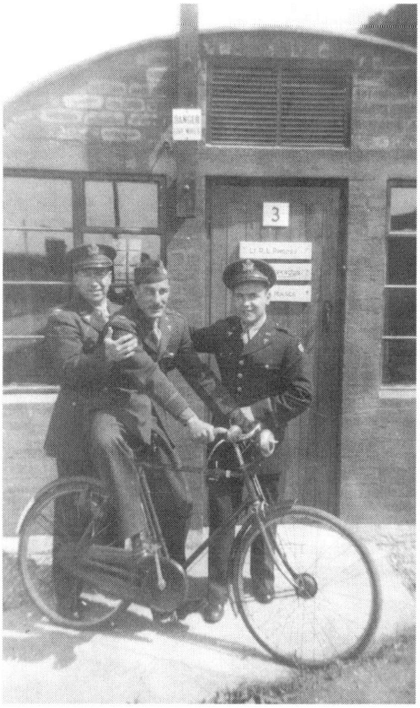

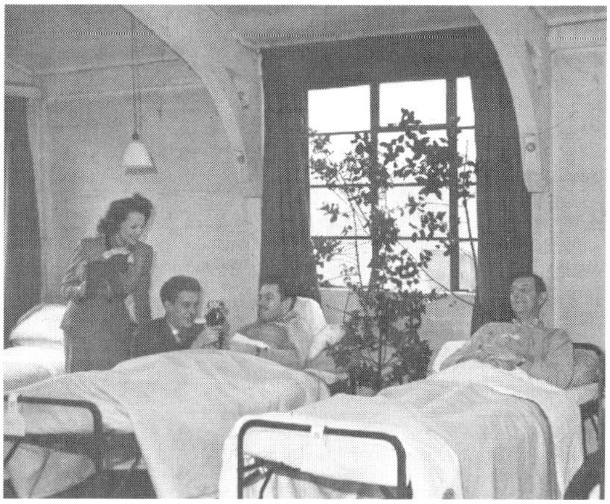

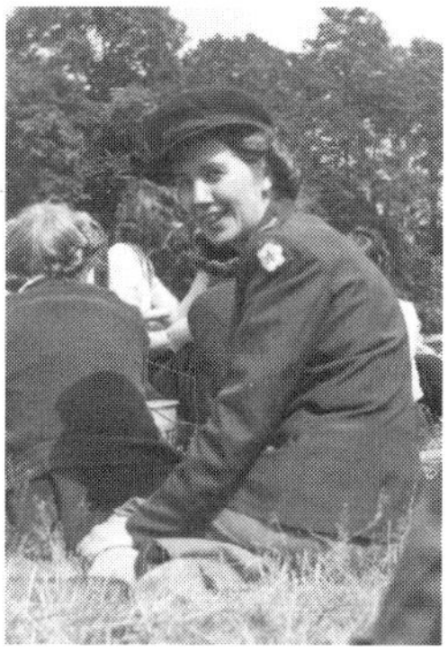

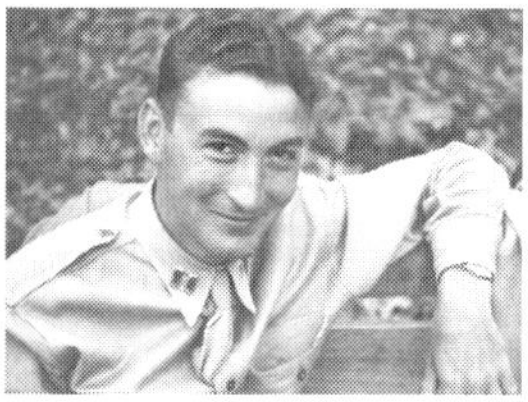

Clockwise from center: head nurse Ivy Wadsworth; the BBC interviewing patients in a specially prepared room; Arthur E. Harris, Class of 1935; (right to left) Wadsworth, Foster C. Rulison, Class of 1918, McNerney, surgeon G. Gowing Broad, and an enlisted man celebrate Christmas 1943; Wardner D. Ayer; Floyd R. Parker, Class of 1928 (left) and Eugene W. Anthony, Class of 1937 (right); (left to right) Raymond L. Rhodes, Class of 1938, John B. Stevens, Class of 1927, and George M. Kirkwood, Class of 1938.

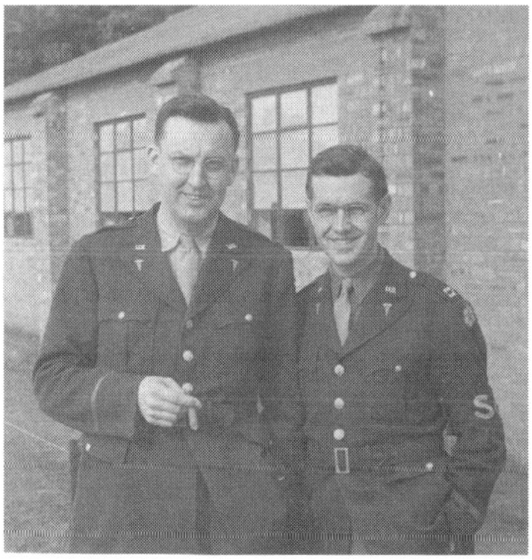

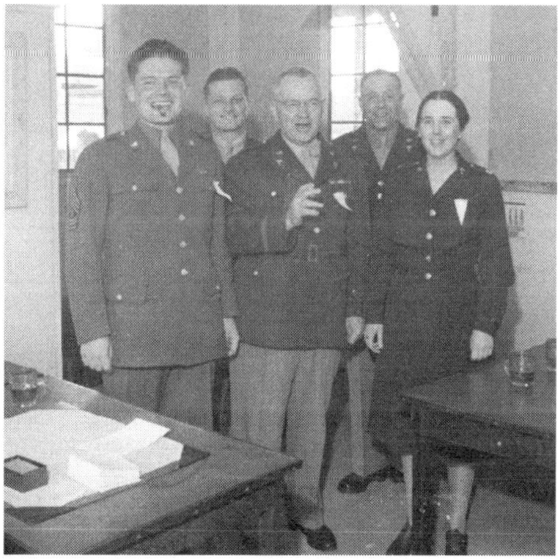

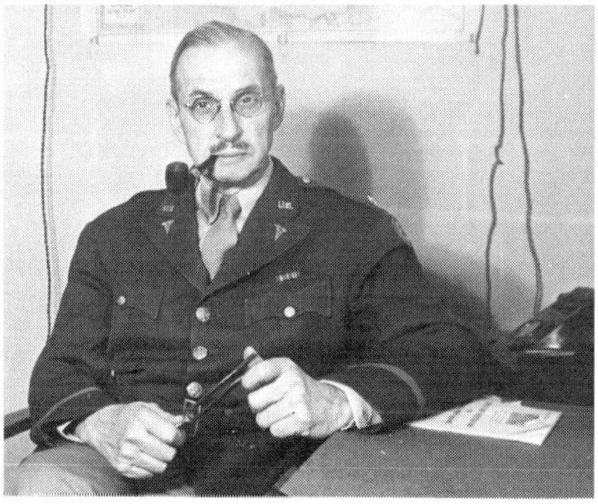

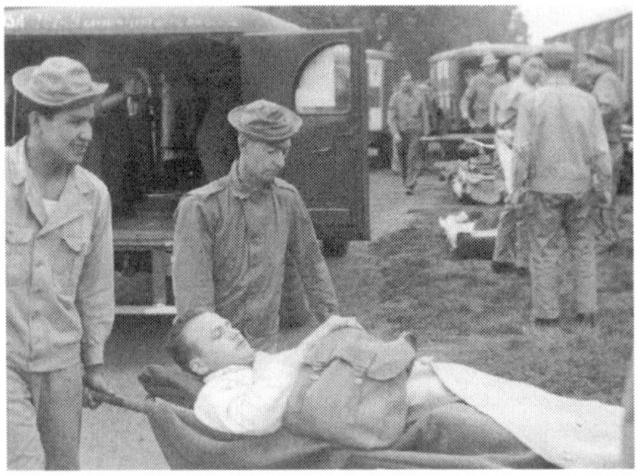

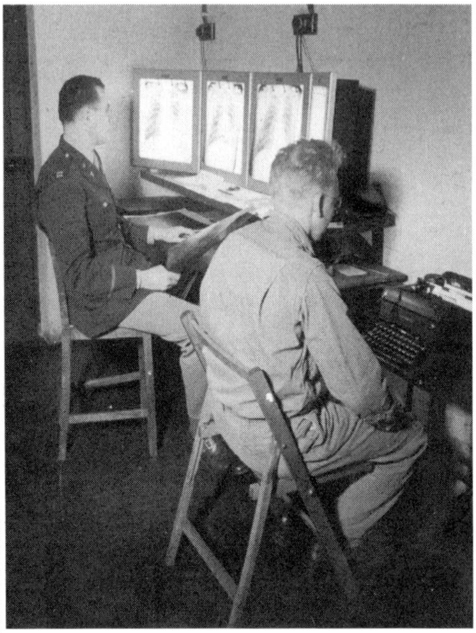

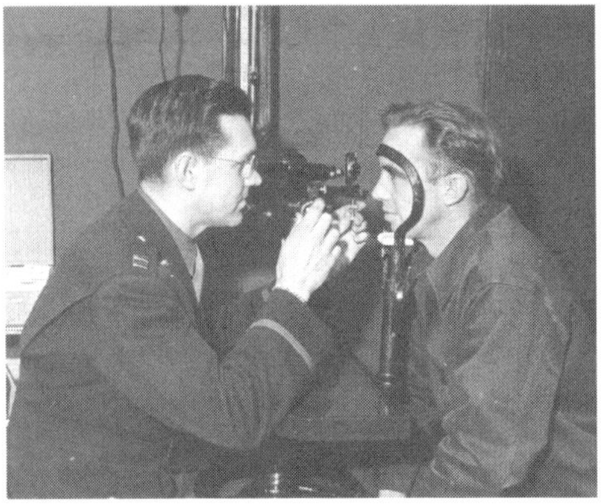

The Army assigned Brewer (above), an otolaryngologist, to radiology, and Wyatt (below), a pediatrician, to pathology.

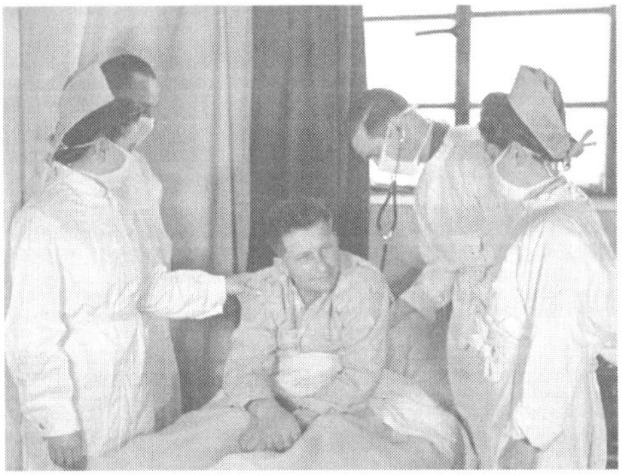

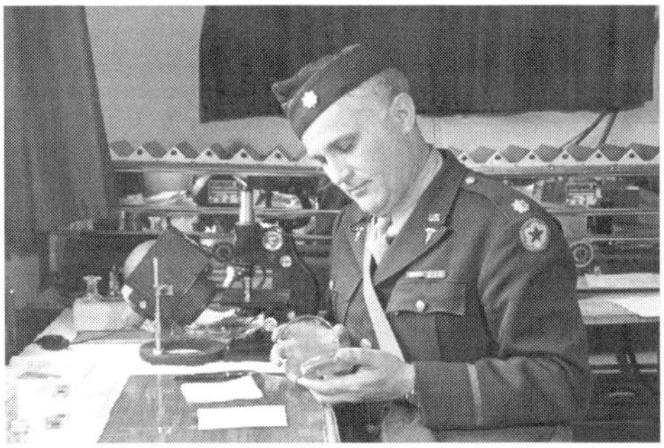

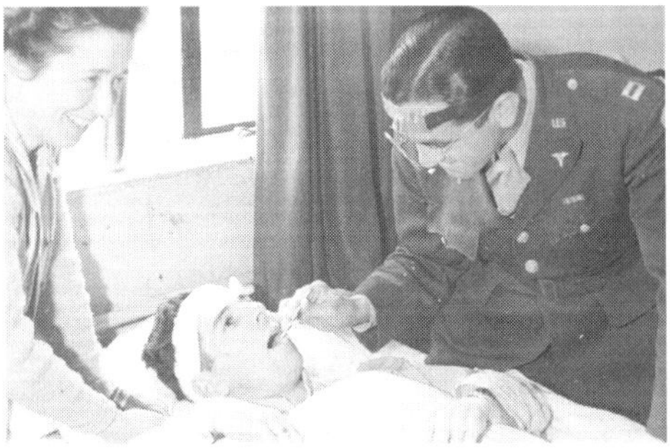

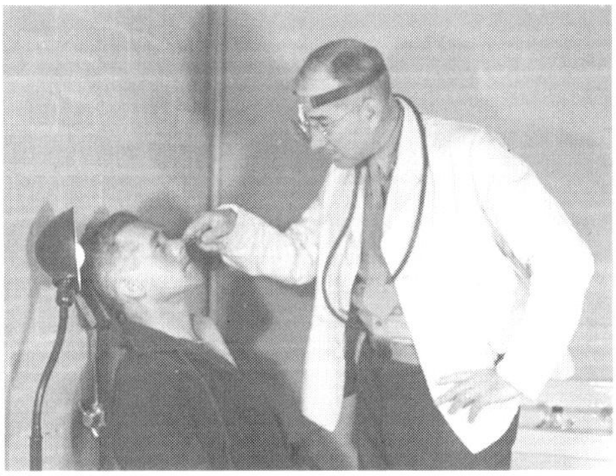

New patients arrived by truck and stretcher. Anthony (upper left); William D. Alsever, Class of 1939 (center left); Samuel C. Bregande, Class of 1937 (lower left); and Gordon D. Hoople, Class of 1919 (lower right), examined them.

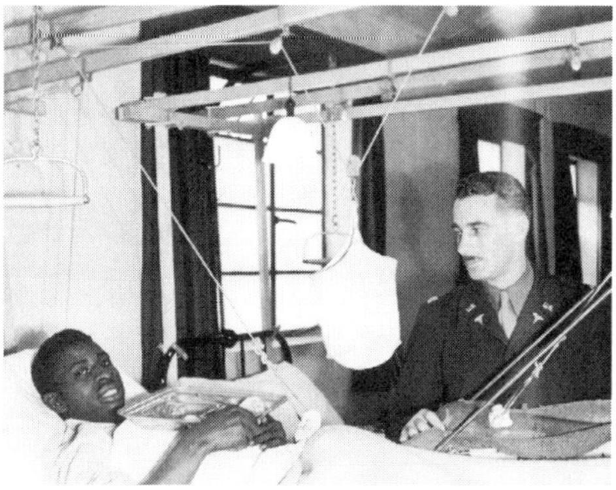

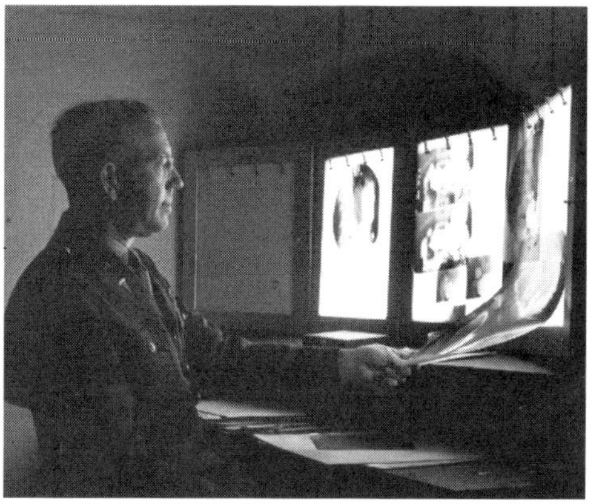

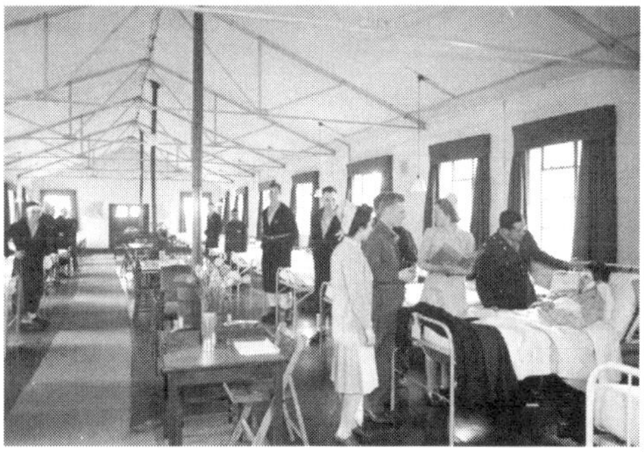

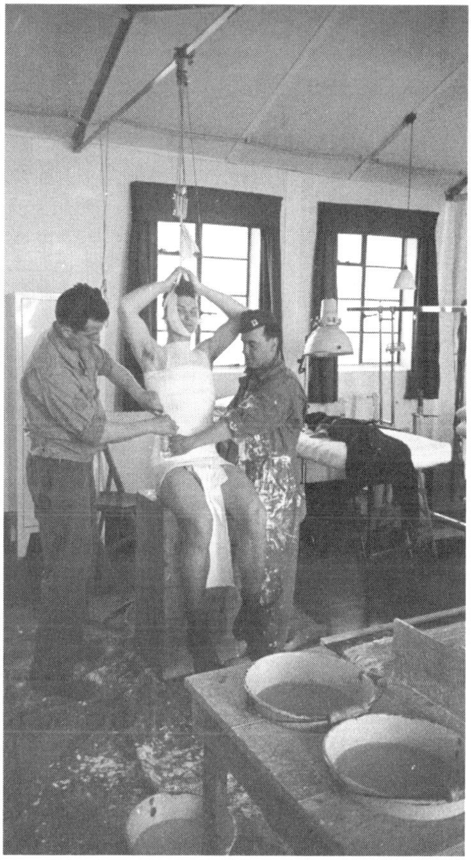

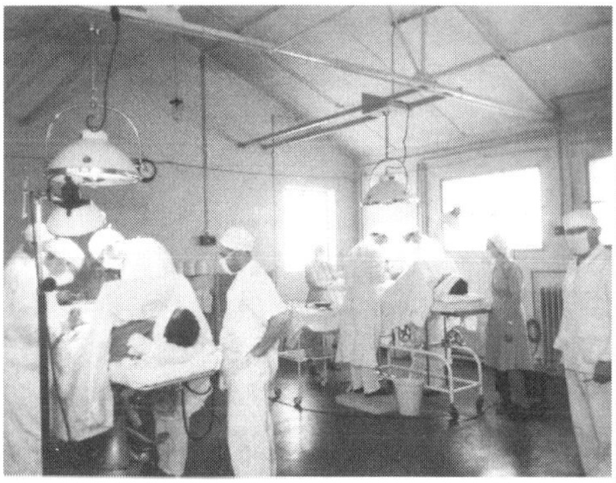

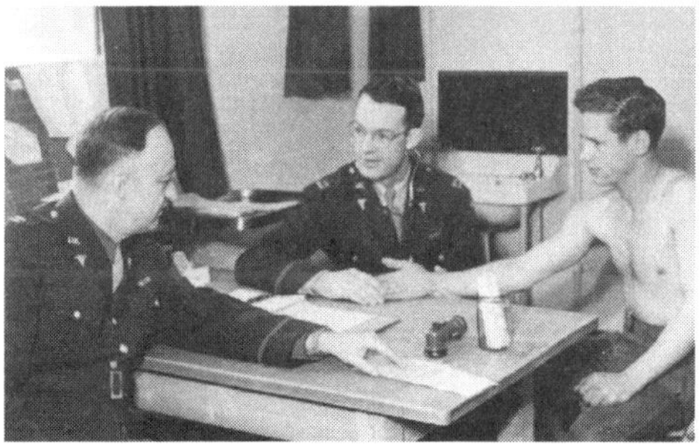

Clockwise from top left: Stevens visiting a patient in the segregated ward; Rulison studying x-rays; Kirkwood (right) molding a full body cast; Leonard E. Nichols, Class of 1922 (left), and John W. Rowlingson, Class of 1940 (right) consulting with a patient; Rowlingson (left) and Robert O. Gregg, Class of 1934 (right), performing surgery on the patient in the left foreground with Martin E. Melamed, Class of 1931, serving as anesthesiologist; Bregande making rounds.

Upstate Medical University has sent personnel to every American conflict since its founding in 1834, but its first official mission of this kind was in World War I when Syracuse University supplied physicians for U.S. Army Base Hospital 31, Medical Unit G, stationed in Contrexeville, France. Even before the United States entered the war on April 6, 1917, George Washington Crile, the surgeon who had become famous in the 1890s for controlling hemorrhage in the operating room, was negotiating in Ohio with the American Red Cross and the Allied Expeditionary Force to establish military hospitals in Europe. The Youngstown Hospital Association organized such a hospital on March 25, 1917, but in April the authority for these overseas operations shifted from the Red Cross to the U.S. Army. Volunteer physicians would thereafter apply through the Red Cross for commissions in the Army Officer Reserve Corps.

Base Hospital 31 arrived in Contrexeville on January 1, 1918. Meanwhile, in Syracuse, surgeon Edward Van Duyn, Class of 1897, was recruiting orthopedist Clarence E. Coon, Class of 1898; internists William Dewey Alsever, Class of 1900, Henry Burton Doust, Class of 1900, and Earl V. Sweet; surgeon and otologist George S. Britten, Class of 1900; dermatologist Henry A. McGruer; surgeons Clyde Orrin Barney, Class of 1910, Murray A. Cain, Class of 1910, J. Herbert Irish, and Arthur D. Meyers; bacteriologist Walden E. Muns; twenty-one nurses from Good Shepherd; and, from about 250 applicants, mostly Syracuse University students, forty-eight enlisted men. This medical detachment, Unit G, was organized in June 1917, mobilized in December, and ordered to France in February 1918. Assigned to Base Hospital 31, it got to Contrexeville on March 13, where it served until the Army closed the hospital on February 2, 1919.

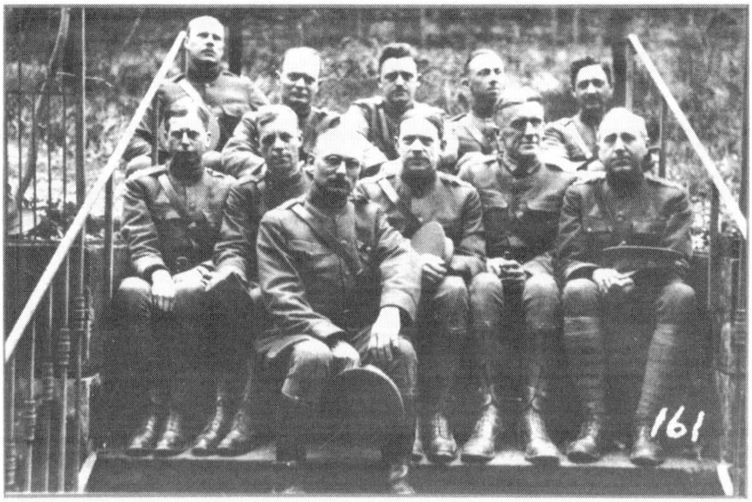

UNIT G···SYRACUSE UNIVERSITY MEDICAL COLLEGE
MAJOR E.S. VAN DUYN – COMMANDING
CONTREXEVILLE, FRANCE 1918

Top Row–Walden E. Munns 1st Lt., George S. Britten Capt., Arthur Meyers 1st Lt., Murray A. Cain 1st Lt., Clyde O. Barney 1st Lt., Bottom Row–H. Burton Doust Capt., Edward S. Van Duyn Maj., Earl V. Sweet 1st Lt., Henry MacGruer Capt., Clarence Coon Capt. Dewey Alsever Capt.

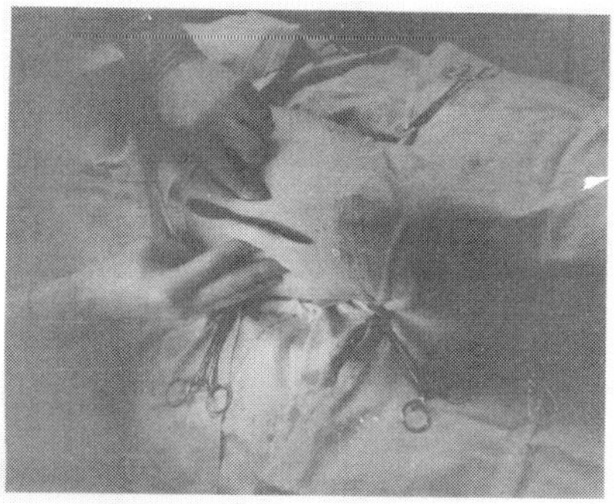

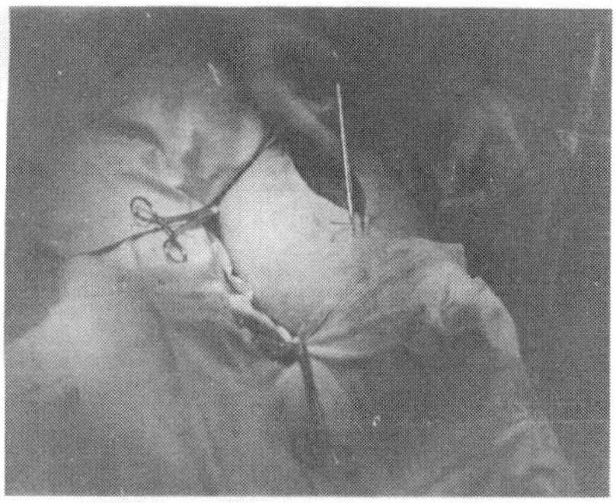

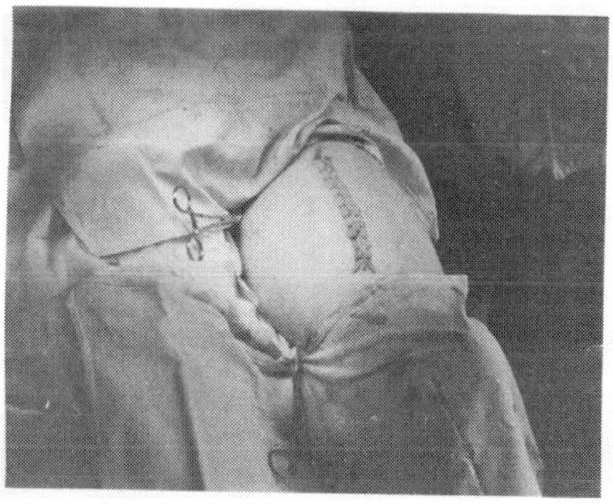

The 52nd admitted its first patient on April 15, 1943. There were many psychiatric and infectious cases, but few trauma patients before D-Day. The first battle casualties from Normandy arrived the second week of June 1944. From then until early 1945 the beds were filled nearly to capacity. The busiest and most difficult time was when the Nazis almost blunted the Allied invasion at the Battle of the Bulge in December 1944, but the load steadily lightened in 1945. By V-E Day only 300 patients remained. Altogether the 52nd treated more than 21,000.

The 52nd was one of the best military hospitals in World War II. In March 1944 Surgeon General of the Army Norman T. Kirk inspected the 52nd and ranked it near the top among U.S. Army affiliated hospitals in the European Theater of Operations (ETO).

Surgery always advances in time of war as surgeons are forced to confront dramatic new presentations. Beyond the usual surgical skills, military surgery demands innovation, speed, efficiency, keen analysis, and a degree of luck. Shortcuts and risks may be taken where they would not be tolerated in civilian practice, especially when the influx of trauma patients overwhelms the team. Within the 52nd, ophthalmologist Anthony and neurosurgeon Ecker were among the most innovative and were known throughout the ETO. The Nazis even spied on Ecker to learn surgical techniques.

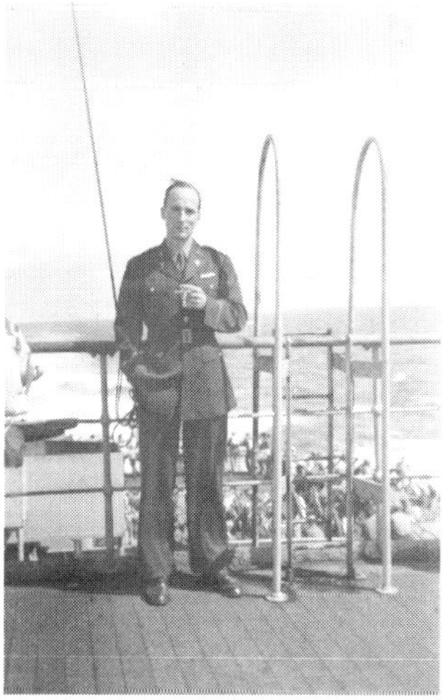

Many of its members were reassigned to other units, especially after D-Day, but the 52nd remained at Wolverley until June 26, 1945, then was transferred to Bristol and finally, in September, home to be disbanded. Of course, the best part of war is going home. Internist Kenneth J. ("Jack") McDermott, a Syracuse physician who served elsewhere in Great Britain, is homebound aboard the *Queen Elizabeth* in August 1945.

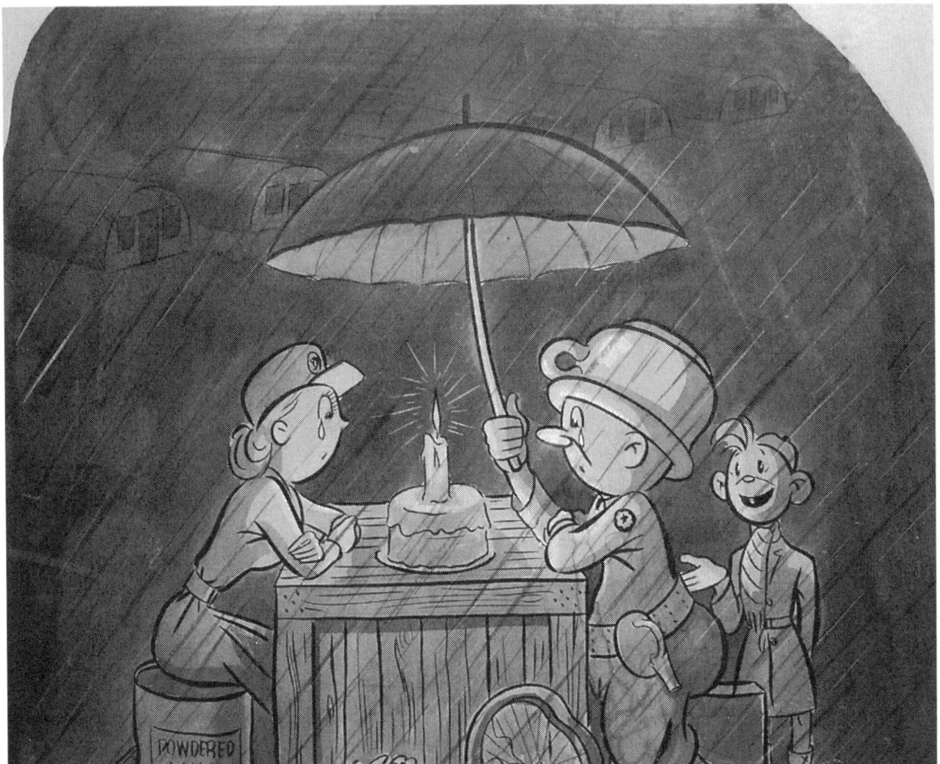

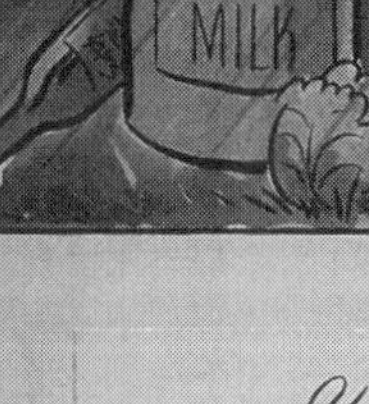

SEASONS
GREETINGS

FROM
THE 52nd GENERAL HOSPITAL
SOMEWHERE IN ENGLAND

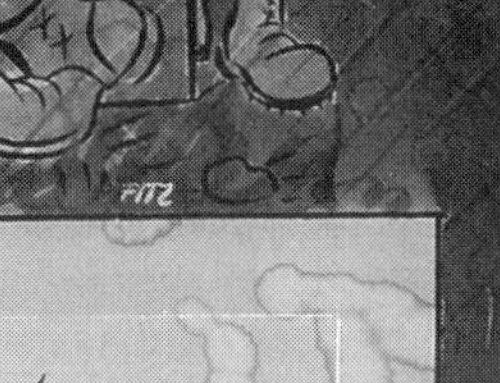

8

New York State Takes Over

On June 1, 1950, Syracuse University sold its medical education resources and transferred its medical faculty to the two-year-old State University of New York, which re-established the medical school as part of SUNY.

The hallmark of the 1950s was the administration's deliberate and mostly successful attempt to improve the quality of science at Upstate. Certainly Weiskotten had been committed to science, but the new dean, William R. Willard (left), proved to be even more energetic in this direction. Weiskotten announced over a year in advance that he would retire on June 30, 1951. In preparation for retirement, he had laid solid groundwork for his successor, even to the point of hiring architects Francis Day Rogers and Jonathan Fairchild Butler in January 1951 to design the basic sciences addition to the College of Medicine building. SUNY approved their plans on May 19, 1951.

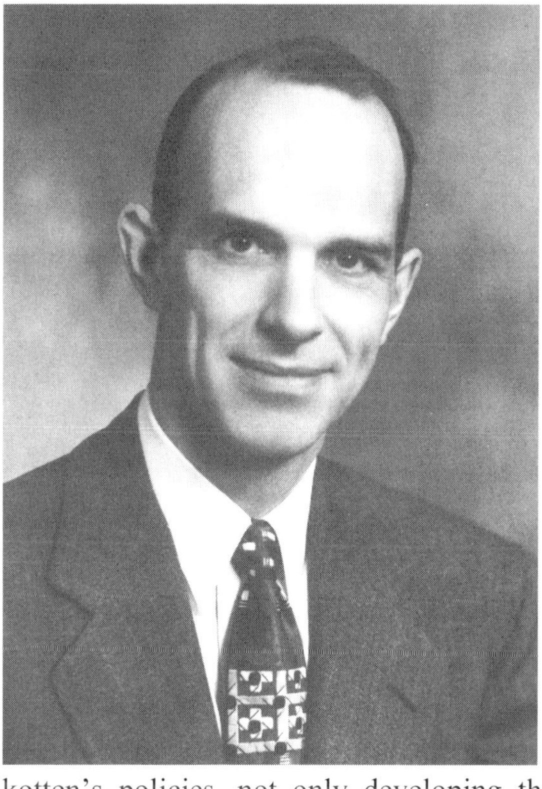

Willard, who earned his M.D. at Yale in 1934, was appointed dean on June 19, 1951, and took office on July 1. He supported and continued Weiskotten's policies, not only developing the basic sciences, but also expanding facilities for the clinical sciences, especially surgery; arranging for increases in the number of students; and beginning the graduate degree program. He resigned on August 31, 1956, to become the founding vice president of the University of Kentucky Medical Center and the founding dean of its medical school. He left a remarkable legacy at the University of Kentucky, where the main medical education building and several professorships and awards are named for him.

By the late 1940s Syracuse University had become anxious to divest itself of its expensive medical school, but it wanted the best of both worlds. On the one hand, it expected the sale agreement to stipulate that the state would pay off the medical school's debts, especially those of Good Shepherd, and thereafter contribute the lion's share of the medical school's operating expenses, which were then about $400,000 a year (about $3,250,000 in 2005 dollars); while on the other hand, it wanted to maintain a close working relationship with the medical school, similar to what it had enjoyed with the New York State College of Forestry since its founding in 1911. The SUNY administration, for its part, wanted its new medical school in Central New York to become completely independent of Syracuse University as soon as possible. Its aim was for the Long Island College Hospital in Brooklyn and the Syracuse University College of Medicine, including Good Shepherd, to come into the SUNY system simultaneously as sister institutions, SUNY Downstate and SUNY Upstate. This aim was achieved, but negotiations were long and difficult. Much credit belongs to State Senator John H. Hughes* — an Onondaga County Republican who represented four different districts in Central New York from 1947 to 1972 — for ensuring that the deal was successfully brokered.

Various arms of SUNY, both from local offices and from central administration in Albany, pressured Syracuse University to relinquish full control of the medical school, to release all medical endowment funds, to transfer all medically related educational materials such as library books and laboratory equipment to the state, and to allow the transformation of the University Hospital of the Good Shepherd into Upstate University Hospital. As this process continued throughout the 1950s, the transition of the medical school and Good Shepherd from private to public management was at best gradual and more commonly piecemeal. After the state's legal objectives were accomplished, Syracuse University complied in good faith. Yet there remained gaps, omissions, and oversights, all of which Syracuse University rectified as soon as each was discovered. Even as late as the mid-1990s Syracuse University librarians would still occasionally find medical books in library storage and immediately transfer them to Upstate.

The first public hearing on the proposed combined acquisition of what would become SUNY Downstate and SUNY Upstate occurred in New York City on January 10, 1949. SUNY already planned to increase the student population at both schools dramatically without any dilution of the high quality of teaching that the private medical schools in Brooklyn and Syracuse had established. On June 16, 1949, the SUNY Trustees and the SUNY Committee on Medical Education made this announcement official.

---

* The State Office Building in Syracuse is named for Senator Hughes.

The formal transfer of the College of Medicine from Syracuse University to SUNY occurred on June 26, 1950. The state assumed the $640,000 mortgage on the property and agreed to offset a maximum of $100,000 of Good Shepherd's expenses for fiscal year 1950-1951; Syracuse University donated the land and Yates Castle. The official name of the new institution was the SUNY College of Medicine at Syracuse, but in January 1953, because of its continuing close relations with Good Shepherd and other clinical facilities, because the state intended to push vigorously toward Weiskotten's goal of a comprehensive academic medical center, and because plans were already afoot to begin offering other professional degrees besides the M.D., it became the SUNY Upstate Medical Center.

In the spring of 1954 SUNY, Yates Castle's new owner, demolished the already crumbling edifice to make room for the southeast wing to the College of Medicine building.

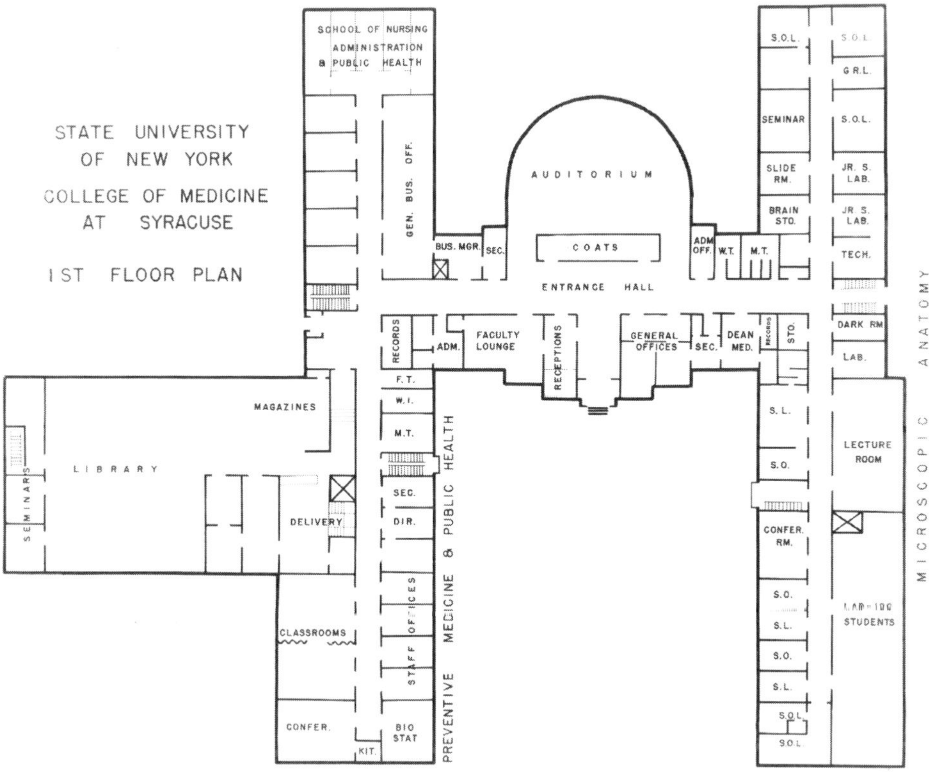

As soon as it took over, the state mandated and encouraged rapid expansion of all medical school departments, particularly the basic science departments. This was welcome news to the professors in these departments, who had typically felt hamstrung as employees of Syracuse University, unable to pursue the research they wanted or to have enough faculty colleagues to teach their students properly. Now under SUNY administration they were not only free, but also financially supported, to rebuild their respective departments as first-rate scientific enterprises. Growth was rapid indeed and the success rate was high.

The expansion of basic science programs and the increased emphasis on science in clinical programs were advantageous for Upstate in many ways throughout the 1950s. Distinguished scientists chaired Upstate departments in this era, and their leadership and national reputations attracted to Upstate other scientists who would continue these advantages into the 1960s. Scientific learning was not confined to the laboratories and formal classrooms. The spirit of inquiry was hale and hearty across the institution.

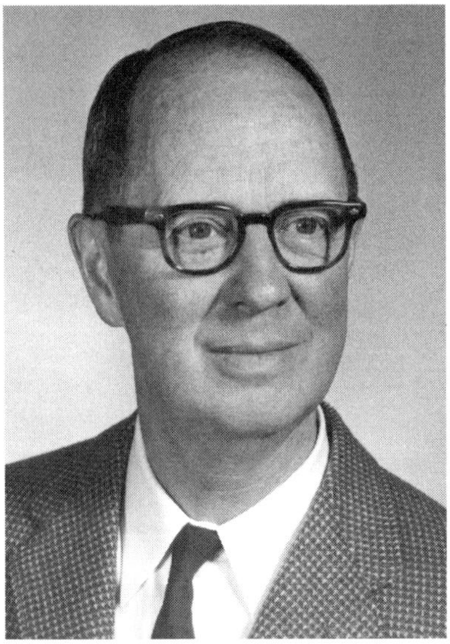

Many professors in the 1950s held noncredit seminars open to anyone on campus who wished to explore scientific topics.

Philip B. Armstrong (left) succeeded Stiles as Professor and Chair of Anatomy in 1938 and served until he retired in 1966. Under his leadership the time for teaching anatomy to first-year medical students was reduced from 1056 to 660 hours but, since at least the same amount of material was covered, the course became more rigorous. Armstrong began to create anatomical and cell biology research programs in the 1940s, but these did not become strong components of the department until the early 1950s when the state gave him more financial and administrative leeway than Syracuse University had. By 1956 Upstate was able to offer a Ph.D. in anatomy.

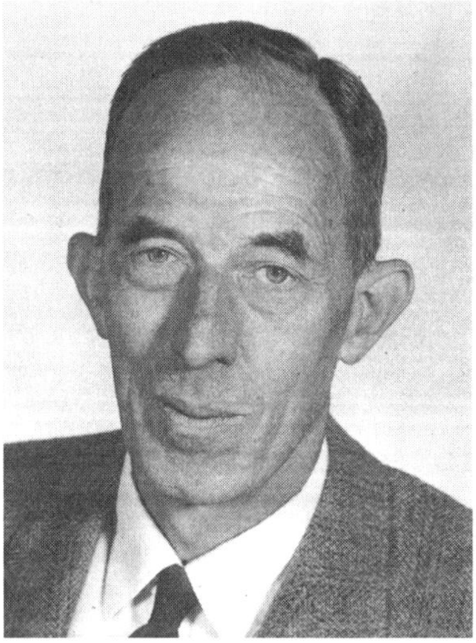

Chester L. Yntema (right), who earned his Ph.D. at Yale in 1930, already had a national scientific reputation in comparative anatomy when he became a member of the faculty in 1946. He achieved his greatest renown for his studies of the embryology of the snapping turtle, especially "A Series of Stages in the Embryonic Development of *Chelydra Serpentina*," which appeared in *The Journal of Morphology* in 1968 and remains fundamental for all reptilian embryology. Despite this achievement, Yntema himself regarded his work on the origin of the sympathetic nervous system of the chicken from the neural crest as more important.

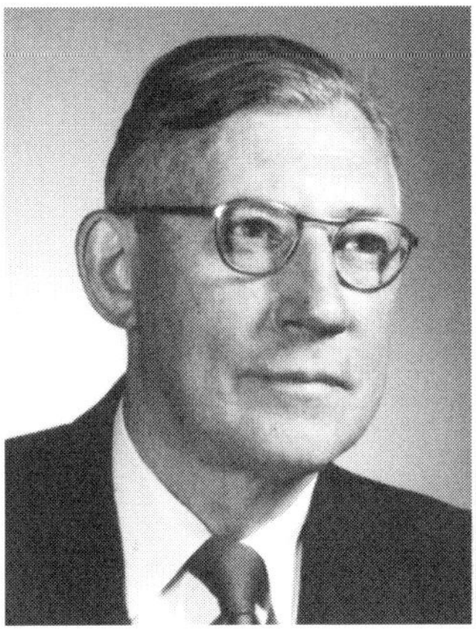 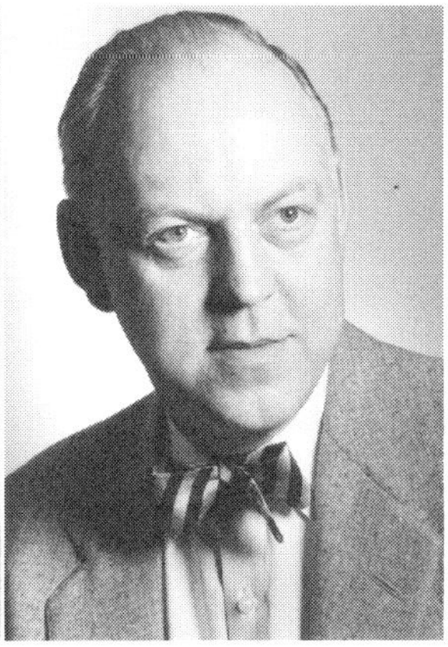 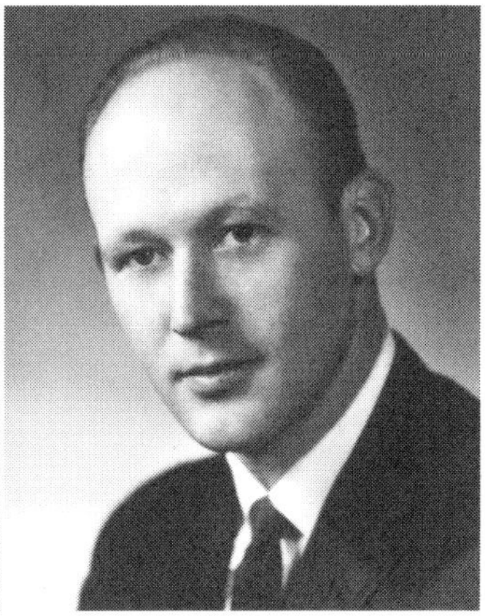

Orren Chapman (left) chaired the Department of Microbiology from 1943 to 1959, presiding over its name change from Bacteriology and Parasitology to Microbiology in 1954. Justus Mueller acted as chair from 1954 to 1956 while Chapman was in Jordan on a public health development mission sponsored by the International Cooperation Administration of the U.S. State Department. Paul F. Wehrle, a pediatrician whose main research concerned infectious diseases, acted as Chair of Microbiology from 1959 until he left Upstate in 1961 to chair the Department of Pediatrics at the University of Southern California. While at Upstate he had helped to develop the Salk polio vaccine and in the 1960s and 1970s he contributed in a major way toward the World Health Organization's successful campaign to eradicate smallpox.

Gordon K. Moe (center) received his Ph.D. in physiology from the University of Minnesota in 1940 and his M.D. from Harvard in 1943. After teaching pharmacology at the University of Michigan for six years, he came to Upstate in 1950 as Professor and Chair of Physiology. He held this position until 1960, when, through the intercession of Syracuse cardiologist J.G. Fred Hiss, Class of 1917, he became Director of Research at the Masonic Medical Research Laboratory in Utica. Specializing in cardiac electrophysiology, Moe sowed the seeds in Central New York for research in cardiology that would later bear excellent fruit in the work of one of Moe's protégés, José Jalife.

James Benson Preston (right) received his M.D. from the University of Cincinnati in 1952, taught pharmacology at the University of Illinois, then came to Upstate in 1954 as Instructor in Physiology. He was promoted in 1956 to assistant professor and in 1960, at the age of only 34, to Professor and Chair of Physiology, posts which he held until his retirement in 1991. Like Moe, Preston was interested in cardiac electrophysiology, but most of his published research concerned the primate motor cortex, especially as regards impulses to the hand.

After Marion Dooley retired in 1945, Allan D. Bass arrived in Syracuse from Army duty to chair the Department of Pharmacology until 1952, when he left Upstate to chair the department at Vanderbilt University. During his tenure in Central New York, the major issue for pharmacology was developing the commercial potential of penicillin, sulfonamides, and other

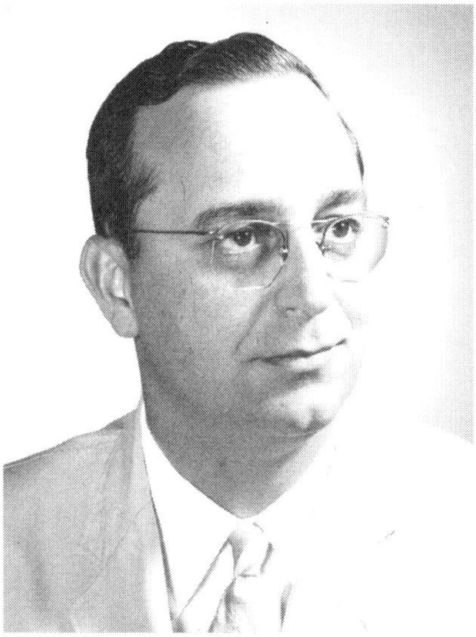

"wonder drugs," many of which were manufactured at the Bristol-Myers plant in Syracuse. Bass's departure put Upstate in a classic win-win situation, because Alfred E. Farah (left) and Jay Tepperman, the two insider candidates to succeed him as chair, each had solid national reputations. Farah was chosen on the grounds that he was more purely a pharmacologist while Tepperman's research involved a good measure of physiology. Farah served as chair from 1953 until 1968, when he resigned to become director of the Biological Division of the Sterling-Winthrop Research Institute.

Having such outstanding investigators as Armstrong, Yntema, Moe, Mueller, Farah, Westerfeld, and Wehrle on Upstate's basic science faculty lent great strength and prestige to their respective departments in the 1950s and to the medical center in general. The talent was in place to begin reputable graduate education. On December 10, 1953, the central SUNY administration approved a plan to develop programs to award M.S. and Ph.D. degrees in the various biosciences at its two medical schools. The next year graduate studies began at Upstate, with eighteen students and new courses in anatomy, biochemistry, microbiology, pathology, pharmacology, and physiology. The Syracuse University College of Medicine had actually begun graduate education in the biosciences on this campus in 1947 by offering the Ph.D. in biochemistry, but that degree was given by the university as a whole, not by the medical school. In 1957, under the joint administration of the Graduate Executive Committee, which consisted of Westerfeld (chair), Yntema, Mueller, Farah, Moe, and administrator Joseph K. Hill, the Graduate Program in Medical Sciences became the School of Graduate Studies. It acquired its own dean, Westerfeld, in 1961, and in 1973 was renamed the College of Graduate Studies. In June 1958 it awarded its first M.S. and in June 1959 its first Ph.D. — to Arthur A. Iodice, in biochemistry, with a dissertation entitled "Purification and Properties of δ-Aminolevulinic Acid Dehydrase," directed by Dan A. Richert and Martin P. Schulman.

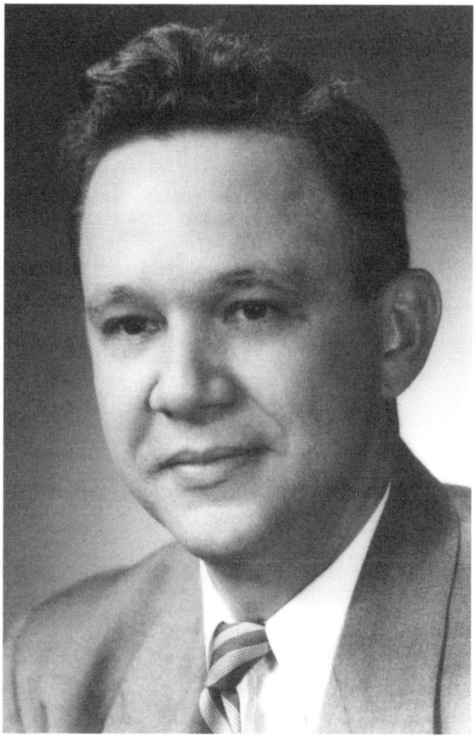

Westerfeld (right) became interim dean on September 1, 1956, following Willard's resignation. As Professor and Chair of Biochemistry for a remarkable thirty-four years from 1945 to 1979 except for a brief period in 1967 and 1968 when he was interim president, he led the shift in biochemical emphasis from "test tube studies" to molecular biology. Devoted to creating and nourishing the various graduate degree programs in the biosciences, he served from 1961 to 1965 as Associate Dean for Graduate Education and Research and from 1965 to 1967 as Dean for Graduate Education in Sciences Basic to Medicine.

After earning his Ph.D. in biochemistry at St. Louis University in 1938, Westerfeld held positions at Oxford, Columbia, and Harvard before coming to Syracuse at Weiskotten's personal behest in 1945. Weiskotten had "discovered" Westerfeld during one of his visits to Harvard. Westerfeld wanted to stay at Harvard, but his department chair, A. Baird Hastings, believed that working for Weiskotten would be good for his career. Weiskotten, Armstrong, Chapman, and even Chancellor Tolley all contributed to entice him to Syracuse. He agreed only when he was allowed to bring in Richert and John M. McKibbin to add a research dimension to the department.

While plans were advancing to close Good Shepherd on Marshall Street and reopen it as Upstate University Hospital in a new facility on Adams Street, Syracuse University, which had not included either the buildings or the land of the McBride Street campus in the 1950 deal, announced in 1954 that Upstate would soon have to vacate the Dispensary building on Fayette Street. Syracuse University had already renovated the 1896 medical school building on McBride Street, renamed it in honor of Jesse T. Peck, and used it since 1947 for University College, which had evolved in 1946 from the Syracuse University School of Extension, founded in 1902. Now Syracuse University wanted to remodel the Dispensary building similarly, rename it after the Rev. John Morrison Reid, an early trustee and benefactor of the university, and use it also for University College. This was accomplished in 1957. The Dispensary relocated to offices rented in the State Building at 333 East Washington Street.

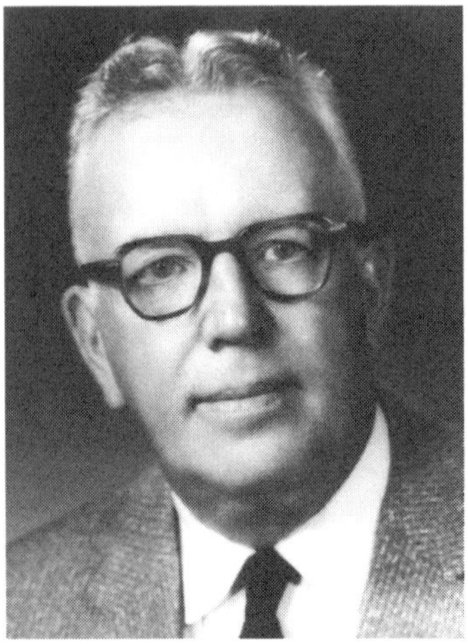

Radiology achieved full departmental status under Donald S. Childs, Class of 1909, who taught radiology from 1920 and chaired the department until 1948. When one of the best loved and most respected physicians in the history of Syracuse, Foster Rulison (left), the chief of radiology in the 52nd General Hospital, returned home from the war, the College of Medicine made him professor of radiology and promoted him to department chair upon Childs's retirement. Rulison's radiological expertise was unquestioned, and even though his term as chair lasted only three years until he retired, he and his successor, Clayton H. Hale, Class of 1939, were together largely responsible for laying the groundwork of the continued excellence of the department.

The Department of Surgery was chaired from 1946 to 1953 by Arthur B. Raffl and from 1953 to 1956 by Robert O. Gregg, Class of 1934. Both were veterans of the 52nd General Hospital, Raffl as Chief of Surgical Service at the rank of lieutenant colonel. Raffl received his M.D. at Washington University in 1919, interned at the Cleveland Clinic, was already recognized as an expert in thyroid surgery when he came to Syracuse in 1926, and co-founded the American Board of Surgery in 1937. Gregg began as a pathologist, but in 1935 he decided to be a surgeon instead. After earning an M.S. in surgery from the Mayo Clinic in 1939, he returned to Syracuse and became well known as both a teacher of general surgery and a practitioner of vascular surgery. He resigned as chair, but not as professor, in 1956 to give more time to his practice.

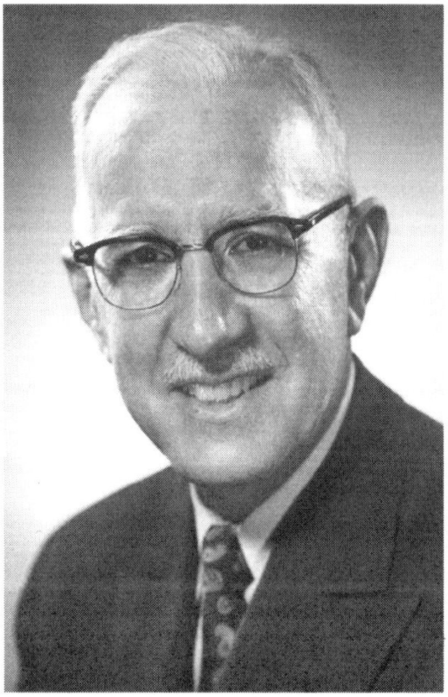

In 1956 Gordon Hoople (right), who chaired the Department of Otolaryngology from 1946 to 1953, began a three-year term as President of the American Board of Otolaryngology. Other high points of his career included chairing the Syracuse University Board of Trustees and founding the Hoople Hearing and Speech Center and the Gebbie Speech-Language Hearing Clinics in the Communication Sciences and Disorders Program of the Syracuse University School of Education.

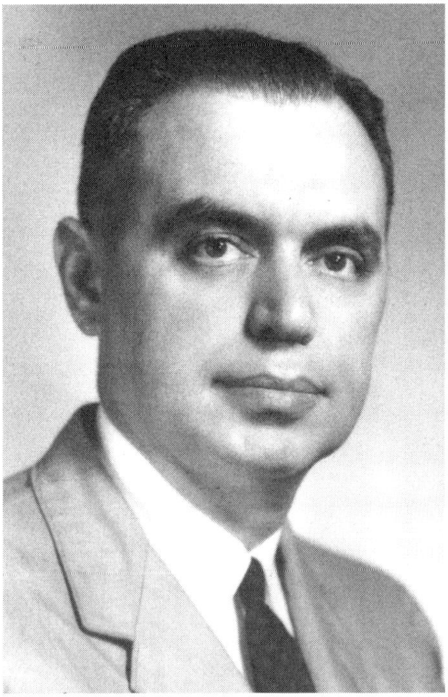

In June 1953 Julius B. Richmond (left), became Upstate's first full-time Professor of Pediatrics and, except for a period of illness in 1967, chaired the department until 1970, even while serving as Dean of the College of Medicine from 1965 to 1970. In the 1960s his collaboration with early childhood expert Bettye M. Caldwell, Ph.D., Research Associate at Upstate from 1959 to 1965 and Professor of Education at Syracuse University from 1965 to 1969, led to the creation of the federal Head Start program. After President Lyndon Johnson appointed him to the Office of Economic Opportunity as Project Director of Head Start in early 1965, Richmond spent a year and a half commuting between Syracuse and Washington, doing three jobs. He was also instrumental in establishing the Young Mothers Education and Development (YMED) program in the Syracuse City School District to help teenage mothers earn their high school diplomas by providing day care and psychological support.

In 1970 Richmond left for Boston to become Professor of Child Psychiatry and Human Development at Harvard Medical School and Director of the Judge Baker Guidance Center. In 1971 he became Chair of the Department of Preventive and Social Medicine at Harvard. In 1977 President Jimmy Carter appointed him U.S. Surgeon General and Assistant Secretary for Health in the Department of Health and Human Services.

Weiskotten, though retired from Upstate, remained active in medicine both locally and nationally throughout the 1950s. On December 17, 1953, the business tycoon Howard R. Hughes chartered the Howard Hughes Medical Institute (HHMI) as a non-profit philanthropic foundation to promote bioscientific and medical research. Hughes hired Weiskotten, Verne R. Mason, M.D., of the University of Southern California, Hugh Morgan, M.D., of Vanderbilt University, and George Thorn, M.D., of Harvard University in 1954 to plan the institute. These four distinguished medical educators founded its Medical Advisory Board in 1955. Even though Weiskotten and Hughes collaborated on this project, they never actually met. Hughes had become so reclusive by that time in his career that he always worked through intermediaries; so even Weiskotten, like everyone else, could deal only with Hughes's staff.

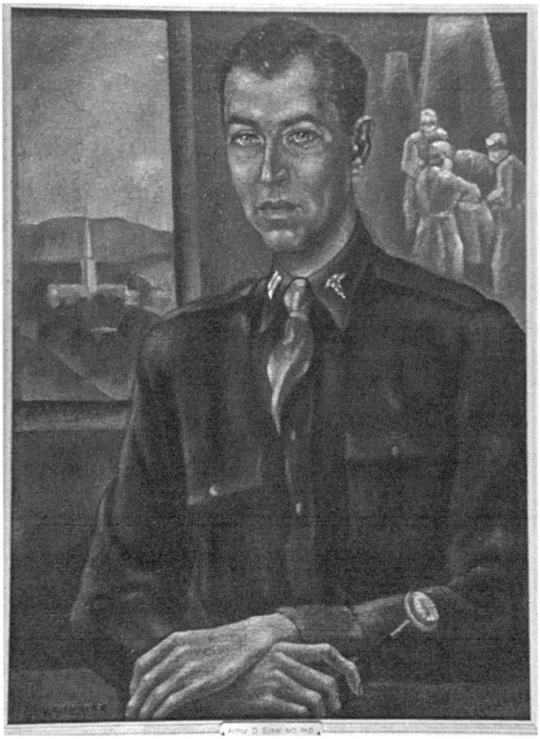

Arthur Ecker was the first neurosurgeon in Syracuse, arriving in 1939. He received his A.B. *summa cum laude* from Dartmouth in 1931 at the age of only eighteen, his M.D. from Johns Hopkins in 1934, and his Ph.D. in neurology from the University of Minnesota in 1938. He held a fellowship in neurology and neurosurgery at the Mayo Clinic from 1935 to 1939, when Weiskotten invited him to the Syracuse University College of Medicine — over the objections of Swift, who believed that general surgeons could handle neurosurgical duties — to found what became in 1966 the Department of Neurosurgery under Robert B. King. Ecker taught at Upstate until 1963 and practiced neurosurgery in Syracuse until he retired in 1988.

As a pioneer of neuroradiology, neurosurgery, and cerebral angiography, Ecker published two books and 120 articles. Among his works are the first demonstration of cerebral vasospasm and, in 1951, *The Normal Cerebral Angiogram*, the first American monograph on cerebral angiography. He was the first to describe upward brain herniation into the foramen magnum and through the tentorial notch. Ecker discovered that placing trigeminal rhizolysis patients in a supine position for the absolute alcohol injection reduces the risk of corneal anesthesia and subsequent keratitis. He and radiologist Theodore Perl, Class of 1941, improved previous radiographic technique to ensure precise injection placement in the Gasserian ganglion for relief of trigeminal neuralgia. This was his clearest success. He said that trigeminal neuralgia patients are the most grateful of all patients, and that his greatest satisfaction as a physician came from finally seeing them smile painlessly for the first time after their long endurance of suffering.

Austrian-British artist Herbert Gurschner painted the above portrait in July 1944 when Ecker was stationed near Salisbury, England, after his transfer from the 52nd General Hospital. Because of wartime shortages of materials in Britain, Gurschner used burlap instead of artist's canvas and either boat paint or linseed-oil-based house paint instead of artist's oil paint. Conservator Peter Schulz restored and stabilized the painting in 1996.

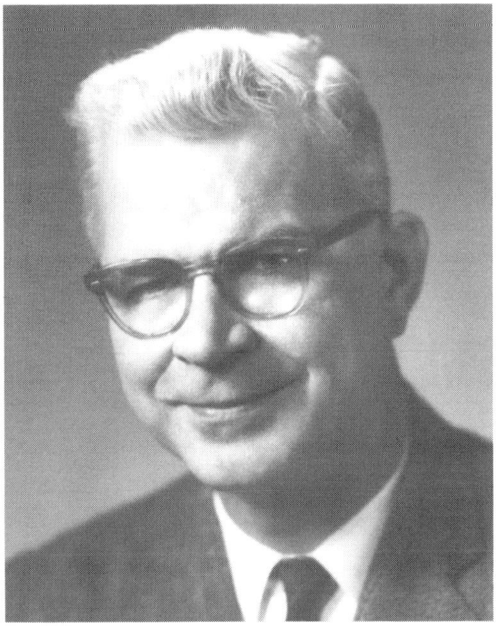

The Department of Medicine received a tremendous boost in 1947 when Richard H. Lyons (right) became chair, succeeding Edward C. Reifenstein and assuming a newly endowed professorship named in honor of his predecessor. Lyons, a 1935 University of Michigan M.D., was the first full-time Professor of Medicine at the Syracuse University College of Medicine. The mainstays of his department were Paul A. Bunn; Ellery Allen; Eugene L. Lozner; J.G. Fred Hiss; Harry Feldman; John Duggan (below); H. Walden Retan, Class of 1921; Maynard E. Holmes, Class of 1918; William Faloon, and J. Howland Auchincloss. Lyons was stubborn in his opinions, but an outstanding clinician, a strong leader, and a very popular teacher. His grand rounds were legendary. When he presented, the largest possible room was necessary; when he was in the audience, his comments were the highlight of the session. He established a close relationship between his department and the clinical staff of the Veterans Administration Hospital, so that as soon as the VA opened in 1953, his students had those teaching services available to them.

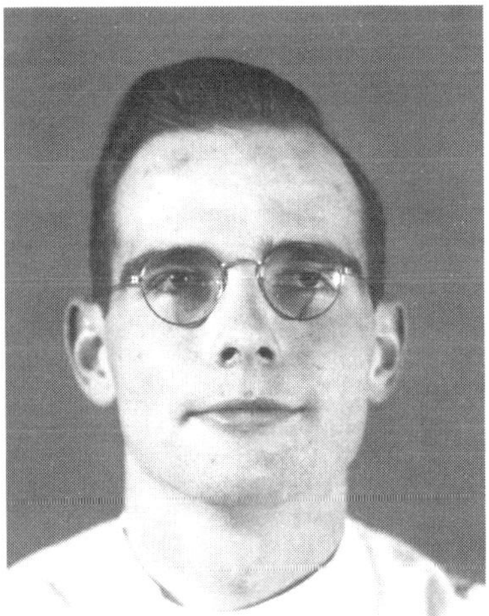

Lyons resigned in 1967 to become Director of the Central New York Regional Medical Program, a joint project of Upstate and the U.S. Department of Health, Education, and Welfare to improve local public health by increasing access to health care. The program existed only from 1967 to 1976 and had only moderate success. Its functions were to some extent taken over by the Central New York Health Systems Agency, which was founded in 1976 as a quasi-private, partially state-funded organization headquartered in Syracuse. According to its mission statement, it serves eleven counties in Central New York "to promote development of health care services, improved access to care, and community health improvement through collaboration, research, data collection, and analysis."

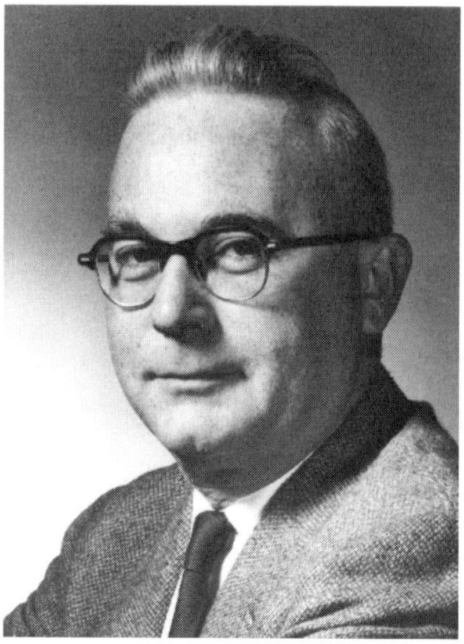

Harry Alfred Feldman (right) was among the premier infectious disease experts of his time. After receiving his M.D. from George Washington University in 1939, he held research fellowships at George Washington, Harvard Medical School, and the Children's Hospital Research Foundation in Cincinnati before coming to Syracuse in 1948 as Associate Professor of Medicine. He became Associate Professor of Preventive Medicine in 1955, full professor in 1956, and chaired the Department of Preventive Medicine from 1957 until his death in 1985.

Feldman published 216 scientific papers between 1938 and 1983. In serology, he co-developed the Sabin-Feldman dye test for toxoplasmosis with Albert B. Sabin. Besides this and other work with *Toxoplasma gondii* and other parasitic protozoans, including *Acanthamoeba*, he achieved international recognition for his research on meningococcal diseases, streptococcal infections, various respiratory diseases, malaria, rubella, measles, and AIDS, all of which had important ramifications for preventive medicine, epidemiology, immunology, and infectious disease control.

Upstate's rigorous emphasis on science throughout the 1950s sustained a competitive atmosphere that arguably fostered among these alumni greater subsequent achievement per capita as clinicians, medical educators, and bioscientists than in any other decade of classes in Upstate's history. The most notable of these achievers was probably Paul Douglas Parkman, Class of 1957 (right), who was part of the team at Walter Reed Army Medical Center that isolated the rubella virus in 1962. As Chief of the General Virology Section in the Laboratory for Viral Immunology in the Division of Biologics Standards at the National Institutes of Health (NIH) from 1963 to 1972, he created a vaccine for rubella, began using it in October 1965, and in September 1966 reported successful clinical trials in *The New England Journal of Medicine*. Mostly thanks to Parkman, the last significant outbreak of rubella in the United States was in 1964.

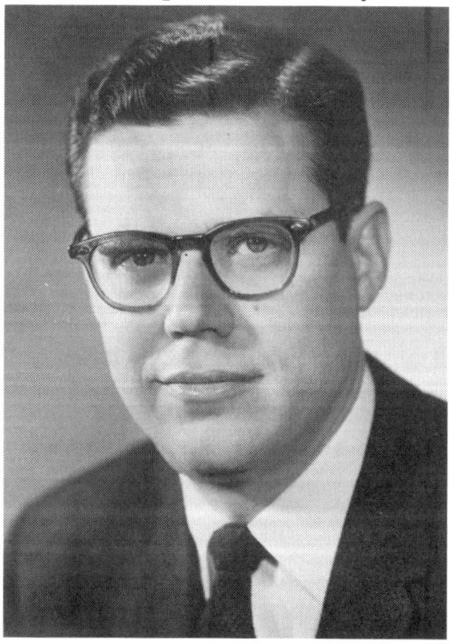

9

Rejuvenation and Expansion

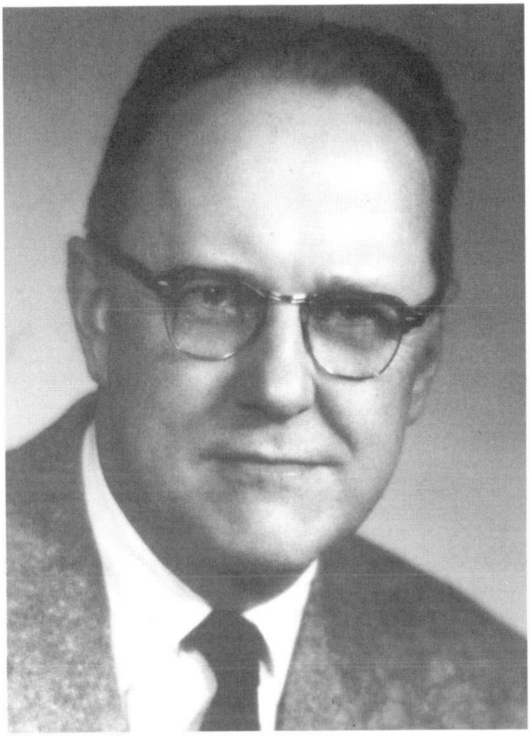

After Willard's departure, Westerfeld acted as interim dean from September 1, 1956, until December 1, 1957, when Carlyle F. Jacobsen, Ph.D. (left), became the first president of the medical center. Given the added responsibilities that had accrued to the deanship since Weiskotten's time, the administration had decided in August 1957 that the chief campus executive would thenceforth be called President of Upstate Medical Center and Dean of the College of Medicine. Jacobsen was appointed to this new position in September but began both sets of duties in December. Creating the presidency further prepared the institution to expand into other kinds of bioscientific education besides training physicians. The presidency and the deanship remained vested in the same person until February 5, 1965, when Jacobsen, remaining as president, appointed Richmond as dean.

Jacobsen received his doctorate in psychology from the University of Minnesota in 1928, then studied anthropoid animals and taught at Yale University, Cornell University, Washington University in St. Louis, and the University of Iowa before joining SUNY in 1950. In Iowa he was Executive Dean for the Health Sciences. Since April 1, 1950, he had been Executive Dean for Medical Education at the SUNY central office in Albany. Before coming to Syracuse he had already acquired superior organizational skills, especially with regard to the techniques of securing grant funding. He knew personally most of the people who influenced American medicine, including medical school deans across the country, elected and appointed politicians, and several top administrators at NIH.

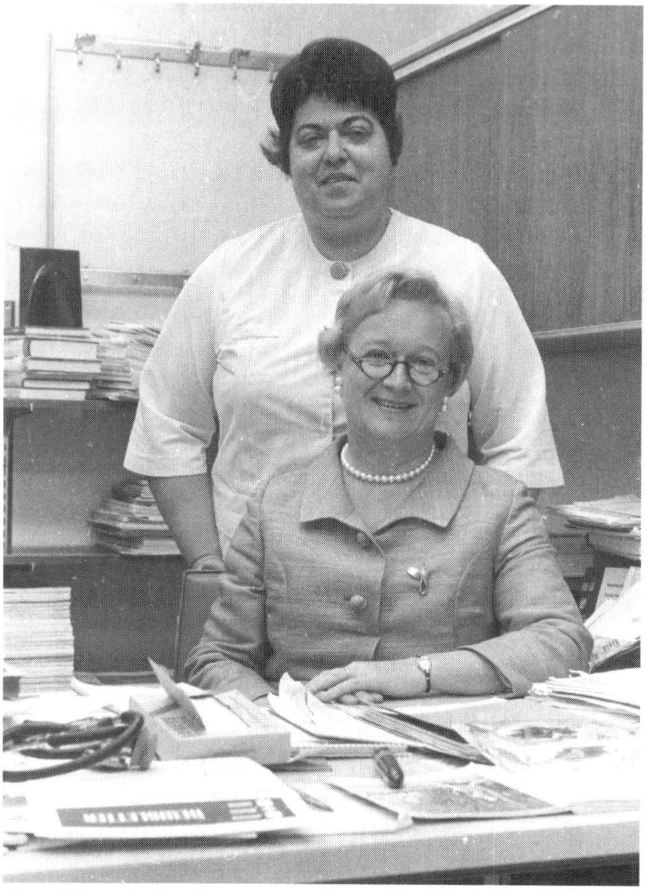

Ellen T. Cook, Class of 1950, married President Jacobsen in 1957. After completing her residency at Upstate she began teaching in the Department of Medicine in 1953 and rose to Associate Professor of Medicine. From 1968 to 1970 she did a second residency at Upstate, this time in psychiatry, and eventually became Associate Professor of Psychiatry. In the 1960s she (foreground) and nurse Shirley Reit (background) ran the Student and Employee Health Service and Diagnostic Office in Room 4800 of University Hospital. As a member of the Department of Psychiatry until she retired in 1990, she worked closely with Eugene A. Kaplan, Class of 1957, son-in-law of Arthur Ecker. Kaplan also did his psychiatric residency at Upstate, then joined Upstate's psychiatric faculty in 1961. As chair of the department from 1986 to 1999, he was nationally recognized as a leader and innovator in psychiatric education.

Upstate's most famous psychiatrist is Thomas S. Szasz, whose international reputation as a libertarian philosopher of medicine is based, despite his prolific output of publications, mostly on just one book, *The Myth of Mental Illness*, which appeared in 1961, five years after he began teaching at Upstate. The swift, multifaceted reaction to this book made Szasz notorious overnight. Traditional psychiatrists and psychologists were generally aghast that a member of their profession would assert that what we call "mental illness" is really a contrivance of the medical, governmental, social, and religious establishments to control, oppress, and manipulate otherwise free individuals. Timothy Leary, the Harvard psychology professor who would soon found the League of Spiritual Discovery (LSD) to promote lysergic acid diethylamide (LSD), wrote in a letter to Szasz on July 17, 1961:

The Myth of Mental Illness is the most important book in the history of psychiatry. I know it is rash and premature to make this early judgment. I reserve the right later to revise and perhaps suggest it is the most important book published in the twentieth century. It is great in so many ways — scholarship, clinical insight, political savvy, common sense, historical sweep, human concern — and most of all for its compassionate, shattering honesty. I have already contacted several of my colleagues and intend that everyone I meet will be exposed to your work. I am in charge of the first year graduate training at this Center and while I don't believe in "required" reading I shall certainly "suggest" with enthusiasm that this book be read and re-read. Your text states most eloquently, convincingly, systematically what a group of us here have been attempting to communicate.

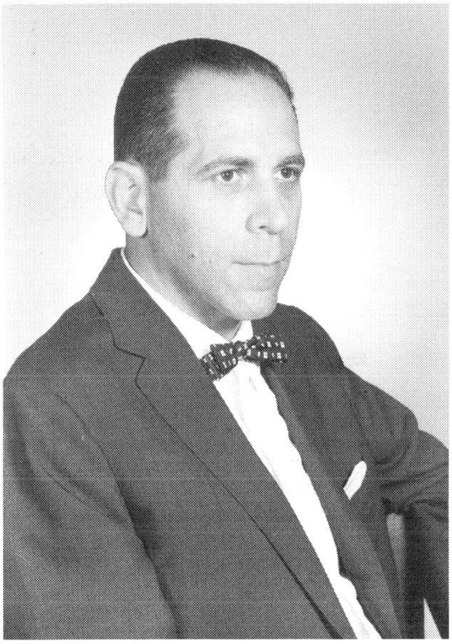

Szasz (left) enjoyed an idyllic childhood in his native Budapest and would have liked to remain there as a Hungarian poet, but his father wisely took the family out of Hungary after the Austrian *Anschluss* in 1938. He earned his baccalaureate with honors in physics in 1941 and his M.D. in 1944, both at the University of Cincinnati, and did postgraduate training in psychiatry at the University of Chicago and in psychoanalysis at the Chicago Institute for Psychoanalysis.

Szasz was acclaimed the most exciting teacher in the Department of Psychiatry from when he arrived at Upstate in 1956 through the 1970s, and was especially popular with the residents. It is said that approximately 25 percent of Upstate's psychiatric residents in that era came to Syracuse specifically to study with him.

Even after retiring in 1990, Szasz remained active with students. At a session in the Medical Alumni Auditorium of Weiskotten Hall on February 22, 2001, jointly sponsored by the Center for Bioethics and Humanities and the student-run Humanistic Lecture Series, he said, when challenged about his disbelief in mental illness: "Show me 100 brain CAT scans, blind, that will show which patients have mental illness as reliably as 100 leg x-rays, again blind, will show which patients have fractures, and then I will believe that there is mental illness." He argues that, because the medical criterion for "illness" is the physical lesion, therefore the mind, not being a physical object like the brain, cannot become "ill."

The last polio epidemic in the United States hit Syracuse in August 1961. Jonas Salk's killed-virus injected vaccine (IPV) had been available since 1955, but millions of injections across the country had brought mixed results. Albert Sabin soon thereafter developed an attenuated-virus oral vaccine (OPV), but endured a long fight to win government approval. Sabin's vaccine was more effective, but it could contain dangerous impurities such as simian virus 40 (SV40) and the weakened virus could mutate and occasionally cause severe complications such as vaccine-associated paralytic polio (VAPP). Nevertheless, after the AMA became critical of IPV in early 1961 and after preliminary reports of the AMA Ad Hoc Committee on Poliovirus Vaccines appeared, the U.S. Public Health Service on August 17, 1961, even before clinical field trials were underway, licensed Pfizer to manufacture OPV. The first life-or-death trial of OPV was in Syracuse.

Local public health officials noticed in the fourth week of August 1961 that 32 new cases of paralytic polio had arisen that month in Onondaga, Madison, and Oneida Counties, including eight in Syracuse. These officials decided to try immediate mass immunization to stop the epidemic. Harry Feldman, a friend of Sabin, contacted the New York State Department of Health, the U.S.P.H.S., and all the other appropriate agencies and individuals to ensure that 350,000 doses of OPV would be available for the emergency clinics that were to be opened in twenty public schools on August 29, 30, and 31. He personally oversaw the delivery, storage, and dilution of these doses. A.C. Silverman, then Director of the Onondaga County Bureau of Communicable Diseases, wrote in the October 1961 *Bulletin of the Onondaga County Medical Society*:

> The response was remarkable. People stood in lines for long periods during the rush hours. The Syracuse population under 50 was estimated at 150,000 but even older ages were not refused. At least 211,000 doses were given and the reports are not yet complete. For the tri-county area nearly 400,000 doses were given. ... The reasons for the remarkable response may be found in the potent publicity supervised by the people from the State Health Department aided by the press, radio and TV. The vaccine was free and was to be distributed in the fixed time of 3 days. Moreover the day before the clinics started a bulbar polio case had died.

Willard claimed in the 1956 *New York State Journal of Medicine* that Upstate's three greatest contributions to American medicine were: being the third medical school in the country to introduce the graded curriculum, bringing women into the profession, and playing a major role in public health. The work of Silverman, Feldman, and their colleagues during the 1961 Syracuse polio crisis is strong evidence for Willard's third point.

Jacobsen's most important accomplishment during his ten years as president was the successful construction of University Hospital, the transfer of its services from Good Shepherd and other superseded facilities, and the addition of new services that made it one of the most elaborate and technologically advanced hospitals of the time. Jacobsen had been working on this project while still in Albany, before his presidency began. It was a complicated process that demanded all his skills negotiating with politicians, architects, medical professionals, hospital administrators, university officials, expert consultants, and other interested parties in Albany and Washington as well as locally and regionally.

Ground was broken for the new University Hospital building in July 1961. On January 20, 1964, the Dispensary moved from the State Office Building to the outpatient clinic affiliated with University Hospital. In March 1964 Upstate terminated its primary affiliation with Memorial Hospital as a teaching facility. All teaching except surgery was transferred to

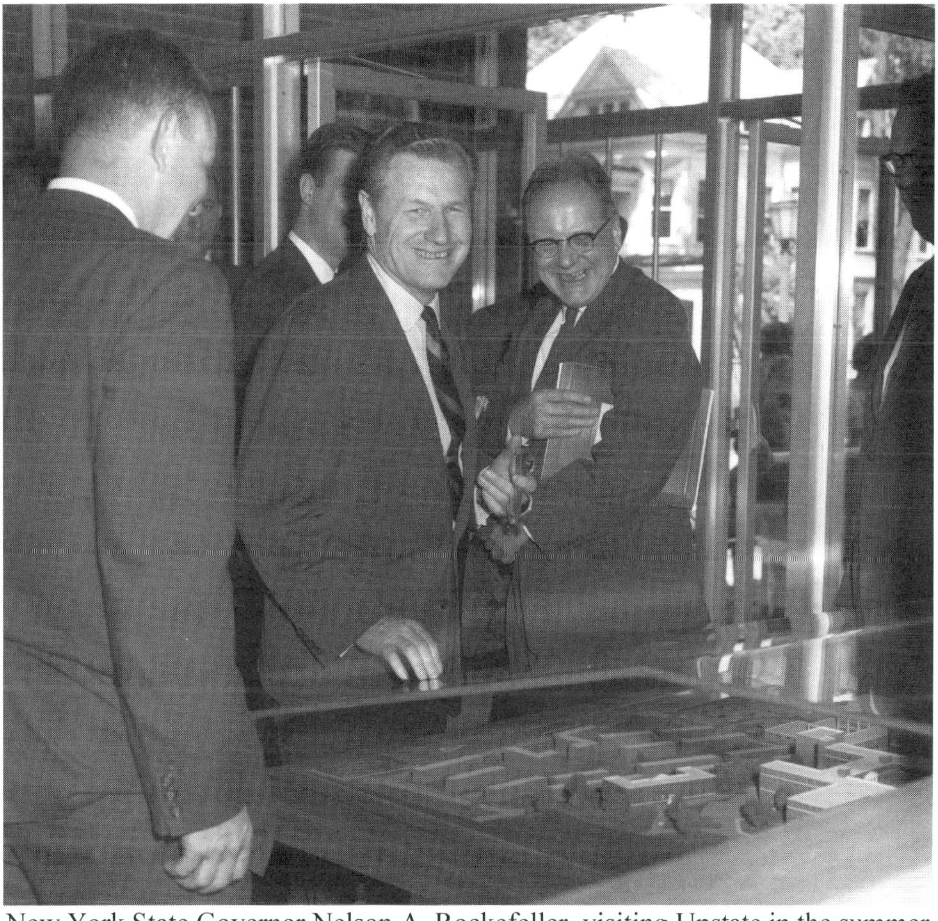

New York State Governor Nelson A. Rockefeller, visiting Upstate in the summer of 1961, with President Jacobsen looking at an architectural model of the campus.

other institutions. Obstetrical, gynecological, and pediatric services had particular difficulty in finding other venues. Crouse-Irving hospital offered Upstate temporary ob/gyn space and eventually ob/gyn instruction for Upstate students was re-established at Crouse Irving Memorial Hospital, but in the meantime Jacobsen acted quickly to provide this component at University Hospital. A seven-year NIH grant that he had secured in 1962 enabled City Hospital to be remodeled and used for pediatric services until the pediatrics unit of University Hospital was ready for occupancy.

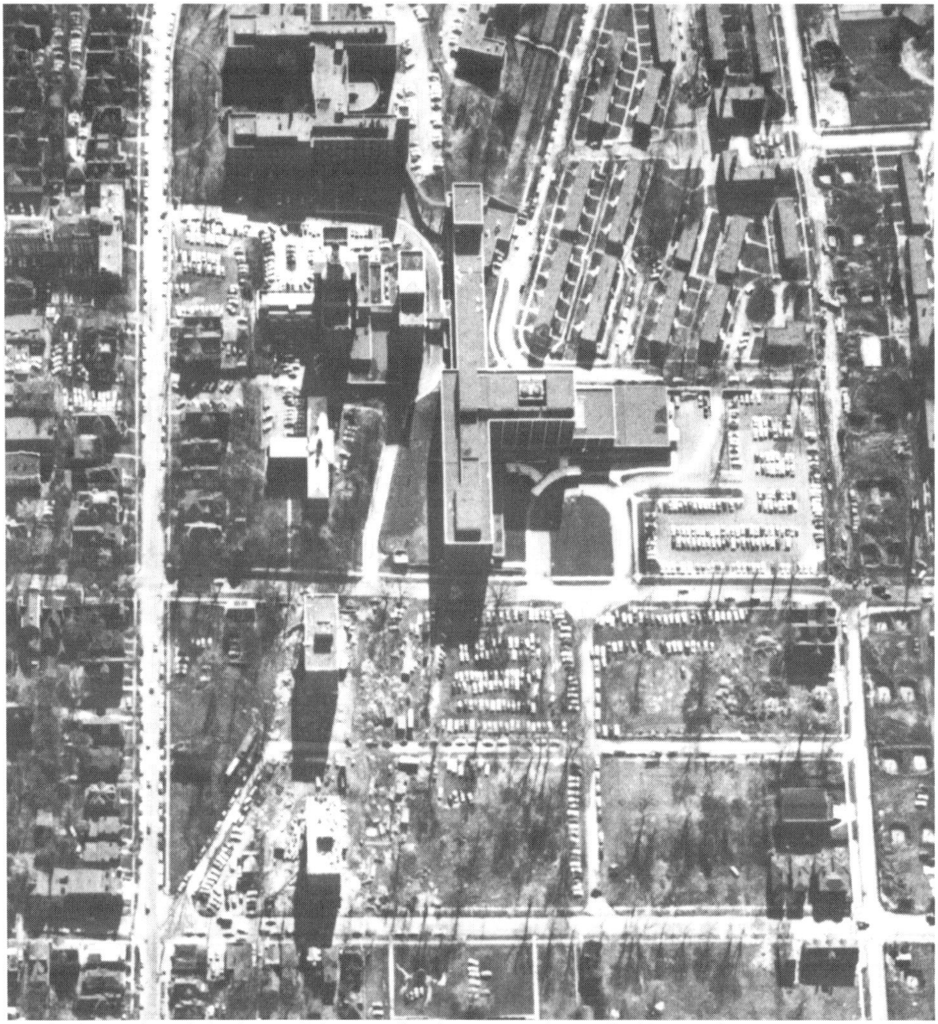

Southward aerial view of the medical campus bounded by Irving Avenue (left), Harrison Street (bottom), and Almond Street (right) in 1966, just as construction was beginning on Interstate Route 81 through Syracuse. University Hospital is in the center. On the left (from top) are the College of Medicine, Syracuse Memorial Hospital, Syracuse Psychiatric Hospital, and the two Gaylord Clark Dormitories, which were completed in 1965. The dormitory closer to Adams Street would later be converted into an office building and renamed in honor of Carlyle Jacobsen.

The three hospitals that Weiskotten brought to University Hill in the 1920s had very different fates. City Hospital was officially renamed A. Clement Silverman Public Health Hospital on May 16, 1969, as it had already been popularly called Silverman Hospital since at least 1968. Until the 1960s it was the major facility in Syracuse for infectious diseases, treating both children and adults, but was dissolved in 1977 because University Hospital had taken over most of its responsibilities. Upstate Medical Center bought the building in 1977, renamed it A. Clement Silverman Hall, and used it to house the College of Health Related Professions. Syracuse Memorial Hospital merged with Crouse Irving Hospital in 1968 to form Crouse Irving Memorial Hospital and subsequently Crouse Hospital. The Syracuse Psychiatric Hospital had evolved by 1972 into the Richard H. Hutchings Psychiatric Center at 620 Madison Street.

University Hospital, with 350 beds, was formally dedicated on May 24, 1965, and its first patients, transfers from Good Shepherd, were admitted on June 11. Almost immediately new procedures became available in Central New York. Kidney transplantation had been done since the 1950s, but was not yet common when the first one at University Hospital was performed on August 2, 1968.

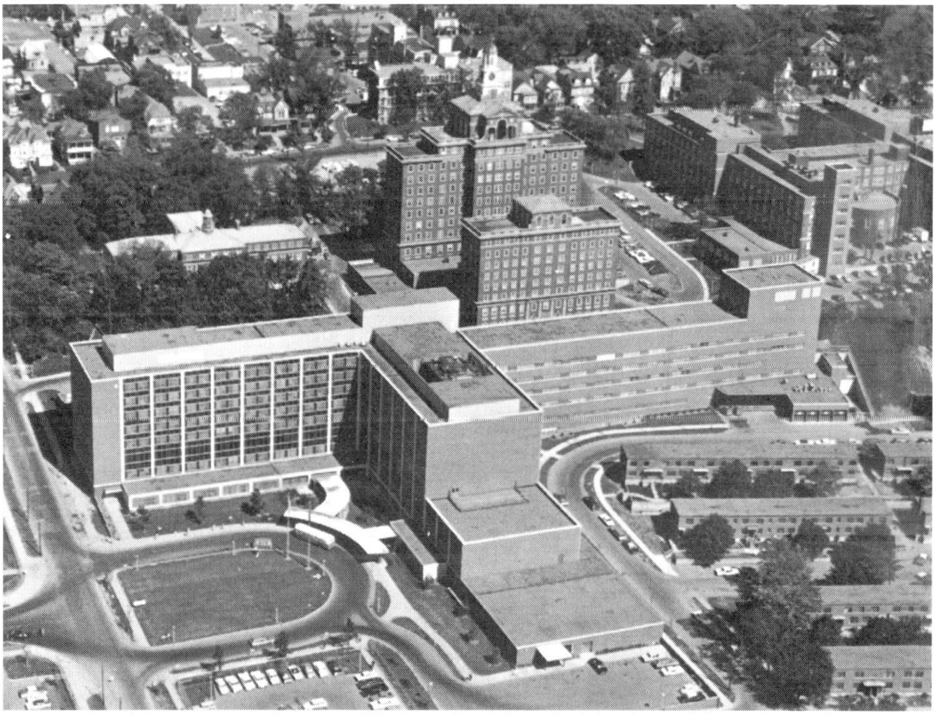

Looking east at the new University Hospital in the mid-1960s, with (left to right) the Syracuse Psychiatric Hospital, Syracuse Memorial Hospital, and the College of Medicine building. Crouse Irving Hospital is across Irving Avenue from Syracuse Memorial.

The College of Health Professions can trace its origins to 1956 when a few students enrolled in a certificate program in cytotechnology. New allied health curricula gradually emerged in response to demand, including x-ray technology (below). The School of Allied Health Professions opened in 1965, authorized to grant the B.S. in medical technology, the associate of applied science (A.A.S.) in radiation technology, and the A.A.S. in radiation therapy technology. In 1967 it added the A.A.S. in inhalation therapy, in 1968 the M.S. in medical technology, in 1970 the B.S. in physical therapy, and in 1972 the B.S. in cytotechnology and the B.S. in respiratory therapy. A. Geno Andreatta directed the school from the late 1960s until John Bernard Henry took over in 1971 to become the first Dean of the College of Health Related Professions, as it was then renamed. Subsequent deans have been Mary Jane Brennan Schneider, 1977 to 1978 and 1981 to 1982; John Herbert Morrison, 1978 to 1980; G. Bruce Dearing (left), 1980 to 1981; Donald C. Goodman, 1983 to 1995; and Hugh W. Bonner since 1995. The word "Related" was dropped from the name of the college in 1996.

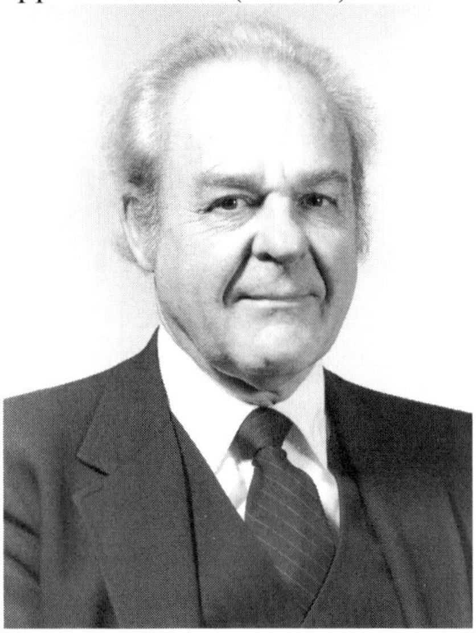

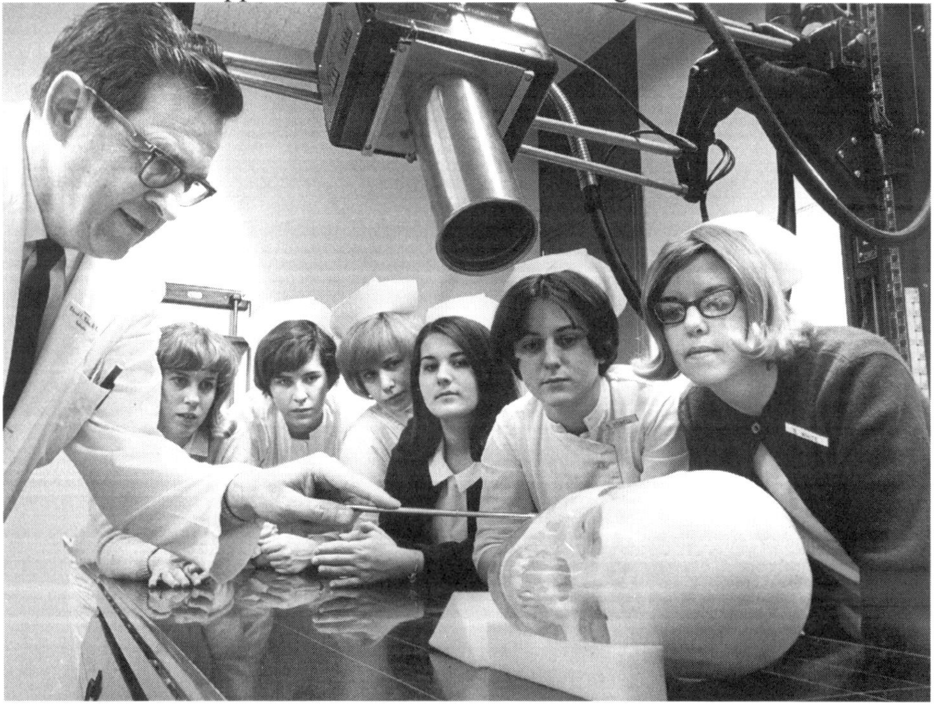

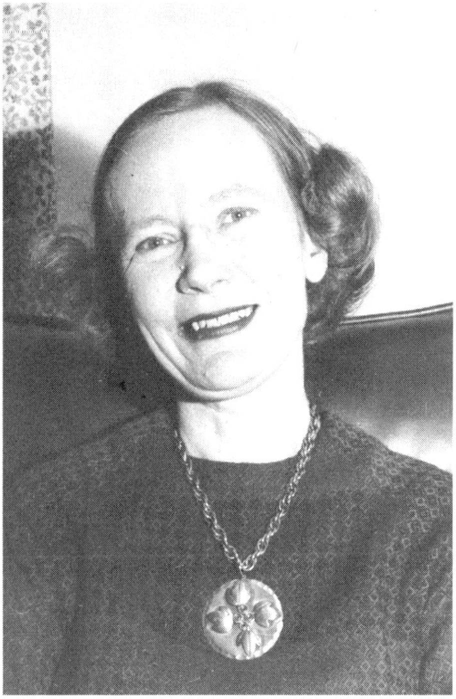

In September 1959 the newly founded School of Nursing admitted its first class to study for the A.A.S. in nursing. Maja C. Anderson (right), who had her master's degree in nursing from Yale University, directed the school from its inception until she retired in 1975. She was the author of two textbooks: *Basic Patient Care: A Programed Introduction to Nursing Fundamentals* (1965) and *Basic Nursing Techniques: A Programed Introduction to Nursing Fundamentals* (1968). It graduated seven in its first class in 1961 and altogether graduated about 500 nurses.

Facing competition and objections from the two-year SUNY colleges if it kept its associate's program, and from Syracuse University if it developed a baccalaureate program, Upstate decided to get out of the business of training nurses in 1976. Instead, it began in January 1975 to train nurse practitioners through the College of Health Related Professions under the direction of Margaret D. Sovie. This program graduated about 300 nurse practitioners before it was superseded by the Nursing Education Program, which M. Janice Nelson, Ed.D., R.N., Director of Nursing at University Hospital from 1980 to 1986, created in 1984 to offer a combined B.S. and M.S. in nursing. This new program became the College of Nursing in 1986, with Nelson serving as its first dean until 1996. Elvira Szigeti, Ph.D., R.N., succeeded her as dean.

One of the most prominent professors in the College of Nursing, Susan Bastable, Ed.D., R.N., wrote *Nurse as Educator: Principles of Teaching and Learning for Nursing Practice*, which *The American Journal of Nursing* honored as its Book of the Year in 1997. She left her faculty position at Upstate in 2003 to found the baccalaureate program in nursing at Le Moyne College.

Upstate's first African-American nursing graduate, Gwendolyn Snellings Lipscomb, earned her A.A.S. in 1968 and went on to earn further degrees, enjoy a distinguished career, and eventually rise to be Director of the Division of Minority Health in the Alabama Department of Public Health. She and M. Elizabeth Carnegie, author of *The Path We Tread: Blacks in Nursing, 1854-1990*, were Upstate's guests of honor on February 21, 2001, as part of the annual Black History Month celebrations.

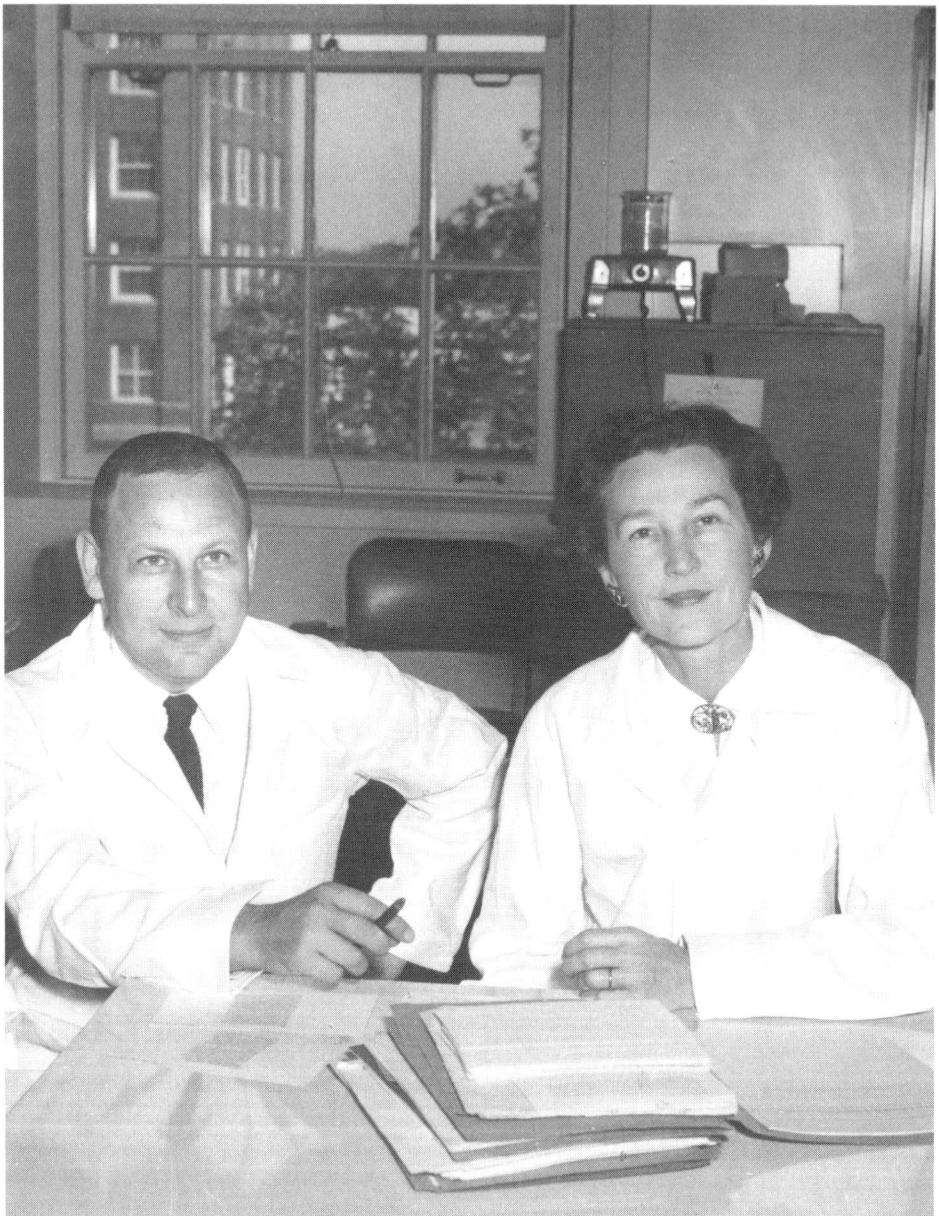

In 1962 the husband and wife team of pharmacologists, Jay Tepperman and Helen M. Tepperman, published the first of five editions of *Metabolic and Endocrine Physiology*, the standard textbook in that field for three decades. He received his A.B. at the University of Pennsylvania in 1933 and his M.D. at Columbia in 1938. After graduating *summa cum laude* from Mount Holyoke College in 1938, she earned her Ph.D. in physiological chemistry at Yale in 1942. They met at Yale, married in 1943, came to the Syracuse University College of Medicine in 1946, and retired in 1985.

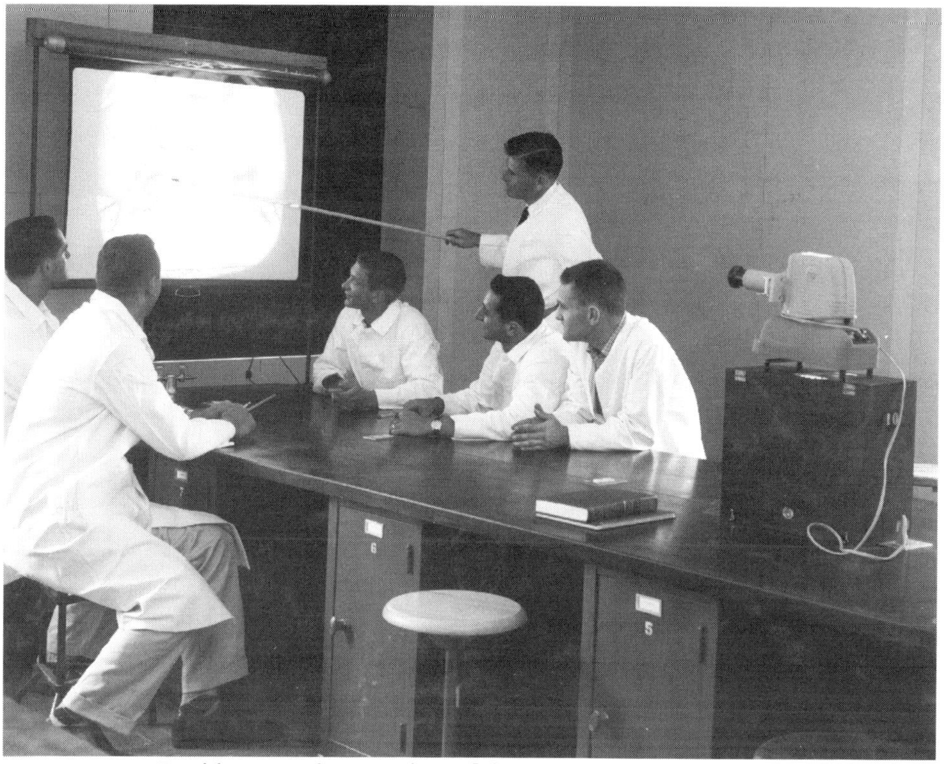

Residents study a section of the midbrain in the 1960s.

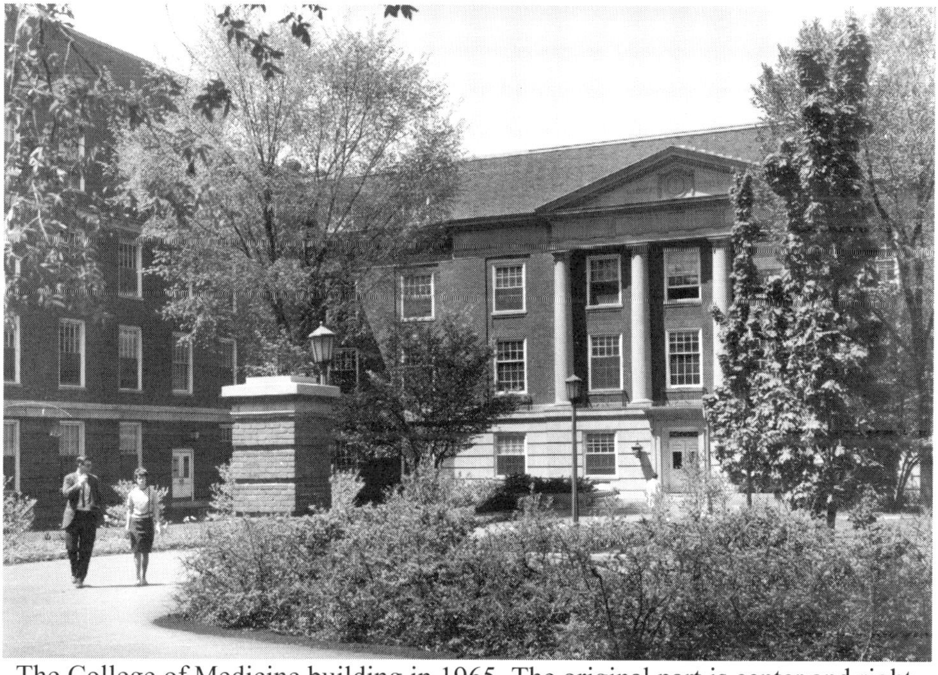

The College of Medicine building in 1965. The original part is center and right. At the left is the southeast addition that replaced Yates Castle in the 1950s.

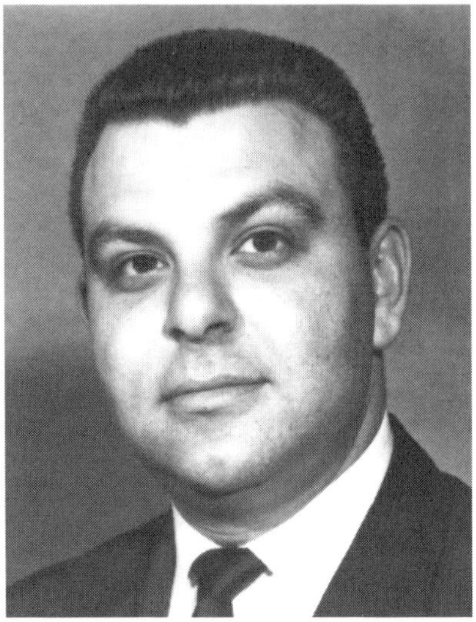

The earliest mention of physical rehabilitation medicine in the Syracuse University College of Medicine records is in the minutes of the June 5, 1902 faculty meeting, where Charles A. Covell, Class of 1894, a medical chemist, was appointed the first electrotherapist at Good Shepherd. Subsequently Clifford Mercer, Jacob Levy, Class of 1903, Lee A. Hadley, Class of 1917, and Thomas E. Walsh, Class of 1920, explored various possibilities for practicing and teaching physical therapy. The independent Department of Physical Medicine and Rehabilitation arose in 1949. The new chair, George M. Raus, Class of 1936, worked with Hadley and Walsh to develop a modern curriculum in this field. Raus's initiative received a boost in 1959 when Leo Jivoff (above) arrived in Syracuse to direct the new rehabilitation annex at Good Shepherd, which had just been built with Ford Foundation and federal money. The department lost its independent status from 1957 to 1966, but when Jivoff's Good Shepherd unit was transferred to the new University Hospital in 1965, impetus grew to restore the department as a separate entity. Jivoff chaired it from 1966 to 1987.

The Jacobsen years were marked by tremendous growth, not only in buildings and budget, but especially in personnel. Many essential teaching positions that had formerly been taken by part-timers whose main business was their clinical practice were now transformed into full-time professorial appointments. While all the basic sciences had been established with full-time chairs between 1892 and 1919, the clinical departments did not begin to have full-time leaders until 1947, when Lyons was hired for the Department of Medicine. The Departments of Psychiatry, Pediatrics, and Surgery each hired their first full-time professors and chairs in the 1950s, and between 1960 and 1966 all other then-existing departments followed suit. Allen B. Dobkin became Upstate's first full-time professor of anesthesiology in 1960 and Robert E.L. Nesbitt its first full-time professor of obstetrics and gynecology in 1961.

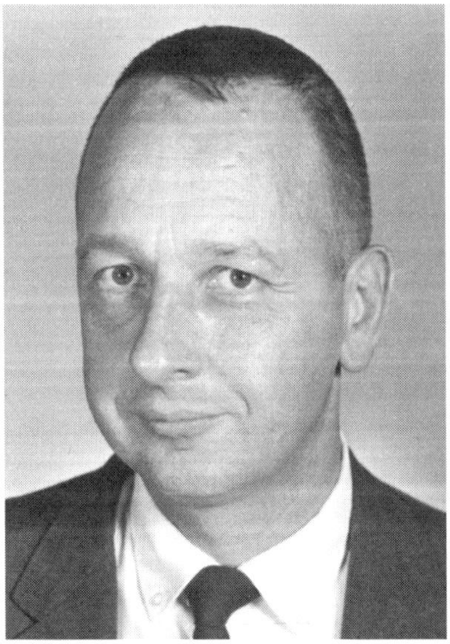

Radiology's first full-time professor was Paul A. Riemenschneider (right), who earned his M.D. at Harvard in 1944, came to Upstate as an instructor in 1950, and was promoted to full professor in 1956. He collaborated with Ecker on several projects, including their jointly authored 1955 book, *Angiographic Localization of Intracranial Masses*. In 1964 he succeeded Hale as Chair of Radiology, but had difficulty juggling conflicting interests between Crouse Irving Hospital and Good Shepherd in planning for the radiological services at the new University Hospital. He resigned in 1965, left academia, and became Chief of Diagnostic Radiology at Santa Barbara Cottage Hospital, California.

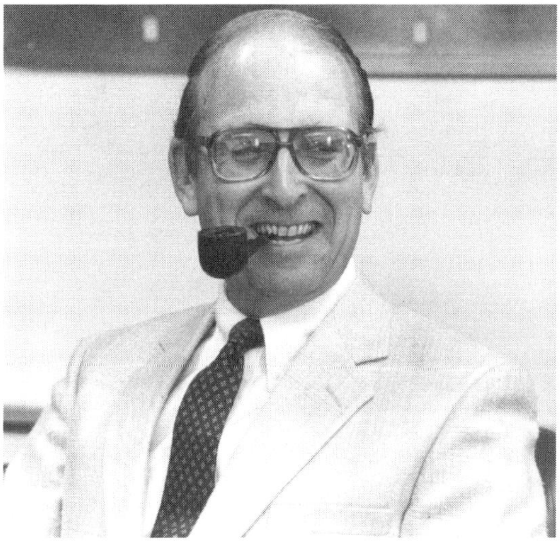

Riemenschneider was followed as chair first by John G. McAfee then in 1974 by one of the most prominent authors and editors in American radiology, Stephen A. Kieffer (left). Another outstanding member of this department was E. Robert Heitzman, Class of 1951, who wrote *The Lung: Radiologic-Pathologic Correlations* (1973, 1984, 1993) and *The Mediastinum: Radiologic Correlations with Anatomy and Pathology* (1977, 1988), both standard textbooks.

George F. Reed, Class of 1946 (below), became in 1965 Upstate's first full-time Professor of Otolaryngology. After interning in Syracuse, he had done postgraduate work at Harvard and his residency at the Massachusetts Eye and Ear Infirmary in Boston before returning to Syracuse in 1952. He chaired the department from 1965 to 1977, succeeding Alfred Doust, who had chaired it since 1955. At various points in his career, Reed was president of the American Board of Otolaryngology, the American Society for Head and Neck Surgery, the Society of University Otolaryngologists, the American Council of Otolaryngology, and the Onondaga County Medical Society. Under him, the Upstate department trained superior otolaryngologists, many of whom would later become department chairs at other institutions. He retained his chair when he became Dean for Graduate Medical and Continuing Education in 1974.

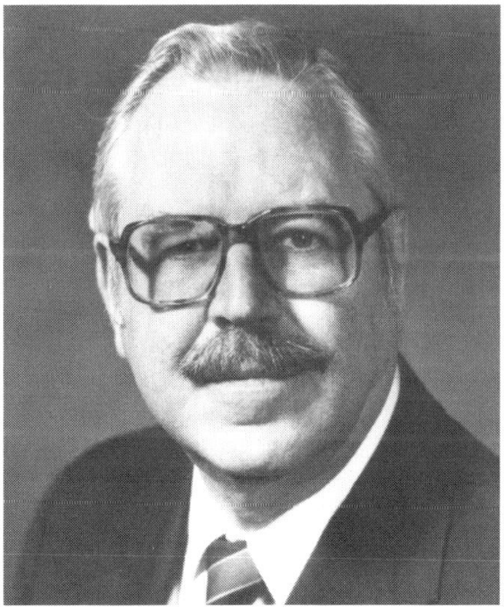

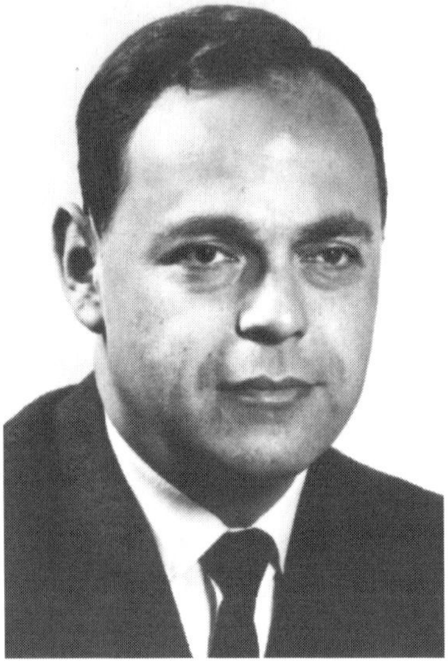

Otto M. Lilien (left) became Upstate's first full-time urologist in 1961 and had been chief of the urology service within the Department of Surgery for three years when the independent Department of Urology was created in 1966. He served as chair from 1966 until 1982, when he resigned to become chief of staff at the Veterans Administration Medical Center. While at Upstate he used time lapse photography to study urodynamics and renal function. In 1984 he published a famous paper in the *Journal of Urology* on the Camey procedure of male human bladder replacement. When the *Journal of Urology* reprinted this article in 2002, Lilien wrote:

> I had a patient with bladder carcinoma who categorically refused a proposed Bricker procedure. When told about the Camey alternative, he insisted on going this route, saying, "… the worst that can happen is that you'll learn something, but I ain't going to wear no bag." The operation was successful, as was a second procedure. Convinced that the surgery was technically feasible, the question of long-term results remained. When I communicated this reservation to Camey, he invited me back to Paris, where I spent 3 months analyzing his 25-year experience. This article was the product of that review.

David G. Murray (right) chaired the Department of Orthopedic Surgery from its founding in 1966 until 1986 and again from 1990 to 2000. An important pioneer in total hip and total knee replacement surgery, he chaired the NIH Consensus Development Conference on Total Hip Replacement in 1994. He is an Honorary Fellow of the Royal College of Surgeons and was president of the American Academy of Orthopaedic Surgeons from 1982 to 1983, the Knee Society from 1988 to 1989, the Onondaga County Medical Society from 1992 to 1993, and the American College of Surgeons from 1996 to 1997.

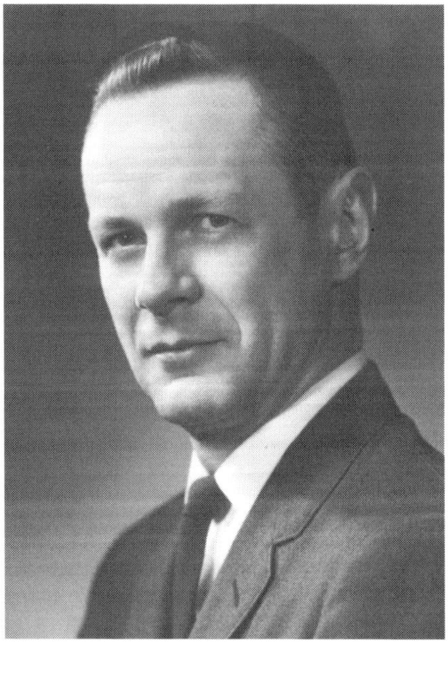

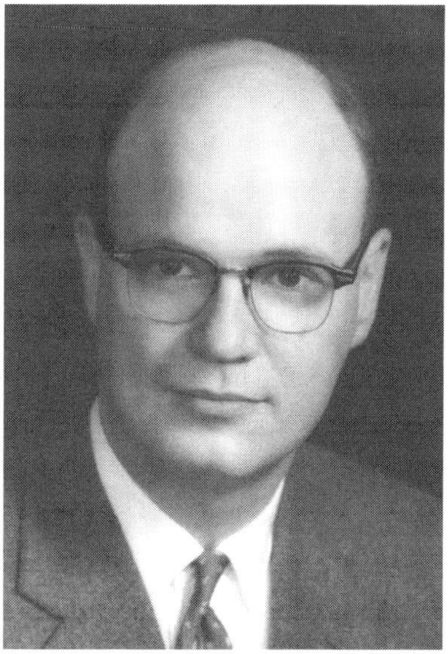

Robert B. King (right) chaired the Department of Neurosurgery from 1966 to 1987. After earning his M.D. *cum laude* at the University of Rochester in 1946, he interned in general surgery and did a neurosurgery residency at Barnes Hospital, St. Louis, then was Assistant Chief of Neurosurgery at Walter Reed Army Medical Center. While a Markle Scholar at Washington University from 1951 to 1956, he held a fellowship at National Hospital, Queen's Square, London, from 1952 to 1953. Shortly after coming to Upstate as Professor of Neurosurgery in 1957, he achieved national prominence for his work in neurosurgical education. In 1968 he organized and was the first chair of the American Association of Neurological Surgeons (AANS) Education Committee and in 1981 founded the AANS Research and Education Foundation. His presidencies included not only the AANS from 1980 to 1981, but also the Society of Neurological Surgeons from 1977 to 1978, the American Academy of Neurological Surgeons from 1979 to 1980, and the American Board of Medical Specialties from 1988 to 1990. King also co-founded the Research Society of Neurological Surgeons, an amorphous group that presents a scholarly conference each year at the home institution of one of its members.

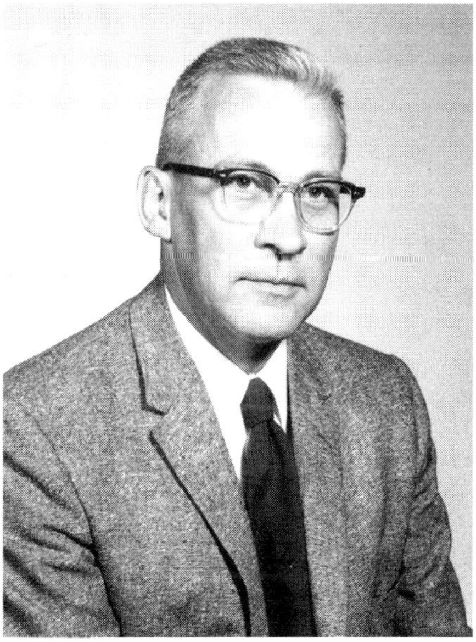

C. Barber Mueller (left) came to Syracuse from Washington University in 1956 to become Upstate's first full-time Professor and Chair of the Department of Surgery. As chair, he managed occasional tensions between general surgeons and specialists and between salaried academic faculty and volunteer clinical faculty. He encouraged rapid development and diversification of surgical services, presiding over the emergence of Neurosurgery, Anesthesiology, Urology, and Orthopedic Surgery as separate departments. He resigned in 1967 to become chair at McMaster University, where he contributed to create the "problem-based learning" (PBL) method of medical education, which has influenced medical schools and residency programs around the world.

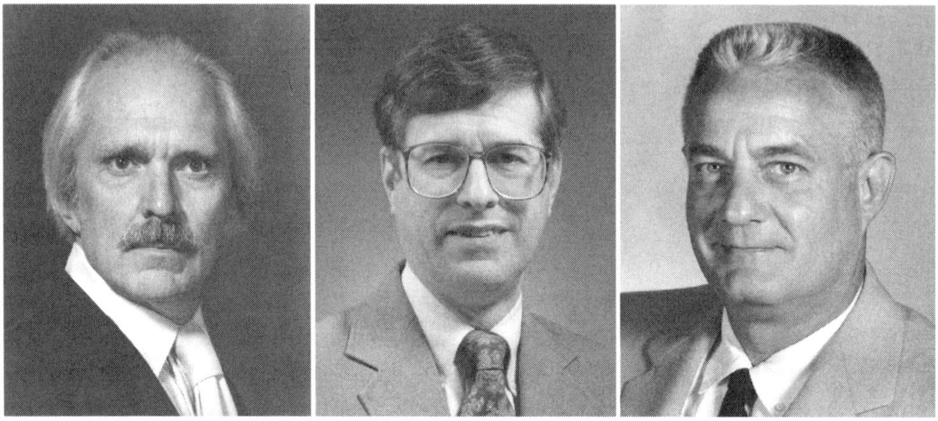

In 1964 Ferguson brought clinical pathology out of the Department of Medicine back into the Department of Pathology with John B. Henry as chief of that division. Henry's medical classmate at the University of Rochester, Rolla B. Hill (left), succeeded Ferguson as chair in 1969 and served until 1986. Hill had a national reputation in pathology, co-authoring or co-editing several influential publications. After Gerald B. Gordon served two years as interim chair, Frederick R. Davey, Class of 1964 (center), chaired the department from 1988 until 2001. Gordon's main research interest was the ultrastructural pathology of cell injury; Davey's was hematopathology and immunohematology.

Paul A. Bunn (right) served as acting chair of the Department of Medicine for two years between the long terms of Lyons and William J. Williams, who was inspired to become a physician by Sinclair Lewis's *Arrowsmith.* His two real-life role models were surgeon I.S. Ravdin and internist Francis C. Wood at the University of Pennsylvania, who mentored him as a medical student and resident. Williams, chair from 1969 to 1992, is best known outside Upstate for creating what served North American medical schools as the standard textbook in hematology for over three decades. The first edition of *Hematology* appeared in 1972, a massive volume of 1480 pages edited by a team led by Williams. The second edition, 1755 pages, appeared in 1977; the third, 1728 pages, in 1983; and the fourth, 1882 pages, in 1990. The 1881-page fifth edition, the first to be titled *Williams' Hematology*, appeared under chief editor Ernest Beutler in 1995.

Williams's wife, Margaret L. Williams, was Upstate's first neonatologist. She received her M.D. at the University of Pennsylvania in 1949 then served at several hospitals in Philadelphia, most notably at Philadelphia General Hospital from 1961 to 1969 as Director of Newborn Services. In 1969 she established Upstate's neonatological and developmental care program and in 1970 began clinical work also at Crouse Irving Memorial Hospital, where she soon became Chief of Neonatology and Co-Director of the Perinatal Center.

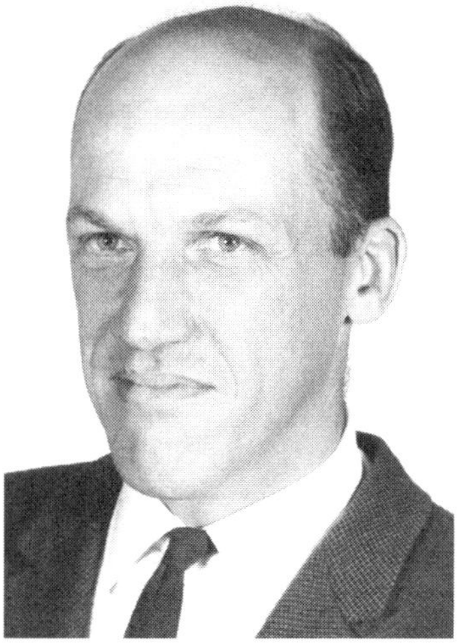

George G. Holz (right) chaired the Department of Microbiology from 1962 to 1989. He specialized in invertebrate zoology, received his Ph.D. in zoology from the University of California at Los Angeles in 1952, then joined the Syracuse University Department of Zoology in 1953 and remained there until coming to Upstate. His main research interest was the protozoan membrane and from 1963 to 1964 he was president of the Society of Protozoologists.

After eight years at Johns Hopkins and two in the Department of Molecular Biology at Albert Einstein College of Medicine, Irwin M. ("Ike") Weiner, Class of 1956, came to Upstate as an associate professor in 1966. He was Chair of Pharmacology from 1968 to 1987, Vice President for Research from 1982 to 1988, and Dean of the College of Medicine from 1987 until he resigned in 1991 to become Dean of the SUNY Health Science Center at Brooklyn (SUNY Downstate) College of Medicine.

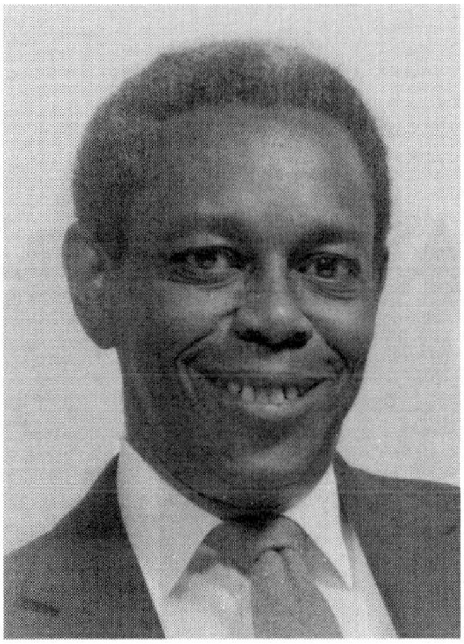

Charles R. Ross (left), Dean of the College of Graduate Studies from 1982 until his untimely death from cancer in 1989, was the first African-American to achieve the rank of dean at Upstate. A man of impeccable character, keen scientific skills, and genuine friendliness, he was among the best liked of all faculty members. Ross, whose main area of research was renal pharmacology, earned his Ph.D. at the University of Michigan in 1963 then came to Upstate as a postdoctoral fellow to work in Farah's laboratory. He became assistant professor in 1966, associate professor in 1970, and full professor in 1978. His project, "Renal Transport for Organic Compounds," received thirty-two consecutive years of NIH funding and resulted in fifty-two published scientific papers and thirty-seven abstracts. In June 1988, just before illness forced Ross to leave his job, President Henry appointed him Vice President for Research.

Maxwell M. Mozell succeeded Ross as Dean of Graduate Studies in 1990. A physiologist specializing in olfactory neurophysiology, Mozell received his Ph.D. at Brown University in 1956, came to Upstate in 1961 as an assistant professor, was promoted to associate professor in 1966 and to full professor in 1970, and became Associate Dean for Academic Program Development in 1971.

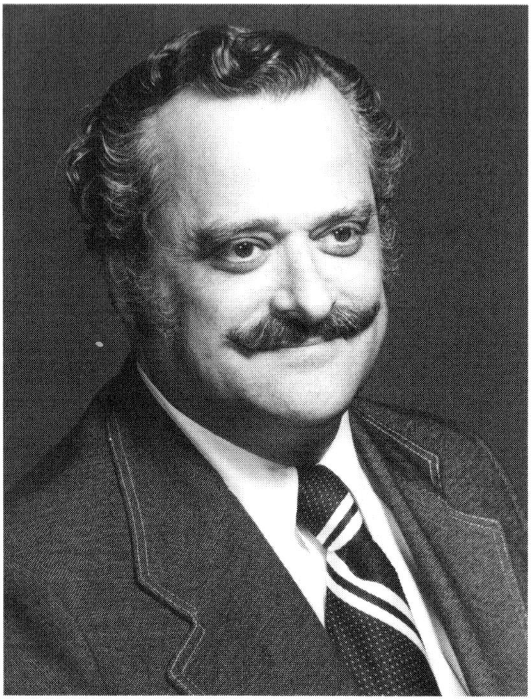

Donald Charles Goodman (left) received his Ph.D. in zoology from the University of Illinois in 1954, then taught anatomy at the University of Pennsylvania and the University of Florida before coming to Upstate in 1968 as Professor and Chair of Anatomy. A worthy successor of the colorful James Webster, Goodman was noted for his jovial and sometimes earthy sense of humor. He remained Chair of Anatomy while he held several other administrative positions at Upstate, but in 1982 he relinquished this position to Elinor Spring-Mills as acting chair. Larry F. Lemanski then chaired the department from 1983 until 1997, when he left to become Associate Vice President for Research and Professor of Medical Physiology and Biology at Texas A&M University and subsequently, in 2001, Vice President for Research at Florida Atlantic University.

As Dean of the College of Graduate Studies from 1973 to 1982, Vice President for Research from 1978 to 1982, Vice President for Academic Affairs from 1976 to 1982 and again from 1983 to 1985, and Provost from 1985 to 1995, Goodman pushed hard to gain budgetary and extrabudgetary funding to enable research, to improve curriculum, and to provide for the library, the medical humanities, and other services and programs essential for comprehensive medical education. He was briefly Vice President for Academic Affairs at East Tennessee State University in 1982, but, at President Schmidt's request, returned to Upstate as Dean of the College of Health Related Professions from 1983 to 1995. This experience all combined to qualify him to serve as interim president from 1992 to 1993.

Goodman was always known as a friend of the faculty and a vigorous promoter of faculty development, but ironically he saw this great asset as his greatest failure. He wrote in the *CHRP Alumni News* in 1995, just before he retired: "My single major regret is that I was never able to provide enough support for creative inquiry by our faculty that I felt they needed. Although much has been accomplished in research/creative activity by our faculty, I would have liked to have provided more time in the busy teaching schedules to be devoted to research projects."

In December 1966, even though SUNY had offered special dispensation for one more year, Jacobsen announced that he would comply with the mandatory retirement age of 65 and leave the presidency on June 30, 1967. Westerfeld was appointed in April 1967 to act as interim president effective July 1.

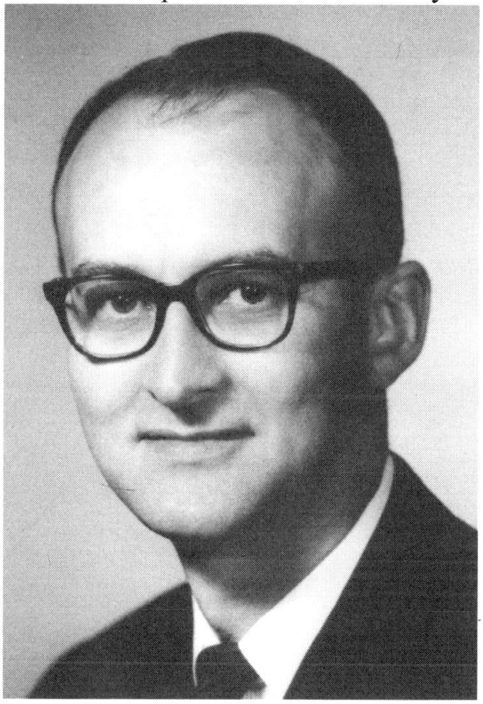

Lewis W. ("Bill") Bluemle (right) became Upstate's second president on November 1, 1968. Former U.S. Surgeon General Luther Terry was among those who spoke at the inauguration at Loew's State Theatre (later called the Landmark Theatre) at 362 South Salina Street on September 26, 1969. The same day Upstate dedicated the Campus Activities Building (CAB) on Irving Avenue, which Jacobsen had conceived in 1964 as a student union and which had opened in July 1969.

A member of the Johns Hopkins medical class of 1946, Bluemle was a nephrologist at the University of Pennsylvania before coming to Upstate. In 1951 he established the first dialysis unit in Philadelphia, one of the first in the nation, and served until 1968 as chief of that unit. In 1961 he founded the Clinical Research Center at the Hospital of the University of Pennsylvania. His pioneering research on dialysis produced about thirty articles in the 1950s and 1960s. He holds several patents on artificial kidneys and blood pumps, including U.S. Pat. No. 3,362,540, issued on January 9, 1968, for a flat plate dialyzer.

Perhaps Bluemle's greatest contribution to Upstate was in 1969, recruiting William and Margaret Williams, both of whom had been his colleagues at the University of Pennsylvania. William Williams wrote in 1992, when Upstate awarded Bluemle an honorary D.Sc., that "what made him such an effective administrator was that he was an excellent listener. He was always able to put himself in the other person's place and because of that he came up with thoughtful, well-reasoned positions ... His short time in Syracuse will go down as the most ambitious faculty development period in the history of the Center. By the time he left we had a new generation of faculty leadership in place."

After leaving Syracuse, Bluemle was president of the University of Oregon Health Sciences Center in Portland, Thomas Jefferson University, and the College of Physicians of Philadelphia.

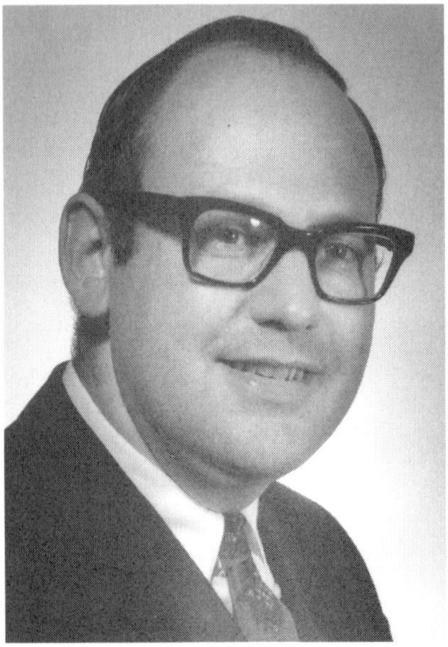

A vital milestone in library automation in general and medical informatics in particular was achieved in the fall of 1968 when the Library of SUNY Upstate Medical Center became the site of the world's first interactive online bibliographic retrieval service. Irwin H. Pizer (left), Library Director from 1964 to 1969, made history by instituting the SUNY Biomedical Communication Network (BCN) on campus. This network appeared a year before the Online Computer Library Center (OCLC), then called the Ohio College Library Center, went live. BCN eventually included thirty-two libraries, including the National Library of Medicine (NLM). It ran until January 1977, but had evolved by December 1976 into the famous commercial network, Bibliographic Retrieval Services (BRS), which was sold in 1980 to the Thyssen-Bornemisza Group and in 1989 to Maxwell Online, a division of Macmillan. In 1992 Maxwell Online became InfoPro Technologies, which sold BRS Online Products to CD Plus Technologies in 1994. CD Plus changed its name in 1995 to Ovid Technologies, which in 1998 became a subsidiary of Wolters Kluwer.

Much has been written in praise of Pizer and BCN. One scholar noted that "the SUNY Biomedical Communication Network was designed from the beginning as a user-friendly (then termed user-oriented) system."[*] Such emphasis on user-friendliness may been unusual at the time to computer scientists, but not to librarians, for whom service is paramount.

The SUNY Upstate Health Sciences Library continues to receive high marks for its service, both online and in-person. Always mindful of the lofty standards of excellence set by Pizer, it has remained in the forefront of automated medical librarianship, especially through the efforts of innovative directors like Suzanne H. Murray, who served from 1985 to 1995. In the early 1990s it became one of the first medical libraries to create offsite instant access to its CD-ROM databases.[†] This popular feature, "CDLink," was state-of-the-art until access via the Internet replaced it in the late 1990s.

---

[*] Carolyn E. Lipscomb, "SUNY Biomedical Communication Network: Irwin Pizer," *Bulletin of the Medical Library Association* 89, 2 (April 2001): 231-234.

[†] Patricia W. Onsi, James A. Capodagli, and Diane K. Hawkins, "Dial-In Access to CD-ROM Databases: Beyond the Local Area Network," *Bulletin of the Medical Library Association* 80, 4 (October 1992): 376-379.

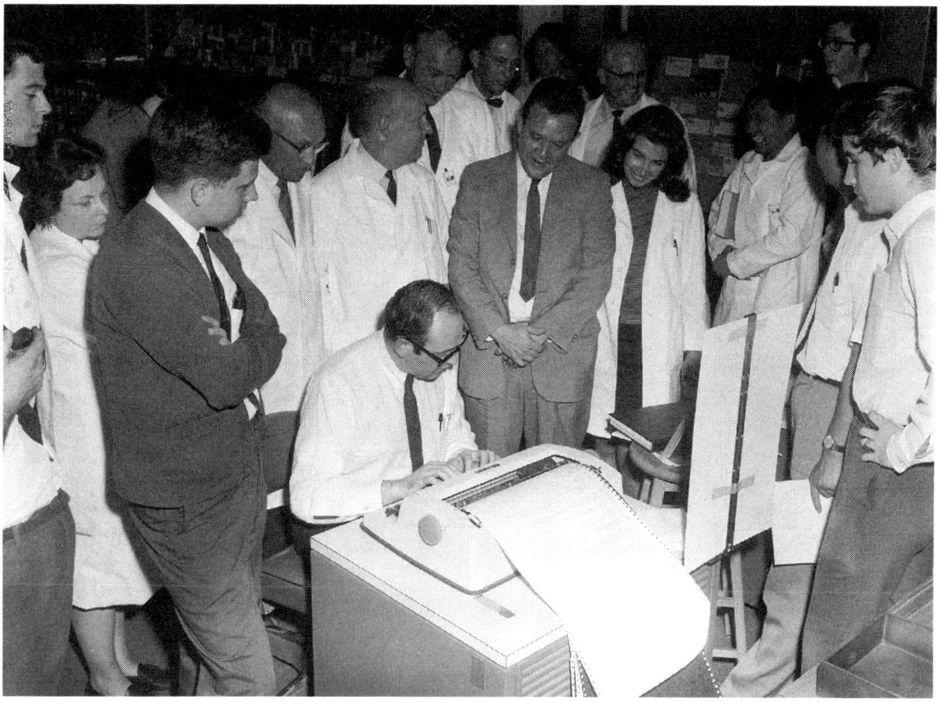

Pizer teaches BCN to Interim President Westerfeld, faculty, and students.

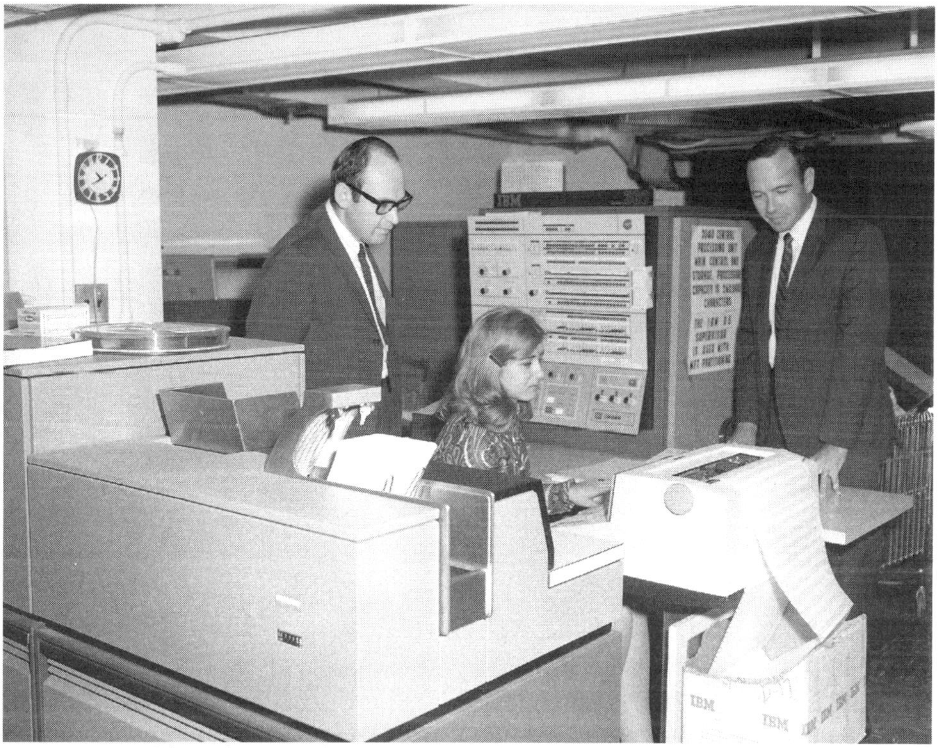

Pizer, keypunch operator Bertha V. Izyk, and computer manager Richard N. Fenzl at the BCN console.

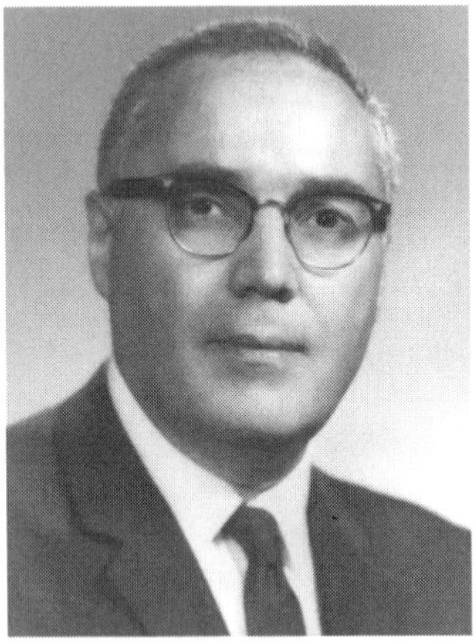

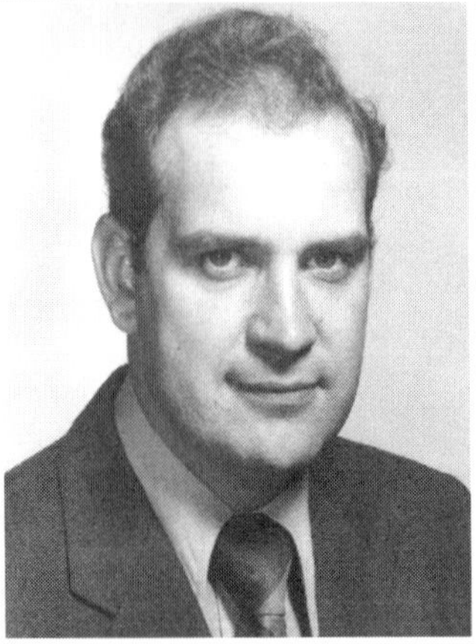

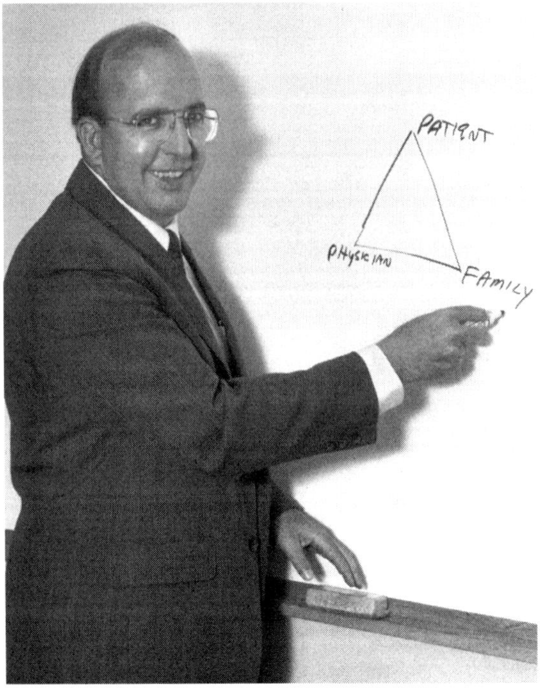

On March 26, 1969, Governor Rockefeller signed into law a bill that required Upstate to create a Department of Family Practice. The initiative was put into effect immediately, with Francis Salvatore Caliva, Class of 1948 (top), as chair. Upstate had already established a pilot three-year residency program in family practice (then called "general practice") at St. Joseph's in 1963. This program became fully accredited in 1969.

Caliva's death in November 1972, at the age of only 48, left a wide hole in the Upstate fabric. John B. Henry, then Dean of the College of Health Related Professions, stepped in to guide the department until Bernard A. Bernstein succeeded him as acting chair in January 1973. L. Thomas Wolff (center) became chair in August 1973 and served until 1985. A graduate of Albany Medical College and the St. Joseph's residency program and a fellow of the American Academy of Family Physicians, Wolff was president of the Society of Teachers of Family Medicine from 1985 to 1986 and president of the American Board of Family Medicine from 2003 to 2004. In 1988 the department's name changed from Family Practice to Family Medicine and its offices moved from St. Joseph's to the Madison Irving Medical Center.

In 1989 Wolff and Macaran Baird (bottom), who had been chair since 1987, cofounded the Rural Medical Education (RMED) program, whose purpose — and success — is to provide nine-month clerkships in underserved areas, thus creating a symbiotic relationship between the rural physicians, who need the personnel, and the students, who need the clinical experience.

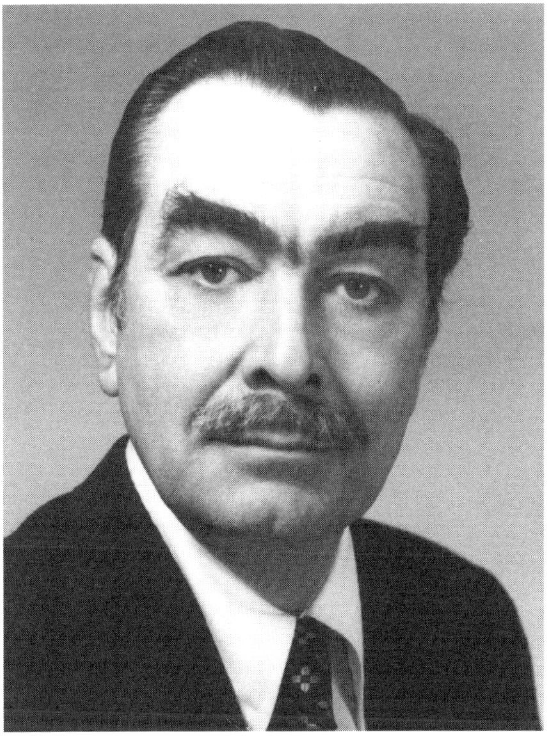

In 1975 Richard P. Schmidt (left) was inaugurated as Upstate's third President. Schmidt earned his M.D. at the University of Louisville in 1945, did a residency in neurology in Louisville and one in psychiatry in Cincinnati, then held a fellowship in neurology in Louisville. He taught neurology at Louisville, the University of Washington, and the University of Florida, becoming known as an expert on epilepsy. He chaired the Department of Medicine at the University of Florida from 1962 to 1965 and was the associate dean of its medical school from 1965 until he came to Upstate as Dean of the College of Medicine and Vice President for Academic Affairs in 1970.

The Schmidt presidential years were difficult, not only for Upstate, but also for academic medical enterprises nationwide. Economic pressures, decreasing budgets, and increasing governmental regulation created unprecedented dilemmas for medical school administrators. Throughout this protracted crisis, Schmidt fought like a hero, sometimes succeeding, and sometimes ending up discouraged. A story is told that once, upon returning from meetings in the state capital, he said to a colleague whom he happened across, "I have good news and bad news. The good news is that I made it home safely from Albany. The bad news is that that's all the good news."

Despite these problems, Schmidt managed some noteworthy gains. In 1976, responding to the growing need for primary care physicians, the College of Medicine launched the Binghamton Clinical Campus. In 1972 Bluemle had begun negotiations with SUNY central administration and SUNY Binghamton University to establish a clinical facility in Binghamton for Upstate students. University Hospital opened its burn treatment center in 1979, began offering hyperbaric oxygen therapy in 1981, started a pediatric emergency unit in 1981, and opened the Regional Oncology Center as the main care facility for outpatient cancer treatments in 1984.

Schmidt was also visible in the larger community as, for example, president of the Metropolitan Development Association of Syracuse and Central New York and chair of the University Hill Corporation.

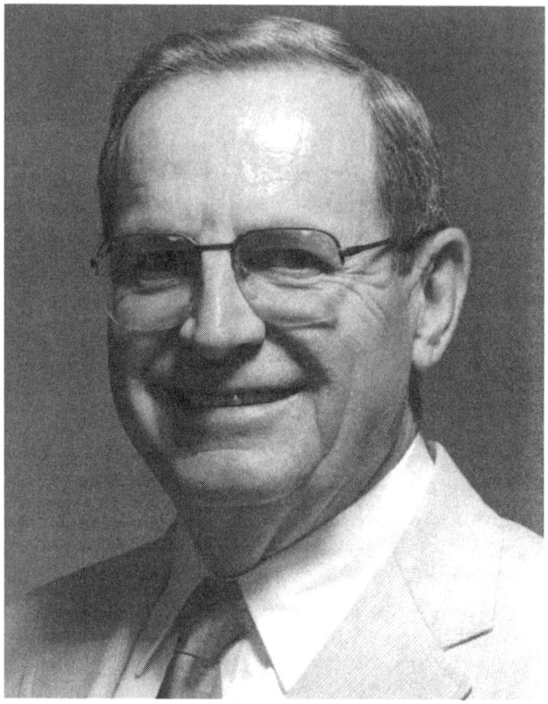

Professor of Pathology John Bernard Henry became the fourth president in 1985. He is best known as the editor of *Clinical Diagnosis and Management by Laboratory Methods*, a standard work that was first published in 1908 as *A Manual of Clinical Diagnosis* by James C. Todd and appeared in its twentieth edition in 2001. His research includes enzymology, hematology, and transplantation immunohematology. By 2004 he had 263 scientific publications.

After receiving his A.B. from Cornell in 1951 and his M.D. in 1955 from the University of Rochester, Henry studied and taught pathology at Washington University, Columbia University, the National Cancer Institute, Harvard Medical School, and the University of Florida, where he served from 1960 to 1964 as director of the blood bank and clinical laboratories in Gainesville. He came to Upstate in 1964 as Professor of Pathology and Director of Clinical Pathology and served also as Dean of the College of Health Related Professions from 1971 to 1977, Acting Chair of the Department of Family Practice from 1972 to 1973, and Acting Chair of the Department of Pathology in 1974. He was president of the American Association of Blood Banks from 1970 to 1971, the American Board of Pathology from 1976 to 1978, the American Blood Commission from 1978 to 1980, and the American Society of Clinical Pathologists from 1980 to 1981.

He left Syracuse in 1979 to become Dean of the Georgetown University School of Medicine and director of several laboratories at the Georgetown University Hospital and Medical Center, but in the fall of 1984 he accepted Upstate's invitation to return as president. One of his first innovations was to rename SUNY Upstate Medical Center as the SUNY Health Science Center at Syracuse (SUNY HSC), in order to reflect more accurately the diversity of services and programs offered.

Keenly aware that no institution can do its best without adequate space, President Henry pursued an aggressive policy of growth and development. He acquired the land bounded by Irving Avenue, South Crouse Avenue, Harrison Street, and Madison Street upon which the Institute for

Human Performance (IHP) would be built between 1996 and 2000. His administration added several new facilities, including a day care center for employees' children; began construction of the new Health Sciences Library building and the East Wing of University Hospital (the Concentrated Care Center); and secured the funding to plan and erect the IHP.

Henry maintained strong ties to the armed services throughout his career. He served as a hospital corpsman in the U.S. Navy from 1946 to 1948, then as a medical officer in the U.S. Naval Reserve (USNR) from 1958 to 1995, achieving the rank of captain in 1974. While dean at Georgetown in 1985, he contributed to the establishment of the first of about sixty Physician Reservists in Medical Universities and Schools (PRIMUS) units in the USNR. The purpose of these units was to provide the Navy with easily mobilized medical personnel to care for naval casualties in case of war or other national emergency. In 1986 he created a PRIMUS unit at the SUNY Health Science Center at Syracuse and commanded it from 1987 to 1991.

Never afraid to try an innovation, Henry boldly introduced new programs and plans. In 1988 the College of Medicine and the College of Graduate Studies began a successful seven-year M.D.-Ph.D. program to educate physician-scientists. In 1990 Henry started a combined M.D.-M.B.A. program with SUNY Binghamton University, similar to what many other medical schools use to train patient care advocates and medical managers, but it graduated only one student and faded away from lack of interest.

Henry was a strong supporter of using computers in medicine and developing high-tech solutions to problems in medical informatics. Between 1990 and 2003 he recorded thirty-six talks and presentations on computer courseware, mostly about pathology, but also about medical education, medical literature, and medical computing. On April 11, 1995, as part of the dedication ceremony for the new Health Sciences Library building, the John Bernard Henry Microcomputer Learning Center was named and opened in the Media Services Department on the second floor of the Library and soon became one of the Library's most heavily used resources.

Henry claimed that his five main values were, in order of priority: God, country, family, profession, and community. He devoted tremendous energy to all five. In an April 2005 self-assessment he listed his strengths as integrity, capacity for hard work, attention to detail, thoroughness, seriousness, sensitivity to human needs, task-orientedness, loyalty, kindness, leadership, decisiveness, ability to act on intuition while rejecting political pressure, commitment to the technological future, and physical fitness. In the same statement he listed his weaknesses as impatience, stubbornness, short attention span, parsimony, difficulty in saying no, tendency to overextend himself, difficulty in relaxing, inattentiveness to personal appearance, and intolerance of other people's lack of effort.

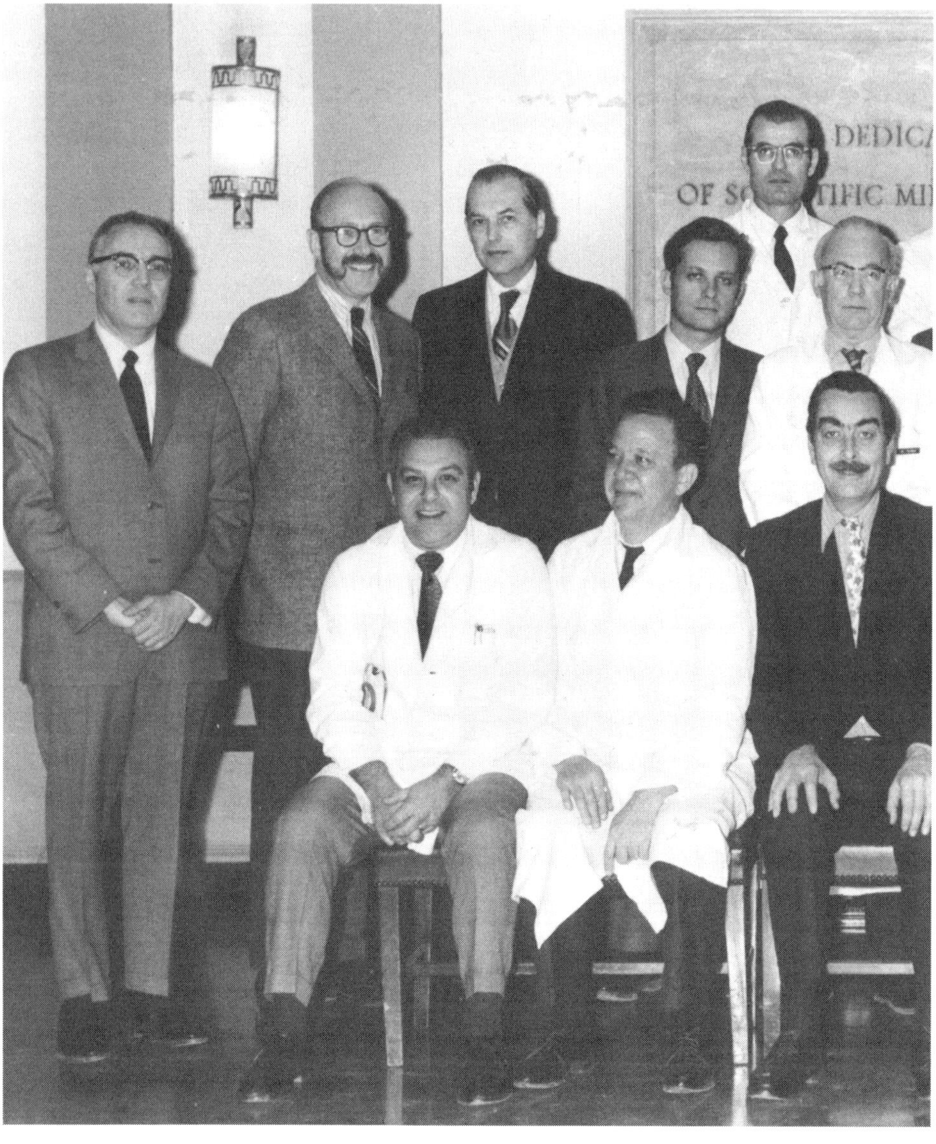

In 1970, the year that Patricia Joy Numann of the Class of 1965 became the first woman surgeon at Upstate, the department chairs and top administrators included: *top row:* Watts R. Webb (surgery), George G. Holz, Jr. (microbiology), Rolla B. Hill, Jr. (pathology), Otto M. Lilien (urology); *middle row:* Francis S. Caliva (family medicine), Donald Oken (psychiatry), Robert E.L. Nesbitt, Jr. (obstetrics and gynecology), Gilbert S. Ross (neurology), Harry A. Feldman (preventive medicine), James L. McGraw (ophthalmology), John G. McAfee (radiology), James B. Preston (physiology), David G. Murray (orthopedic surgery), George F. Reed (otolaryngology); *seated:* Leo Jivoff (rehabilitation medicine), Wilfred W. Westerfeld (biochemistry), Richard P. Schmidt (dean), Lewis W. Bleumle, Jr. (president),

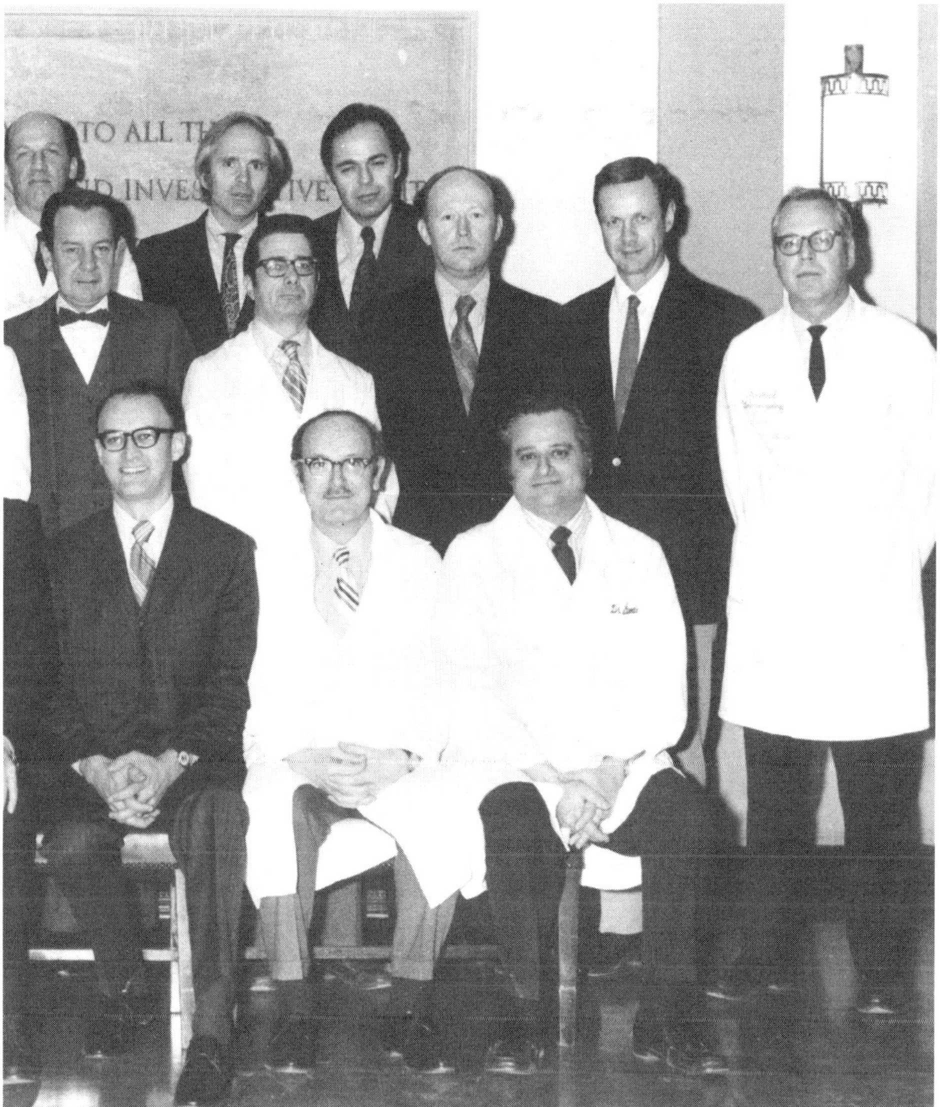

Allen B. Dobkin (anesthesiology), Donald C. Goodman (anatomy); *absent:* John B. Henry (clinical pathology), Robert B. King (neurosurgery), Julius B. Richmond (pediatrics), Irwin M. Weiner (pharmacology), William J. Williams (medicine). They stand in front of the anonymous motto in the main lobby of Weiskotten Hall: "Dedicated to all those of scientific mind and investigative spirit who purpose to serve humanity." This inscribed marble slab was already in place when the Basic Sciences Building, as it was then called, was dedicated on November 22, 1937. Dean Weiskotten was probably either its author or editor, as its sentiment agrees with his personal philosophy of medicine. While he acknowledged that one aspect of medicine is art, he held that science is always the more important aspect.

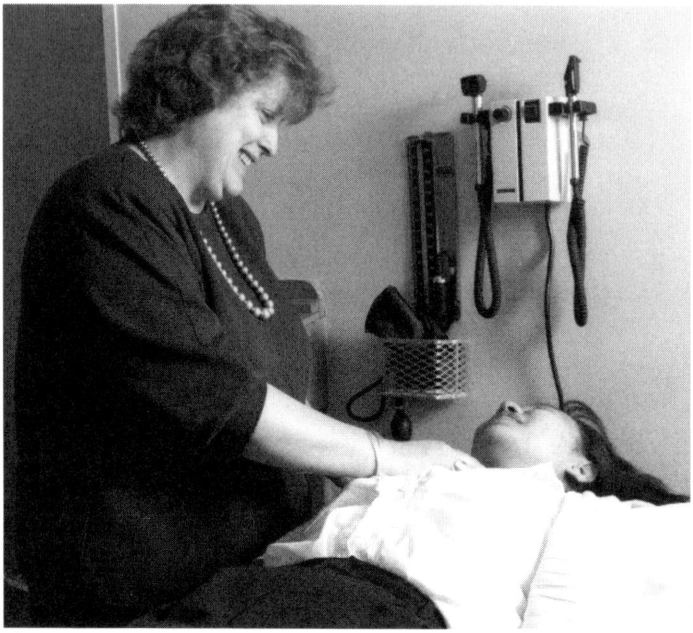

Few medical graduates of Upstate have achieved as much as Patricia Numann. She owns many impressive "firsts" besides being the first woman surgeon at University Hospital. She became in 1978 the first woman Associate Dean of the Upstate College of Medicine, in 1987 the first woman member of the AMA Council on Scientific Affairs, in 1997 the first woman Medical Director of University Hospital, in 1998 the first woman elected Second Vice President of the American College of Surgeons, in 2000 the first Lloyd S. Rogers Professor of Surgery at Upstate Medical University, and in 2001 the first woman to chair the American Board of Surgery. She founded the Association of Women Surgeons in 1981 and University Hospital's Breast Care Center in 1986.

From a poor family in the Catskills, Numann earned her B.A. at the University of Rochester in 1962, did her internship and residency at Upstate, received her surgical certification in 1971, then specialized in endocrine and breast surgery. Her zeal to bring more women into medicine and especially into positions of medical leadership is exceeded only by her legendary devotion to her patients. Her renowned effort to reassure frightened surgical patients eases their burden, gives them strength, and humanizes surgery.

On June 25, 2004, in Washington, D.C., the American Medical Women's Association — founded by obstetrician and surgeon Bertha Van Hoosen in 1915 — inducted Numann into the International Women in Medicine Hall of Fame. At the time of her induction, the twenty-three other honorees of the Hall were Elizabeth Ingram Adamson, Doris Gorka Bartuska, Mary Elizabeth Bates, Patricia E. Bath, Elizabeth Blackwell, Rebecca Lee Crumpler, Jane F. Desforges, M. Joycelyn Elders, Martha Mae Eliot, Jane E. Hodgson, Anandibai Joshi, Leonora Howard King, Louise D. Larimore, Risa J. Lavizzo-Mourey, Mary H. McLean, Alma Dea Morani, Eliza M. Mosher, Antonia C. Novello, Susan La Flesche Picotte, Marion Craig Potter, Barbara B. Stimson, Bertha Van Hoosen, and Martha Welpton.

10

Toward the Future: One University, Nine Names

Gregory L. Eastwood, a gastroenterologist, became the fifth president on January 4, 1993. He once expressed his vision for the medical university in a letter to the chancellor of the State University of New York: "Before coming here I was the dean of the Medical College of Georgia and before that I had pursued a rather typical career in medical academia, running a research laboratory, teaching, and taking care of patients. I have enjoyed everything along the way. I think that is in part because I enjoy dealing with complex things, seeing broadly and integrating, and, most of all, feeling that I am improving the human condition. That is an idealistic sentiment, but something that needs to be articulated. I tell our incoming medical students that I assume that a significant part of the reason they are entering the medical profession is to help humankind and that it is natural and appropriate for their idealism to be tempered by the practicalities of their experience over the coming four years and beyond. I also tell them that unless they retain throughout their life some connection with the ideals that motivated them to become a physician, they are likely to shrivel up and die inside."

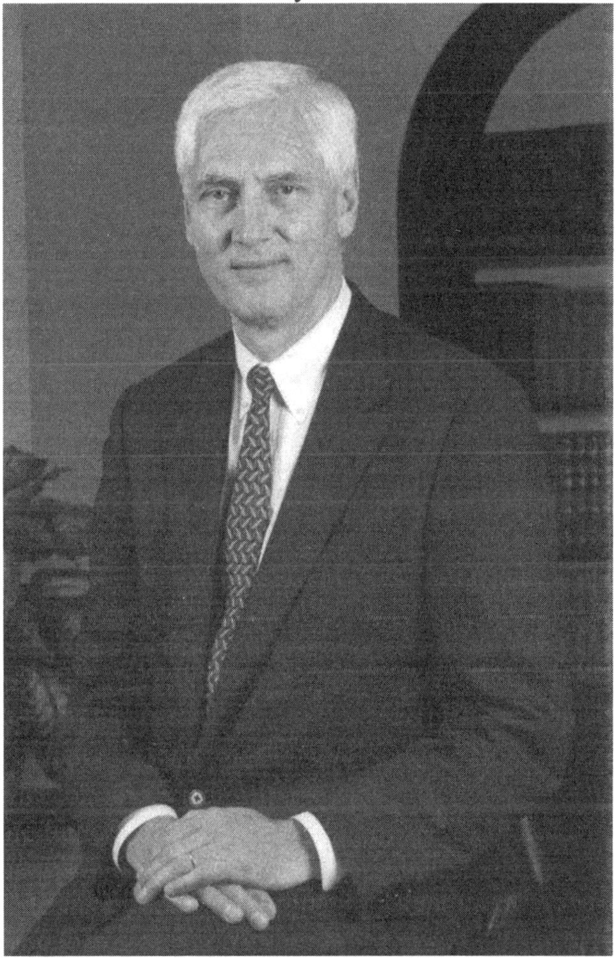

Eastwood's idealism has manifested itself in the first twelve years of his presidency as three main kinds of accomplishments:

1. An increased visibility of Upstate Medical University and especially University Hospital within the greater community of Central New York. As an active member of the University Hill Corporation, a not-for-profit organization of businesses and educational, religious, and medical institutions in the general area of Syracuse University, Eastwood has worked closely with SUNY College of Envrionmental Science and Forestry President Cornelius B. Murphy and Syracuse University Chancellors Kenneth A. Shaw and Nancy Cantor to improve the whole environment for learning and culture in this part of Syracuse. Under his leadership, Upstate faculty, staff, and students have designed and implemented a variety of specific programs to reach out to the community in many important ways.

2. The beginnings of efforts to revitalize and expand the research program, which, among comparable programs at similar medical schools, had fallen below average from its high point in the 1950s and 1960s.

3. Unprecedented capital improvements. While much of the growth that has been realized under Eastwood — notably the East Wing of University Hospital that opened in 1994 and the new Health Sciences Library building that opened in 1995 — was planned during Henry's term, most of it was conceived on Eastwood's watch. Major examples of this growth are the Institute for Cardiovascular Research, the Institute for Human Performance, the Center for Bioethics and Humanities, University Health Care Center, and the forthcoming children's hospital, academic building, and Central New York Biotechnology Research Center.

Eastwood's administration has increased, more than any previous administration, the presence, visibility, and acceptance of the medical humanities on campus. He has given strong personal support to this aspect of medicine. One of his earliest actions when he became president was to enlist psychiatrist Robert W. Daly, Class of 1957, to create the President's Ethics Symposium, a major annual event open to the public. Its topics have included institutional and individual ethics, end-of-life issues, managed care, distributive justice in rationing or triaging health care, relations between regular and alternative medicine, genetic testing, assisted reproduction, drug marketing and other commercial influences on health care providers, stem cell research, and public health policy regarding infectious disease control.

Renowned poet Bonnie St. Andrews, Ph.D. (page 161), whose work appeared in publications as diverse as *The New Yorker* and the *Journal of the American Medical Association*, taught English and writing in the College of Health Professions from 1982 to 2000, then became one of the original faculty members of the Center for Bioethics and Humanities. Always a favorite of students, she was honored as a SUNY Distinguished Teaching

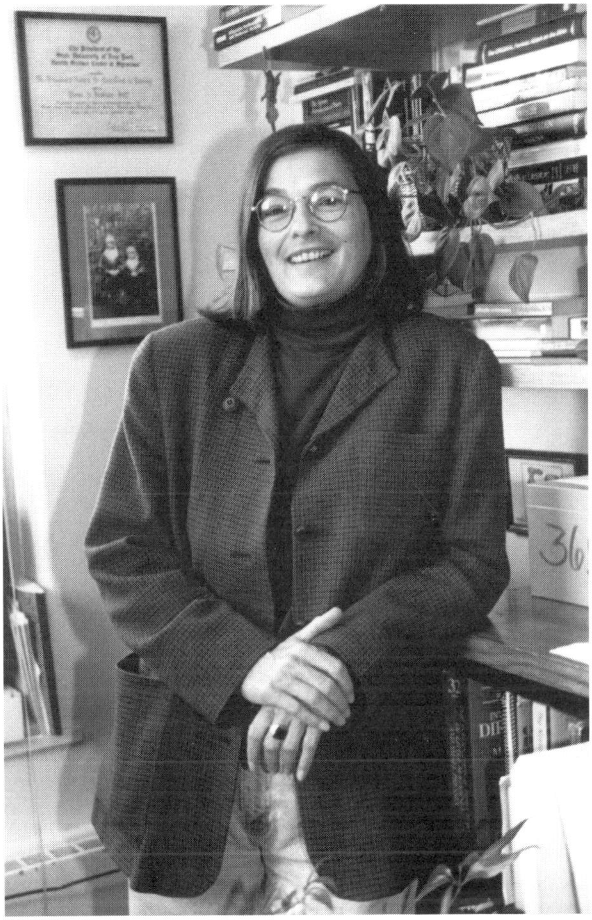

Professor in 1997. She was committed to helping not only students, but everyone connected with health care, to express themselves in writing and other creative activities. At the College of Health Professions she edited intermittently *The Silverman Review* (named after the building in which that college was housed), a literary magazine that consisted mostly of student works. This venture was unsuccessful, but soon after she came to the Center she founded *The Healing Muse*, a more ambitious literary magazine that would solicit contributions both locally and nationally and would accept them for publication only after critical review by an editorial board of professors. *The Healing Muse* has thrived. Since the first annual issue appeared in the fall of 2001, each subsequent issue has been better received than the previous one.

The professorship of the founding director of the Center, Kathy Faber-Langendoen, is endowed by the Medical Alumni Association. From 2001 to 2004 the eminent philosopher Samuel Gorovitz was the first Dearing-Daly Professor of Bioethics and Humanities, honoring both Bruce Dearing and Robert Daly, co-founder in 1978 of the Consortium for Culture and Medicine, a cooperative project of Le Moyne College, Syracuse University, and Upstate.

In 2001 the Medicine and Society course, required of all medical students in their first two years, was replaced by the more rigorous Ethical, Legal, and Social Issues in Medicine (ELSIM) component of the Practice of Medicine (POM) course, which at the same time superseded the required two-year Introduction to Clinical Medicine (ICM) course. Thus the medical humanities — in accordance with AAMC recommendations — have become a robust aspect of the required medical curriculum.

Familiarly known in its three major eras (1834-1871, 1871-1950, and post-1950) as "Geneva," "Syracuse," and "Upstate," respectively, the nine official names of this medical school have been: the Medical Institution of Geneva College (1834-1852); Geneva Medical College (1852-1871); the College of Physicians and Surgeons of the Syracuse University (1871-1875); the College of Medicine of Syracuse University (1875-1887); Syracuse University College of Medicine (1887-1950); the State University of New York College of Medicine at Syracuse (1950-1953); the State University of New York Upstate Medical Center (1953-1986); the State University of New York Health Science Center at Syracuse (1986-1999); and the State University of New York Upstate Medical University (since 1999).

Since 1992 Upstate has been Onondaga County's largest employer. In 2004 it had 6305 employees, compared with 4640 for Syracuse University, the second largest, and 3775 for Wegmans Food Markets, the third largest. In 1995 its 4700 led Carrier Corporation's 4230 and Syracuse University's 3892. In 1991 General Electric was first, Syracuse University second, and Upstate third. Such growth has not come without difficulties.

The institution lost much of its identity and recognition, especially in the local community, during the time when its name was the SUNY Health Science Center at Syracuse. The general public typically continued to call it "Upstate" anyway and few people seemed to know what a "Health Science Center" was. Thus, mainly to alleviate this confusion, on September 8, 1999, at the Fall Faculty Convocation, Eastwood announced that the name would be changed to SUNY Upstate Medical University: "Upstate" to give it a convenient handle; "Medical" to encompass not only physicians, but also nurses, bioscientists, technicians, and all health care professionals; and "University" to let the world know what kind of an institution it is.

Using 2001 AAMC data, the NIH in 2003 ranked Upstate 90th of 121 medical schools in research funding. The National Science Foundation in 2000 ranked Upstate 205th of 641 higher educational institutions in research productivity. NIH data for 1970 showed Upstate ranked 58th of 100 medical schools in research funding. In 2004 Upstate ranked 95th of 123 medical schools in NIH awards received. This slip in extramural funding from the 42nd to the 23rd percentile in thirty-four years is an important area of concern, seriously affecting Upstate's ability to attract and retain top scientists for its faculty. To improve the biomedical research environment in Syracuse is a priority of the Eastwood administration. It is not an insurmountable problem. The school that ranked 99th of 100 in 1970, the University of Massachusetts Medical School in Worcester, improved to 39th of 121 in 2000, thanks in large measure to a concerted administrative effort since the mid-1970s. The Director of the Office for Research at the University of Massachusetts Medical School since 1999 has been John L. Sullivan, an

Upstate alumnus, Class of 1972, who visited Upstate in November 2003 to give a talk called "Building a Biomedical Research Enterprise that Achieves National Distinction" in the Medical Alumni Auditorium of Weiskotten Hall and to offer concrete suggestions in several private meetings.

One of the most important aspects of modern biomedical science is translational research, i.e., the practical study of techniques and policies by which new discoveries are "translated" into commercial products to enhance patient care. The goals of these techniques and policies are speed, efficiency, precision, and safety, all in the service of beneficent global health care delivery. Translational research has become a priority of Upstate's Research Development Office and since 2002 Upstate has hosted an annual conference on translational research. As in any kind of successfully applied science, collaboration is essential. To that end Upstate has become, along with Cornell University, the Ordway Research Institute, Rochester Institute of Technology, Roswell Park Cancer Institute, SUNY University at Buffalo, and the University of Rochester Medical Center, an active member of the Upstate New York Coalition for Biomedical Research (UNYCoR). With its central office on Upstate's campus, UNYCoR is chaired by Upstate's Provost and Vice President for Academic Affairs and Research, Kenneth L. Barker, who holds a Ph.D. in biochemistry from Ohio State University.

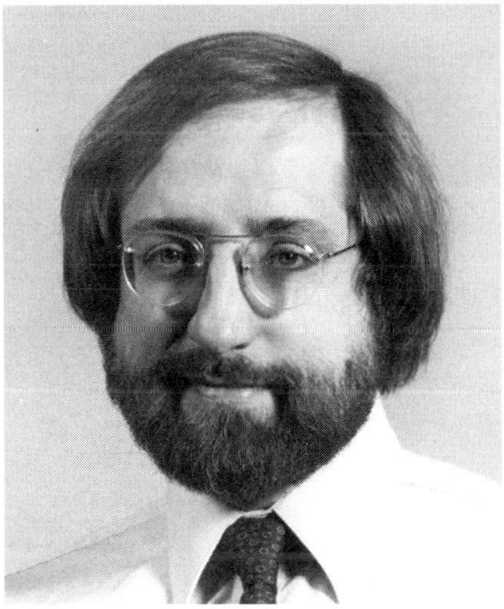

Biochemistry has always been one of the strongest basic science departments in the College of Medicine and the College of Graduate Studies. The legacy of Cutbush, Towler, Smith, Brewer, and Westerfeld has been ably continued by Richard L. Cross (right), a 1970 Yale Ph.D. who joined the Upstate faculty in 1973 and became chair of the department in 1982. From 1970 to 1973 he held a postdoctoral fellowship at the Molecular Biology Institute of the University of California at Los Angeles in the laboratory of Paul D. Boyer, who shared the 1997 Nobel Prize in Chemistry for his "elucidation of the enzymatic mechanism underlying the synthesis of adenosine triphosphate (ATP)." In his official autobiography submitted to the Nobel Foundation, Boyer named Cross among his former assistants and colleagues whose contributions had significantly advanced the knowledge of ATP. Cross has maintained a close collaborative relationship with Boyer since coming to Upstate, including a National Satellite Television Seminar for thousands of science students on April 23, 1998, sponsored by the American Chemical Society.

After Reed retired from his ten-year term as Dean of the College of Medicine in 1986, a succession of short-term deans followed. Weiner served just four years; Williams, as interim, just a few months; then Joseph P. Whalen, Class of 1959, just three years. Whalen, an internationally renowned diagnostic radiologist, brought New York City its first CT, third in the nation, in 1973; its first superconducting MRI, again third in the nation, in 1983; and its first electron beam CT in 1999. He is the author of *Radiology of the Abdomen: Anatomic Basis* (1976), co-author of *Radiation Risks in Medical Imaging* (1984), and co-editor of *Principles of MRI* (1998). He resigned the Upstate deanship in 1995 to return to the radiology faculty of the New York Hospital-Cornell Medical Center, where he had been Radiologist-in-Chief for sixteen years before coming to Upstate in 1992.

Eastwood himself functioned as both dean and president from 1995 until 2001. Anesthesiologist and "Real Age" guru Michael F. Roizen failed to gain the confidence of the faculty and resigned after less than a year. Williams, universally respected, held the reins for two years until a national search could be completed. This search found an insider, Steven Scheinman, who until then had been Chief of Nephrology in the Department of Medicine. Eastwood directed a major reorganization of administrative positions and duties in 2004, with Scheinman being named Executive Vice President as well as Dean, in charge of not only the College of Medicine, but also many other major enterprises, as Eastwood described in his September 8, 2004, State of the Medical University Address:

> In his capacity as Executive Vice President, Dr. Scheinman will function as a campus chief operating officer and the following will report to him: the Vice President for Hospital Affairs and Executive Director of University Hospital; the Dean of the College of Graduate Studies; the Dean of the Binghamton Clinical Campus; the Chief Information Officer; the Provost and VP for Academic Affairs and Research for matters that pertain to research, internal academic affairs, the Colleges of Health Professions and of Nursing, and the Health Sciences Library; and the Vice President of Administration and Finance for matters that pertain to finance and space. In his capacity as Dean of the College of Medicine, the following will report to him: department chairs, the Director of the Center for Bioethics and Humanities, assistant and associate deans, and directors of institutes.

In the fall of 2001, after years of studying complicated options, soliciting and considering feedback from students, and refereeing turf wars among faculty, the College of Medicine inaugurated a new medical curriculum, integrating the basic and clinical sciences, reorganizing the basic science curriculum into an organ-based format, creating the Practice of Medicine course to teach clinical skills and provide patient contact immediately in the first year, emphasizing hands-on, small-group, and online learning while de-emphasizing traditional lectures, and reducing the number of contact hours to allow for more study time. A minority of faculty and students have expressed reservations about the new model, but in general it must be judged a success.

Even more dramatic than the curriculum change has been the gigantic expansion of the physical plant and the accompanying expansion of programs and services.

In 1994 clinical personnel began using the new East Wing of University Hospital according to a phased occupancy plan, bringing state-of-the-art medical and surgical units to Central New York for the concentrated care of burns, emergencies, cardiopulmonary diseases, and neurological disorders, and as well as expanded facilities for endoscopy, imaging, and other diagnostic procedures.

In December 1995 the Health Sciences Library moved without interruption of service into a separate four-floor building attached to Weiskotten Hall. Prior to moving into the new high-tech structure designed by Einhorn, Yaffee, and Prescott, the Library had been housed in substandard facilities in the southeast wing of Weiskotten Hall. Shelving was at well over 100%, all pre-1950 materials were in remote storage, and many of the professional librarians did not even have offices. Despite these physical and logistical limitations, the library staff always bettered the national average when evaluated for its service. The new building has allowed this service to improve even more. For example, in the AAMC *Medical School Graduation Questionnaire* for both 1997 and 1998, SUNY Health Science Center at Syracuse medical students indicated that they were most satisfied with the Library out of all the student support services available on campus. On a Leikert scale of 1 (very satisfied) to 5 (very dissatisfied), the Library received an average score of 1.4. The national average for libraries was 2.0. The Commission on Higher Education of the Middle States Association of Colleges and Schools team that visited the campus on April 25-28, 1999, congratulated Upstate for its magnificent new Library building and praised the Library's consistently high quality of service:

> The Team heard repeatedly in discussions with faculty, students and administrators of the campus-wide pride and appreciation for the new facility, confirming what we read in the self study. The faculty and students universally praise the library staff especially noting their strong customer service orientation. The faculty also commented on the library's willingness to purchase instructional materials to sup-

port their courses. The availability of digital resources in the form of databases, indexes, abstracts, and electronic journals is noteworthy.

Also in December 1995 the Joslin Center for Diabetes opened under the direction of Ruth Weinstock. In April 1997 University Health Care Center opened, bringing many outpatient services together in a single location at the corner of Harrison and Townsend Streets. In 1998 the Central New York Gamma Knife Center opened in University Hospital.

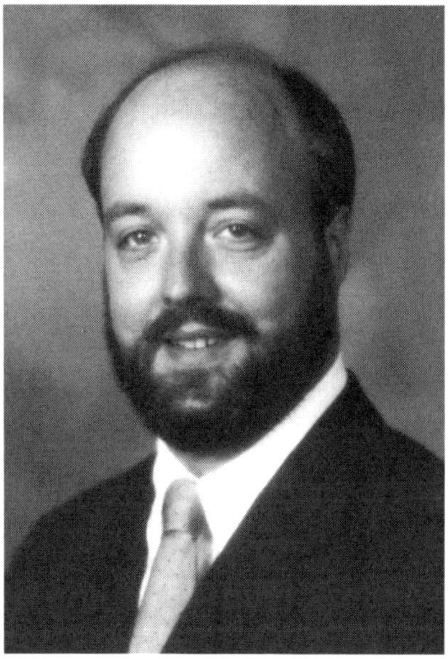

John B. McCabe, Class of 1979 (right), joined the faculty in 1987 to teach critical care and emergency medicine. From 1985 until 1993 he was editor-in-chief of *Resuscitation*, an Elsevier journal started in 1972 to explore both basic scientific and clinical issues in cardiopulmonary acute care. When Upstate founded its Department of Emergency Medicine in 1991, McCabe became its first chair, but left that job in 1996 to become Vice President and Vice Dean for Clinical Affairs.* In 2001 he returned to practicing and teaching emergency medicine.

Richard C. Hunt, who became chair in 1998, organized and coordinated Central New York's response to the great crime of September 11, 2001. He served from 2001 to 2003 as president of the National Association of Emergency Medical Services Physicians (NAEMSP) and, perhaps even more significantly, from 2002 to 2003 as founding president of the Advocates for Emergency Medical Services, which the NAEMSP and the National Association of State EMS Directors created on October 22, 2002, in direct response to the challenge of terrorism, to ensure that all necessary clinical and logistical systems will be immediately ready in case of another attack.

Shortly after Hunt left in January 2004 to become Director of the Division of Injury and Disability Outcomes and Programs in the National Center for Injury Preventions at the Centers for Disease Control in Atlanta, McCabe became chair a second time. He was president of the American College of Emergency Physicians from 1993 to 1994 and of the American Board of Emergency Medicine from 2004 to 2005.

* When Gene Kaplan retired from the Department of Psychiatry in 1999, he joked that medical school professors should always treat their students well because, he said, indicating McCabe, "one of them might come back and be your dean."

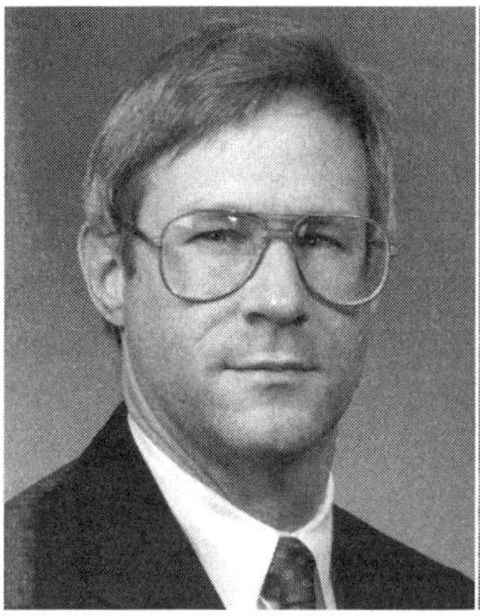
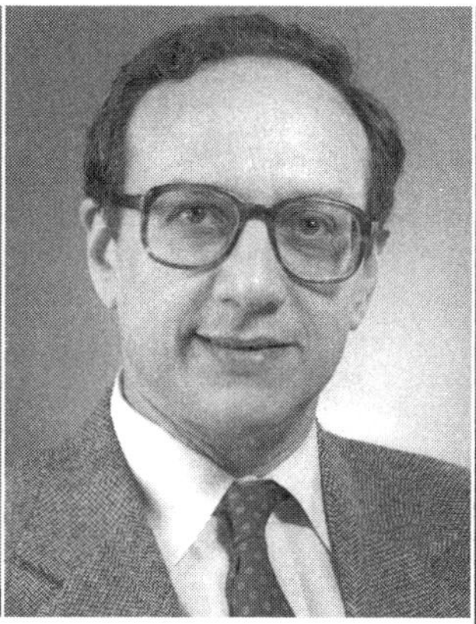
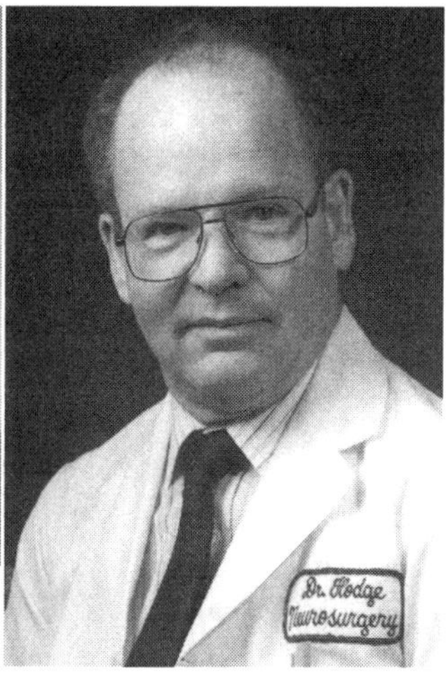

Burk Jubelt (left), whose main research concerns viral infections of the central nervous system, chaired the Department of Neurology from 1989 until 2004. Enrico M. Camporesi (center), Chair of Anesthesiology since 1989 and an expert in hyperbaric medicine, resigned in 2005 to become Chair of Anesthesiology at the University of South Florida. Under his leadership cardiac anesthesia was introduced to Upstate in 1995.

Several long-term department chairs are still serving as this book goes to press. John A. Hoepner became Chair of Ophthalmology in 1984. Charles J. Hodge (right) succeeded King as Chair of Neurosurgery in 1988. John Duggan's son, David B. Duggan, Class of 1979, became Chair of the Department of Medicine in 1993 after a year as interim chair. The separate Department of Radiation Oncology emerged from the Department of Radiology in 1995 with Chung T. Chung as chair. Gabriel P. Haas has chaired Urology since 1995 and Shawky Z.A. Badawy became Chair of Obstetrics and Gynecology in 1998.

On October 8, 1997, University Hospital named its Pediatric Intensive Care Unit after Frank A. Oski, Chair of Pediatrics from 1972 to 1985, author in 1977 of the controversial *Don't Drink Your Milk: The Frightening New Medical Facts about the World's Most Overrated Nutrient*, founder in 1984 of the journal *Contemporary Pediatrics*, and recipient in 1996 of the Lifetime Achievement Award of the American Academy of Pediatrics.

In 2001 Thomas R. Welch, a 1973 McGill M.D. who did his residency at Upstate, succeeded Howard L. Weinberger, Class of 1958, chair from 1991 to 1999, and Leonard B. Weiner, chair from 1999 to 2001, as Chair of Pediatrics. In 2003 Tucson and Syracuse were the only two major American cities without children's hospitals. Because University Hospital is the only tertiary care hospital for a very large area of Central New York and the region's only hospital offering comprehensive pediatric cancer care, pediatric open heart surgery, and dedicated pediatric emergency services, the need for a special facility for pediatrics has been urgent. In September

2003 Eastwood and Welch announced plans to add five floors to the East Wing of University Hospital, including the Central New York Children's Hospital on the top two floors, with state-of-the-art — and kid-friendly — medical and surgical services. Senator Hillary Rodham Clinton, long an advocate of children's rights and improved pediatric health care, visited Upstate on October 7, 2003, to speak in strong support of this initiative.

While most of what Upstate Medical University is, does, advocates, and represents can readily be seen as reflecting the highest aspirations in medical education, one area in which it has remained below AAMC standards is the hiring and retention of women faculty, especially in positions of leadership, such as department chairs. *Women in U.S. Academic Medicine Statistics and Medical School Benchmarking, 2003-2004*, the AAMC report by Diane Magrane *et al.*, showed Upstate, against the national average of 30 percent, with only 23 percent women faculty, tied in this category for fifth from the bottom among all American medical schools; and no women chairs, tied for bottom with thirteen other schools. In 2003 there were 279 women chairs in medical schools nationwide, or ten percent of all chairs.

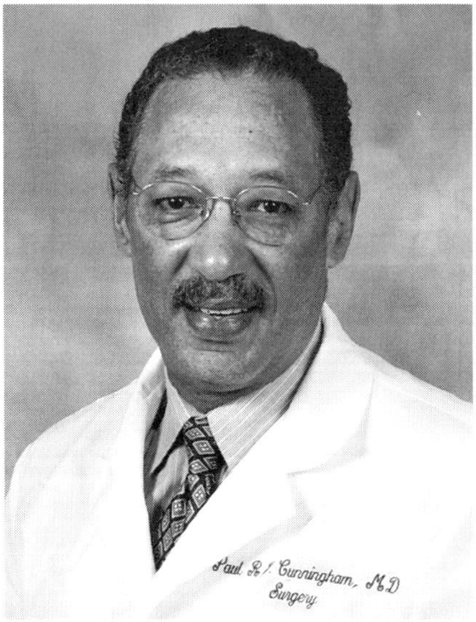

Leslie J. Kohman became Chief of Thoracic Surgery in 1990, Lynn M. Cleary became Associate Dean for Curriculum in 1997 and led the "Curriculum Renewal" movement, Kathy Faber-Langendoen became Director of the Center for Bioethics and Humanities at its founding in August 2000, Vivian Gahtan became Chief of Vascular Surgery in 2003, and a few other women physicians hold or have held some authority at Upstate, but for the most part non-white male minorities have fared better than women on the faculty. Paul R. Cunningham (right) became Chair of the Department of Surgery in 2002 and Gregory A. Threatte, Class of 1973 (shown on page 169 at Match Day 2004 with fourth-year students Tosha Brown [left] and Aashiyana Koreishi [right]), became Chair of the Department of Pathology in 2003.

While the emphasis on improving the status and numbers of women faculty remains nascent, various recent initiatives in research development have shown more promise. Responsibility for expanding Upstate's research presence in the scientific community, not only on campus proper but also through UNYCoR and other more broadly conceived programs, belongs to Provost Kenneth Barker, who arrived at Upstate in 1996 from Texas Tech

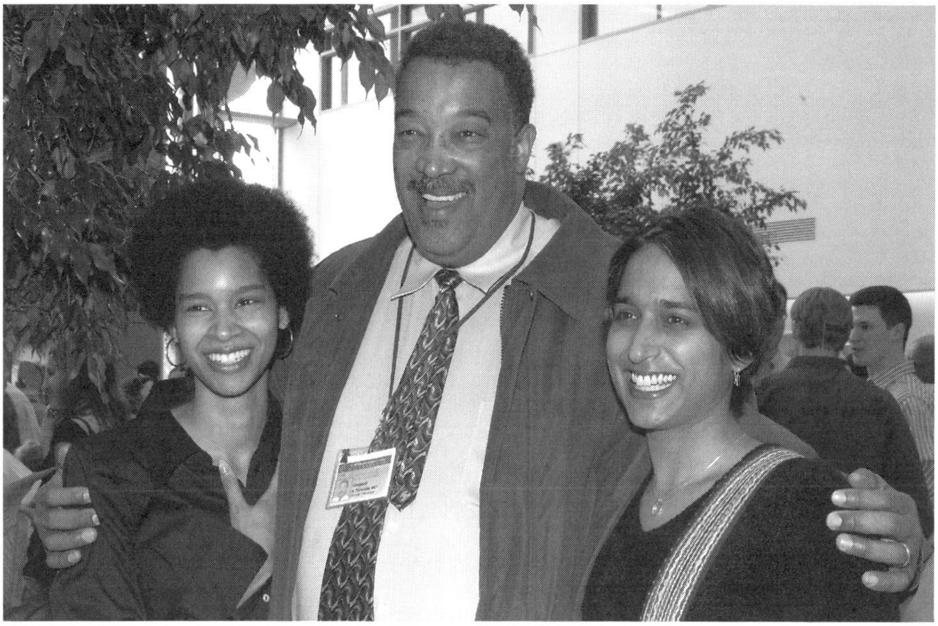

University Health Science Center, where he had been Vice Provost for Research and Dean of the Graduate School for Biomedical Sciences. The revived prominence of research at Upstate has lately been felt in some departments where research had not traditionally been a priority. In 2000, to indicate its research interests beyond the teaching of histology and gross anatomy, the Department of Anatomy and Cell Biology was renamed Cell and Developmental Biology.

In 2000 the $50-million Institute for Human Performance opened. Its biomedical research mission involves discovering not only ways to expand the capabilities and minimize the injuries of athletes, actors, musicians, and other performers, but also ways to improve the rehabilitation and reduce the recovery time of accident and disease victims. Its resources include state-of-the-art gait analysis systems, imaging equipment, exercise and fitness research apparatus, neurological and orthopedic laboratories, and areas for special events.

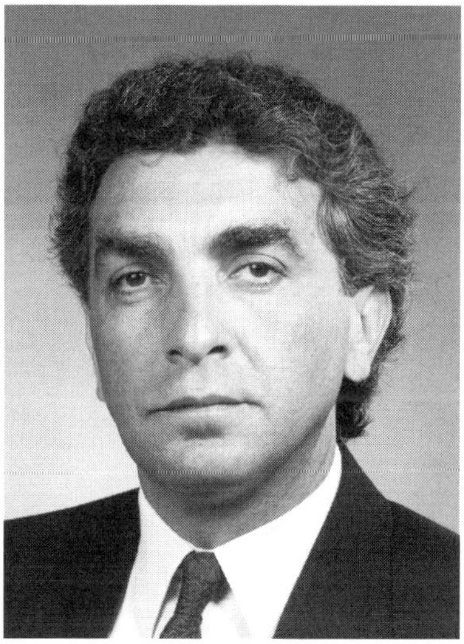

José Jalife (right), who earned his M.D. at the National University of Mexico in 1972, succeeded Weiner as Chair of Pharmacology in 1988. In 2002 the Department of Pharmacology and the Division of Cardiology in the Department of Medicine created the Institute for Cardiovascular Research under his direction. The formal opening of the Institute with forty team members on June 1, 2003, solidified Upstate's two-decade-long reputation as a leader in studies on cardiac arrhythmia. The five divisions of the Institute are Arrhythmia Research, Cellular and Developmental Cardiology, Molecular Cardiology, Clinical Cardiology Research, and Vascular Biology.

On September 23, 2002, Governor George E. Pataki announced in a ceremony on the front lawn of Weiskotten Hall that New York State would commit $20 million toward the $35 million first phase of the projected $80 million Central New York Biotechnology Research Center. A joint venture of Upstate and the SUNY College of Environmental Science and Forestry with support from the Metropolitan Development Association of Syracuse and Central New York, the Syracuse Veterans Administration Medical Center, several large corporations, and local and regional business and political leaders, this new facility should make Syracuse a focal point of high-tech plant and animal research and should hasten the development of the commercial potential of the findings of this research. The 240,000-square-foot building will be erected in three phases on land between Weiskotten Hall and the VA, and may involve demolishing Silverman Hall. The structure will be "green," i.e., environmentally friendly, with solar-powered heating and cooling, rooftop greenhouses, and effective pollution controls. Studies will include genetics, spectrometry, and wood bioconversion.

The Older Adult Service and Information System (OASIS) Institute, a national non-profit organization, contracted with University Hospital and the May Company in 2000 to create a facility in Syracuse. Since opening in 6000 square feet of renovated space in Shoppingtown Mall in 2001, Syracuse OASIS has enriched countless senior citizens' lives with activities involving the arts, the humanities, technology, health care, and wellness.

In August 2004 Eastwood asked K. Bruce Simmons, Class of 1979, Medical Director of the Employee/Student Health Office, to create and chair the *ad hoc* President's Advisory Committee for a Smoke-Free Upstate, whose purpose was to devise ways to implement the new policy that by August 1, 2005, smoking would be banned across the entire campus, indoors and outdoors. In this initiative Upstate joined only a handful of medical centers nationwide, including the Mayo Clinic and the Universities of Arkansas and Michigan. It was the first of the SUNY campuses and among the first educational institutions in New York to adopt this policy. Upstate thus expects to become, like Arkansas, Michigan, and Mayo, a pacesetter for other institutions that may want to ban smoking, especially in New York. Upstate has long recognized the inconsistency between pursuing a health care mission and allowing smoking, and had declared its indoor areas smoke-free on January 1, 1994, over nine years before the New York State Clean Indoor Air Act, which became effective on July 24, 2003.

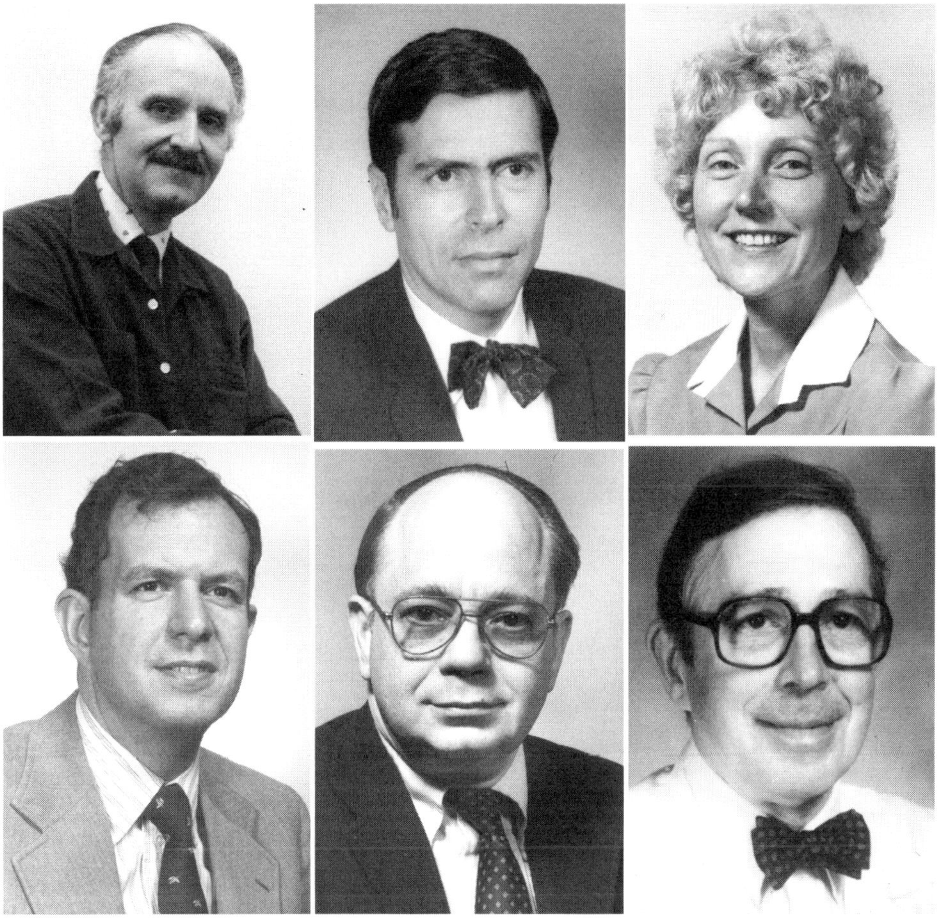

Six high-tech classrooms in the new academic building will be respectively named for six of the most admired teachers in the recent history of Upstate: (clockwise from top left) pathologist Robert F. Rohner, Class of 1952; physiologist Maxwell M. Mozell; anatomist Elinor Spring-Mills; hematologist William J. Williams; pharmacologist Irwin M. Weiner, Class of 1956; and surgeon Frederick B. Parker.

In the first decade of the third millennium, Upstate Medical University's renovation and expansion of laboratory space, its ongoing development of the Institute for Human Performance, its part in the Central New York Biotechnology Research Center, its construction of the new academic building and the children's hospital, its acquisition of state-of-the-art technology such as the da Vinci robotic surgical system and ever faster and more comprehensive medical informatics software, its constant and difficult but often joyous process of curriculum renewal, and many other factors all contribute to ensure and exemplify its commitment to the traditional three-legged stool of the medical profession: biomedical research, teaching, and patient care.

For Further Reading

Alumni Association of Syracuse University. *Alumni Record and General Catalogue of Syracuse University, 1872-1910, including Genesee College, 1852-1871, and Geneva Medical College, 1835-1872*, edited by Frank Smalley (Syracuse: [s.n.], 1911).

Blackwell, Elizabeth. *Pioneer Work in Opening the Medical Profession to Women* (many editions).

Boardman, Andrew. *An Essay on the Means of Improving Medical Education and Elevating Medical Character* (Philadelphia: Haswell, Barrington, and Haswell, 1840).

Boyd, Julia. *The Excellent Doctor Blackwell: The Life of the First Female Physician* (Stroud, Gloucestershire: Sutton, 2005).

Brieger, Gert Henry. *Stephen Smith: Surgeon and Reformer* (Ph.D. dissertation, Johns Hopkins University, 1968).

Corner, Betsy C. "Early Medical Education in Western New York, Geneva and Rochester Areas, 1827 to 1872: I. Early Medical Education Undertaken by Geneva College; II. Early Medicine in Rochester, Rochester's Eclectic Medical College, the Apprentice System as Developed in New York State." *New York State Journal of Medicine* 55, 21 (November 1, 1955): 3156-3164.

Cushing, Harvey. *Pioneer Medical Schools of Central New York: An Address at the Centenary Celebration of the College of Medicine of Syracuse University, June 4, 1934* (Syracuse: [s.n.], 1934).

Dieffenbacher, Jane W. *This Green and Pleasant Land: Fairfield, New York* (Holland Patent, N.Y.: Steffen Publishing, 1996).

Ferguson, J. Howard. "A Chronological Calendar of Events of the College of Medicine of Syracuse, 1872-1968," in Upstate Medical University, Health Sciences Library, Department of Historical Collections, Picture File 2.

Flexner, Abraham. *Medical Education in the United States and Canada: A Report to the Carnegie Foundation for the Advancement of Teaching*. Carnegie Foundation Bulletin No. 4 (New York: [s.n.], 1910).

Francis, Samuel Ward. *Biographical Sketches of Distinguished Living New York Surgeons* (New York: John Bradburn, 1866).

Galpin, William Freeman. *Syracuse University: Volume One, The Pioneer Days; Volume Two: The Growing Years* (Syracuse: Syracuse University Press, 1952-1960).

Galpin, William Freeman; and Barck, Oscar Theodore. *Syracuse University: Volume Three, The Critical Years* (Syracuse: Syracuse University Press, 1984).

Goins, Gregoria Fraser. "Miss Doc," undated typescript in Howard University, Moorland-Spingarn Research Center, Manuscript Department.

Greene, John Robert. *Syracuse University: The Tolley Years, 1942-1969* (Syracuse: Syracuse University Press, 1996).

Hays, Elinor Rice. *Those Extraordinary Blackwells: The Story of a Journey to a Better World* (New York: Harcourt, Brace & World, 1967).

Heffron, John Lorenzo. *Fifty Years of the College of Medicine of Syracuse University* (Syracuse: Syracuse University Press, 1920).

Luft, Eric v.d. "Sarah Loguen Fraser, MD (1850 to 1933): The Fourth African-American Woman Physician." *Journal of the National Medical Association* 92, 3 (March 2000): 149-153.

Miller, Genevieve. "Dr. John Delamater, 'True Physician'." *Journal of Medical Education* 34, 1 (January 1959): 24-31.

Norwood, William Frederick. *Medical Education in the United States Before the Civil War* (Philadelphia: University of Pennsylvania Press, 1944).

Official History: U.S.A. Base Hospital No. 31 of Youngstown, Ohio and Hospital Unit "G" of Syracuse University, edited by Charles Hirsh Kaletzki (Syracuse: Craftsman Press, 1919).

Onondaga County, New York. *Onondaga County Bicentennial, 1794-1994*, edited by Andy Jugan (Syracuse: Extra Points Unlimited, Onondaga County Department of Parks and Recreation, 1994).

Onondaga County Medical Society, 1906-1956, Sesquicentennial. (Syracuse: [s.n.], 1956). [Note: The Society was founded in 1806. This sesquicentennial volume concerns the history of only its third half-century.]

Robbins, Christine Chapman. *David Hosack, Citizen of New York.* Memoirs of the American Philosophical Society, vol. 62. (Philadelphia: APS, 1964).

Sahli, Nancy Ann. *Elizabeth Blackwell, M.D.: A Biography* (Ph.D. dissertation, University of Pennsylvania, 1974).

Smith, Warren Hunting. *Hobart and William Smith: The History of Two Colleges* (Geneva, N.Y.: Hobart College, 1972).

Snyder, Charles McCool. *Dr. Mary Walker: The Little Lady in Pants* (New York: Vantage, 1962).

State University of New York Health Science Center at Syracuse Library. *Thirty-Five Treasures of Special Collections*, edited, ... selected, described, and photographed by Eric v.d. Luft (Kennett Square, Pa.: KNA Press, 1993).

Stookey, Byron. *A History of Colonial Medical Education in the Province of New York, with its Subsequent Development* (Springfield, Illinois: Charles C. Thomas, 1962).

Stringer, Helen Dann. *Millie M.D.: The Story of a Nineteenth-Century Woman, 1846-1927* (Utica, N.Y.: North Country Books, 1992).

Upstate Medical University, Health Sciences Library, Department of Historical Collections, home page <www.upstate.edu/library/history/>.

Walsh, James J. *History of Medicine in New York: Three Centuries of Medical Progress* (New York: National Americana Society, 1919).

Weiskotten, Herman G.; Schwitalla, Alphonse M.; Cutter, William D.; and Anderson, Hamilton H. *Medical Education in the United States, 1934-1939* (Chicago: American Medical Association, Council on Medical Education and Hospitals, 1940).

Westerfeld, Wilfred Wiedey. *The Making of a Medical Center: A Personal History of the Background* (Syracuse: SUNY Health Science Center, 1989), typescript in Upstate Medical University, Health Sciences Library, Department of Historical Collections, Historical-Biographical Folders.

Index

Deans of the Medical School

At Geneva Medical College:

1. Edward Cutbush, M.D., 1834-1839
2. Charles Brodhead Coventry, M.D., 1839-1841
3. Thomas Spencer, M.D., 1841-1845
4. James Webster, M.D., 1845-1847
5. Charles Alfred Lee, M.D., 1847-1853
6. John Towler, M.D., 1853-1872

At the Syracuse University College of Medicine:

7. Frederick Hyde, M.D., 1872-1887
8. Henry Darwin Didama, M.D., 1887-1905
9. Gaylord Parsons Clark, M.D., 1905-1907
10. John Lorenzo Heffron, M.D., 1907-1922
11. Herman Gates Weiskotten, M.D., 1922-1950

At the SUNY College of Medicine at Syracuse:

11. Herman Gates Weiskotten, M.D., 1950-1951
12. William R. Willard, M.D., 1951-1953

At the SUNY Upstate Medical Center:

12. William R. Willard, M.D., 1953-1956
  Wilfred W. Westerfeld, Ph.D., 1956-1957 (interim)
13. Carlyle F. Jacobsen, Ph.D, 1957-1965
14. Julius B. Richmond, M.D., 1965-1970
15. Richard P. Schmidt, M.D., 1970-1975
  Donald C. Goodman, Ph.D., 1975-1976 (interim, basic science departments)

George F. Reed, M.D., 1975-1976 (interim, clinical departments)
16. George F. Reed, M.D., 1976-1986

At the SUNY Health Science Center at Syracuse:

John Bernard Henry, M.D., 1986-1987 (interim)
17. Irwin M. Weiner, M.D., 1987-1991
William J. Williams, M.D., 1991-1992 (interim)
18. Joseph P. Whalen, M.D., 1992-1995
19. Gregory L. Eastwood, M.D., 1995-1999

At SUNY Upstate Medical University:

19. Gregory L. Eastwood, M.D., 1999-2001
20. Michael F. Roizen, M.D., 2001-2002
21. William J. Williams, M.D., 2002-2004
22. Steven J. Scheinman, M.D., 2004-____

Presidents of the Medical Campus

At the SUNY Upstate Medical Center:

1. Carlyle Ferdinand Jacobsen, Ph.D., September 1957 - June 30, 1967
Wilfred W. Westerfeld, Ph.D., 1967 - 1968 (interim)
Julius B. Richmond, M.D., 1968 (interim)
2. Lewis William Bluemle, Jr., M.D., November 1, 1968 - October 30, 1974
Richard Penrose Schmidt, M.D., 1974 - 1975 (interim)
3. Richard Penrose Schmidt, M.D., May 30, 1975 - July 1, 1984
George F. Reed, M.D., 1984 - 1985 (interim)
4. John Bernard Henry, M.D., February 1985 - 1986

At the SUNY Health Science Center at Syracuse:

4. John Bernard Henry, M.D., 1986 - August 27, 1992
Donald C. Goodman, Ph.D., August 28, 1992 - 1993 (interim)
5. Gregory L. Eastwood, M.D., January 4, 1993 - 1999

At SUNY Upstate Medical University:

5. Gregory L. Eastwood, M.D., 1999 - ____

About the Author

Eric v.d. Luft has been Curator of Historical Collections in the Health Sciences Library of SUNY Upstate Medical University since 1987. He received his A.B. magna cum laude in philosophy and religion from Bowdoin College in 1974, his M.A. and Ph.D. in philosophy from Bryn Mawr College in 1977 and 1985, and his M.L.S. from Syracuse University in 1993. He formerly taught philosophy at Villanova University and served as Historical Collections Assistant at the College of Physicians of Philadelphia. He is listed in *Who's Who in America* and *Who's Who in the World*. His approximately 520 publications are mostly encyclopedia articles, but also include three books authored, three books edited, one book translated and edited, 32 peer-reviewed articles in professional journals and anthologies, and frequent contributions to the *Upstate Medical Alumni Journal*. Among the topics of his writing are philosophy, librarianship, clinical medicine, history of medicine, history of science, military history, intellectual and cultural history, popular culture, medieval Iceland, and contract bridge.